PEDIATRIC DERMATOLOGY

DDx Deck

William L. **Weston** | Joseph G. **Morelli**

ELSEVIER

Author Details

WILLIAM L WESTON MD
Emeritus Professor
Departments of Dermatology & Pediatrics
University of Colorado School of Medicine
Aurora, CO
USA

JOSEPH G MORELLI MD
Professor of Dermatology and Pediatrics
University of Colorado School of Medicine
Pediatric Dermatology
Children's Hospital Colorado
Aurora, CO
USA

Content Strategist: Belinda Kuhn
Content Development Specialist: Trinity Hutton
Project Manager: Anne Collett
Design: Christian Bilbow
Illustration Manager: Lesley Frazier
Marketing Manager: Melissa Fogarty

Contents

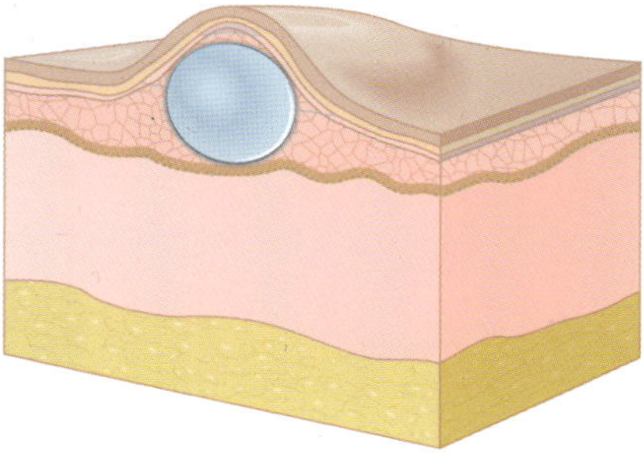

Vesicles. Lesions less than 1 cm, filled with clear fluid.

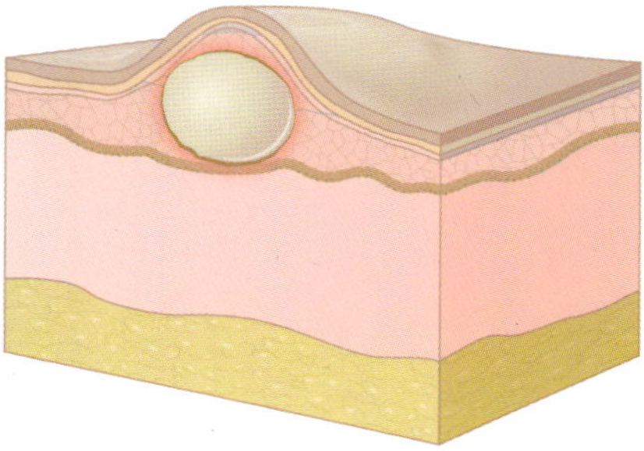

Pustules. Lesions filled with yellow fluid exudate.

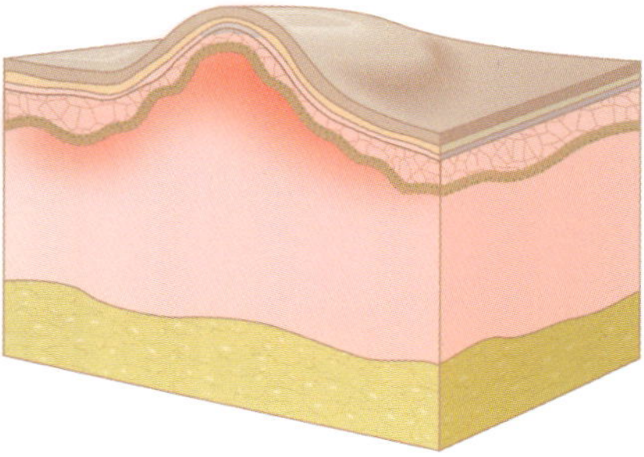

Papules. Solid raised lesions with distinct borders less than 1 cm in diameter.

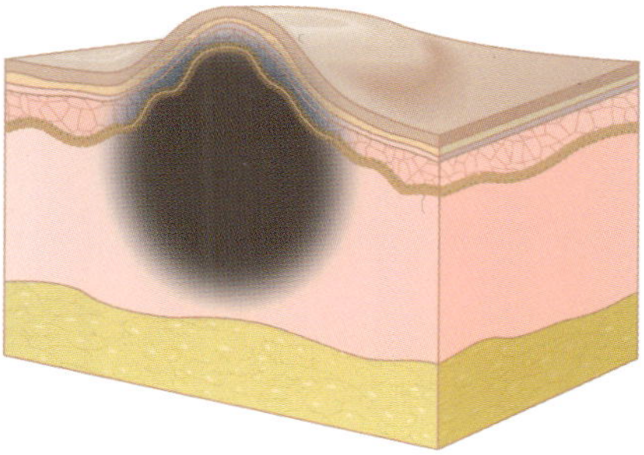

Nodules. Solid raised lesions with indistinct borders and a deep palpable portion.

The morphology of individual skin lesions is the key to diagnosis of skin diseases in pediatric age groups. Identification of the primary lesion should be the first step.

Primary lesions Primary lesions include vesicles (and bullae), pustules, papules (and plaques), nodules, macules, wheals, and cysts.

A **vesicle** is a raised lesion less than 1 cm, filled with clear fluid (topics 1 and 2).

A **bulla** is a blister greater than 1 cm (topics 13 and 18).

A **pustule** is a raised lesion filled with fluid exudates giving it a yellow appearance (topics 23 and 25).

A **papule** is a solid raised lesion with distinct borders and 1 cm or less in diameter (topics 4 and 8).

A **plaque** is a solid lesion greater than 1 cm, often flat-topped resembling a mesa (topics 40, 67, and 72).

A **nodule** is a raised solid lesion with indistinct borders and a deep palpable component. Vascular nodules are compressible (topics 55 and 79).

A **macule** is a color change in the skin that is flat to the surface of the skin and not palpable (topics 49 and 105).

A **wheal** is a flat-topped, slightly raised area of tense edema within the outer layer of skin (topic 48).

A **cyst** is a solid raised dome-shaped lesion with a smooth surface. Some have a palpable sac that skin moves over. Others are within the epidermis and move with the skin (topics 96 and 97).

Additional clues can be obtained from the description of secondary changes, palpation of the lesion, color changes, the arrangement of multiple lesions, and the overall distribution of lesions. Palpation helps determine whether the lesion is solid or cystic and within the dermis or beneath. These contribute to the identification of differential diagnosis groups.

Secondary changes Secondary changes include **erosions**, which are blister bases (topics 2 and 13) and **crusting**, which is the combination of plasma and epidermis as seen in impetigo (topic 5). Erosions are the predominant feature of vesiculobullous diseases on mucous membranes (topic 19). Thus, erosions and crusting in the absence of blisters indicates a vesiculobullous disease. Scaling is seen in papulosquamous conditions and ichthyoses (topic 66, 67, and 70). Lichenification is seen as thickening of the epidermis due to external irritation (topic 79). Fissures are linear splits in the skin, seen as wedge-shaped cracks through the epidermis narrowing in the dermis (topic 79). Scars are fibrous thickenings of the dermis resulting in loss of epidermal ridges. They may be raised as in hypertrophic scars, or flat (topic 39). Atrophy is thinning of the epidermis, dermis, or subcutaneous fat (topics 111 and 139).

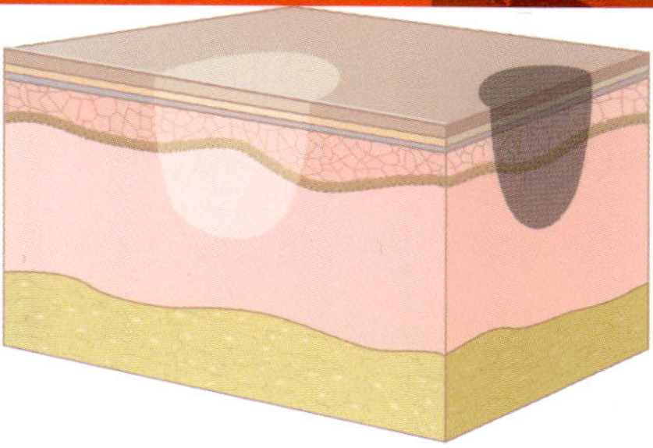

Macules. Color change that is flat to the surface of skin.

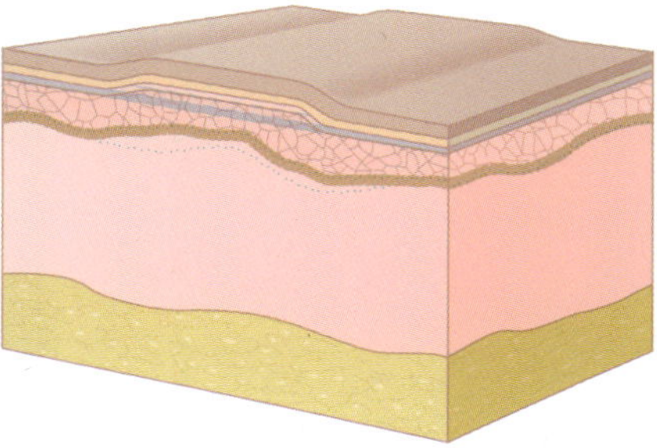

Wheals. Tense edema in the upper dermis with a flat-topped slightly palpable lesion.

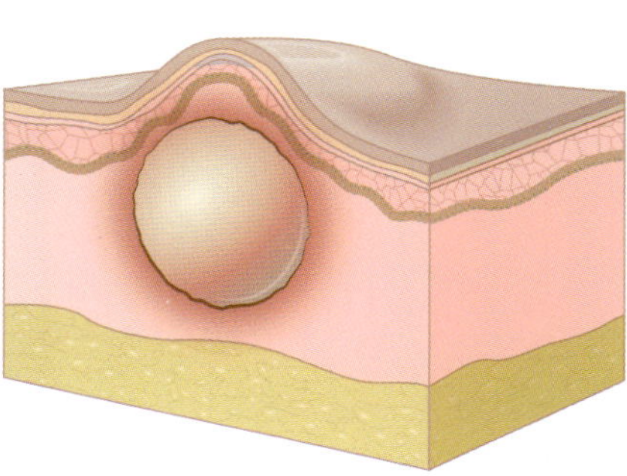

Cysts. Raised solid dome-shaped lesions with a smooth surface. Some have a deep palpable sac where the skin moves over it.

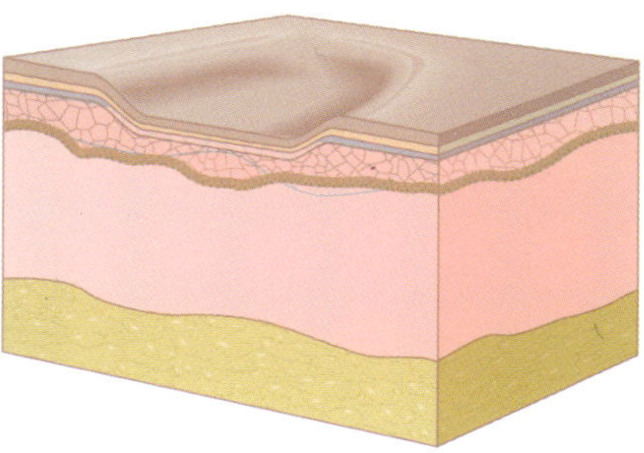

Atrophy. Skin surface is depressed due to thinning or absence of the epidermis, dermis, or subcutaneous fat.

Color Color should be described as unchanged from normal skin color, red, blue, brown, white, tan, or yellow. A red lesion should be compressed to determine whether it is blanching (vascular). If it does not blanch, then it is petechial or purpuric. Melanin is the dominant pigment of skin, as it is located within the outer layer of skin. Very dark skin may be brown, blue-black or black, and obscure other colors such as red or yellow. The exam should first determine the color of normal skin, then compare with the changed color. Some DDx groups are defined by color alone, e.g., white lesions, brown lesions.

Arrangement Arrangement of skin lesions in relation to each other may offer useful clues to diagnosis. Lesions may be **discrete** and separated from one another such as warts. *Curvilinear* skin lesions are found in genetic mosaicism and may have a whorled or parallel pattern (topic 159). The presence of curvilinear lesions should initiate assessment for visual or neurologic abnormalities. **Annular** (circular) arrangements may indicate tinea infections or granuloma annulare (topic 158). **Grouped** lesions such as vesicles may be clues to herpes simplex or zoster.

Distribution Skin lesions can be **generalized** or **localized** to specific skin locations such as acral (hands, feet, buttocks, and face) or **photodistributed** (topics 9 and 156), where sunlight strikes the skin such as cheeks, bridge of the nose, and dorsum of extremities.

Hair and nails Examination of hair abnormalities requires description and timing of changes such as loss of hair being generalized or patchy, congenital or acquired (topics 140 and 145).

Examination of nails should include a description of the type of nail distortion and whether the nail is thick or thin (topics 146 and 152).

USE OF THE DDX DECK

After the first step (identification of the **primary lesion(s)**), diagnostic possibilities are refined by noting secondary changes (e.g., erosions and crusts indicate a vesiculobullous category), papules with scaling, a papulosquamous category. Further clues are obtained from distribution, arrangement, and color. Thus, generalized, discrete, red, scaly papules would describe guttate psoriasis. Within a diagnostic group, one can fan out the images to match the clinical appearance. On the reverse side of the diagnostic image is a description of the clinical features, pathogenesis, and recommended treatment.

N

This symbol indicates a neonatal dermatology image. Text shaded in orange indicates content specific to neonatal patients.

Herpes simplex infections

DDx ref 2 • 8 • 19

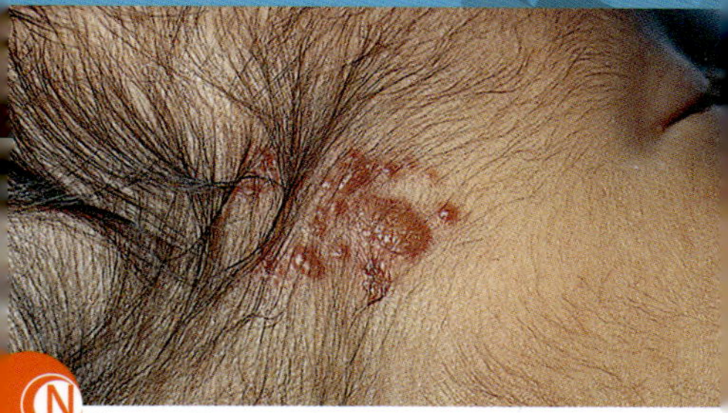

Neonatal herpes. Grouped vesicles on a red base on the scalp of a 9-day-old infant.

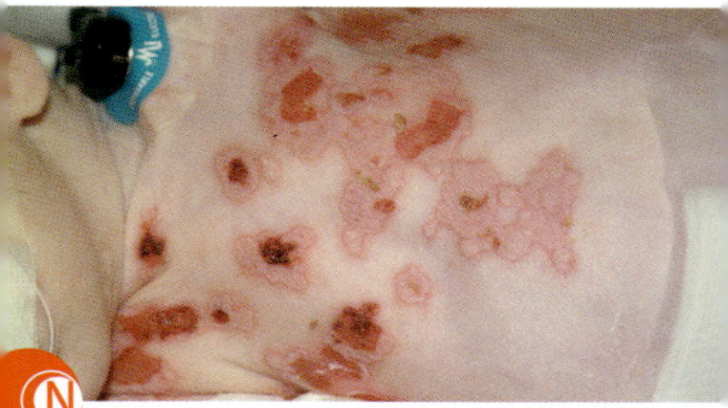

Neonatal herpes. Widespread vesicles and erosions in a 2-day-old infant.

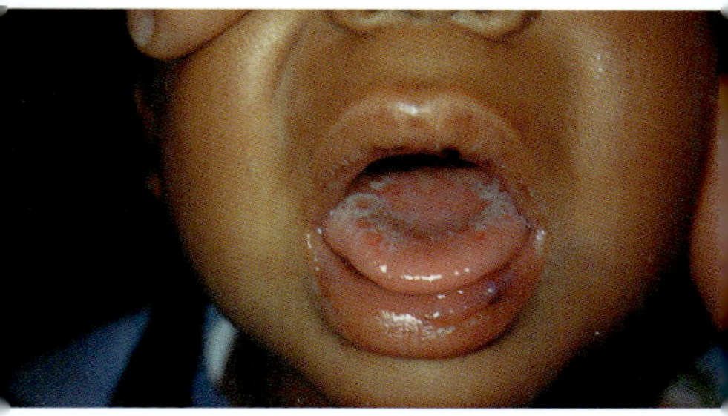

Primary herpes gingivostomatitis. Oral erosions seen in this 3-month-old infant.

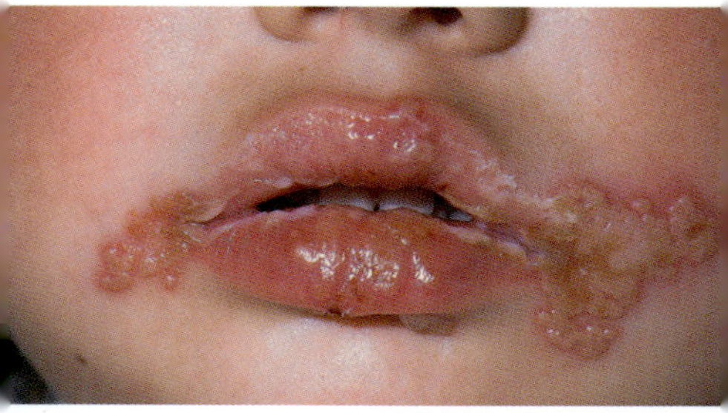

Primary herpes gingivostomatitis. Perioral and lip vesicles in a 10-month-old infant.

CLINICAL FEATURES

Grouped vesicles on a red base are the characteristic lesions of herpes simplex regardless of location on the skin. On mucous membranes, the blister roof is easily shed and erosions are seen. A variety of clinical patterns is seen.

Neonatal herpes simplex Grouped vesicles on a red base may be found anywhere on the skin of a neonate and lesions may be widely scattered. Mucous membrane involvement is common. Vesicles may be present at birth but commonly appear 1–7 days after birth. Historically, HHV-2 has been the predominant cause; the incidence of HHV-1 is increasing. Of mothers with active HHV-2 infections, 10% of their newborns will be affected. The disease may at first be mild skin involvement but systemic disease will eventuate with hypothermia, jaundice, progressive hepatosplenomegaly, and CNS symptoms. With encephalitis, death within 96 hours has been reported.

Primary gingivostomatitis In infants, severe oral erosions and grouped vesicles on lips and gums appear. The child has a high fever, irritability, foul breath, and is unable to eat. The disease lasts 7–14 days. Many infants encountered with HHV-1 result in a mild pharyngitis without characteristic vesicles.

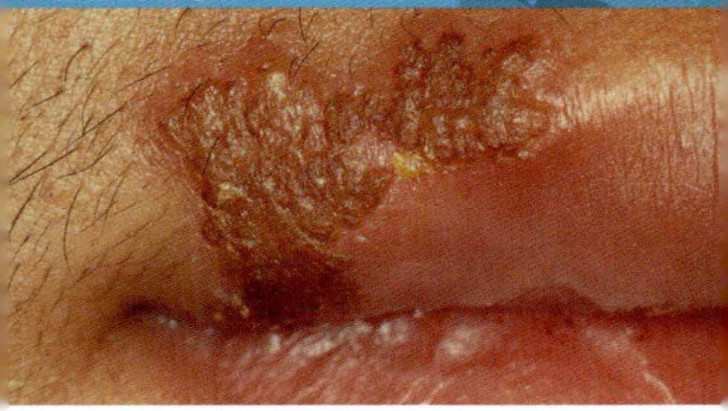

Recurrent herpes labialis with grouped vesicles on upper lip.

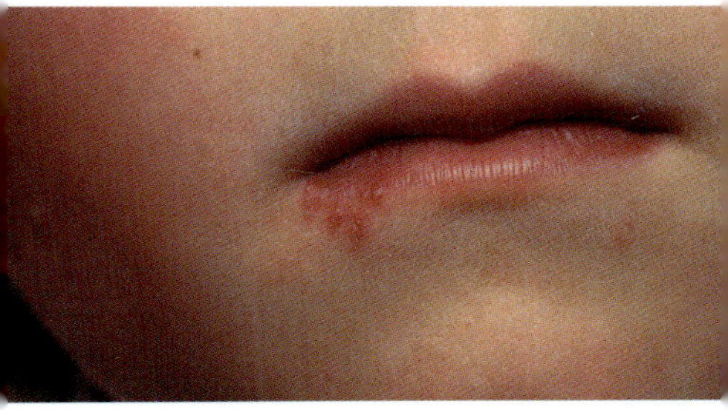

Recurrent herpes labialis with grouped vesicles on lower lip.

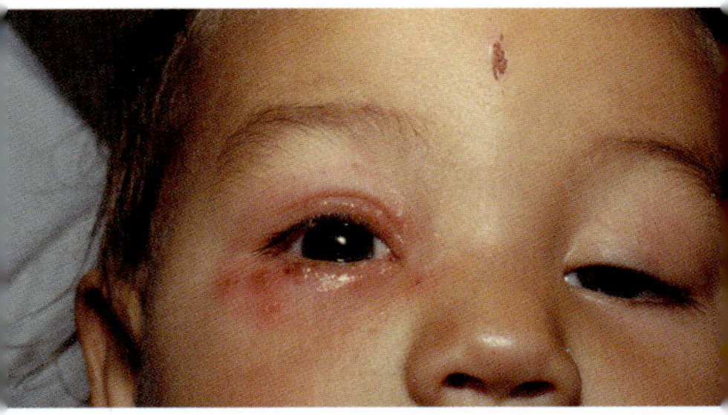

Herpes keratitis. Grouped vesicles on lower eyelid and red eye in child.

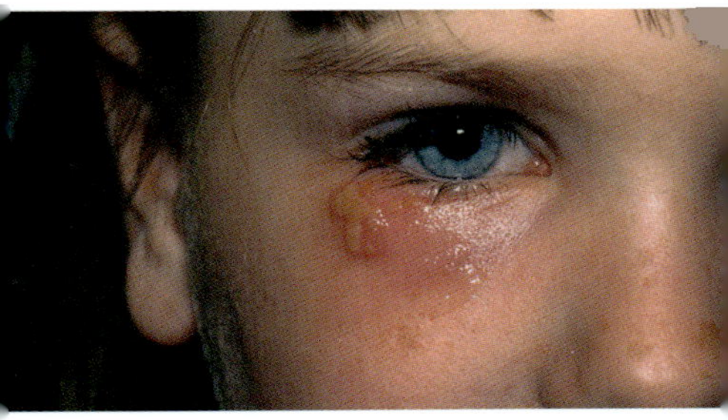

Herpes facialis. Recurrent grouped vesicles on child's cheek. No eye involvement.

Herpes simplex infections

DDx ref 2 • 8 • 19

Recurrent herpes simplex infection Herpes simplex viruses (HSV) may persist in nerve ganglia and reactivate after UV light exposure, fever, trauma, or menses. Vesicles recurring in the same site should be considered to be due to herpes simplex.

Herpes labialis The majority of recurrent HSV infections are on the lips. It occurs in 20% of children who have had primary HSV infection. A prodrome of lower lip pain precedes development of vesicles on a red base on the lip, lasting 8 days.

Herpes keratitis Involvement of the skin around the eye should bring concern about corneal herpes. Dendritic ulceration occurs and may lead to scarring and permanent loss of vision. Periorbital vesicles and a red eye should prompt ophthalmologic consultation.

Herpes facialis Recurrent episodes of grouped vesicles on the forehead or cheek are less common and frequently misdiagnosed.

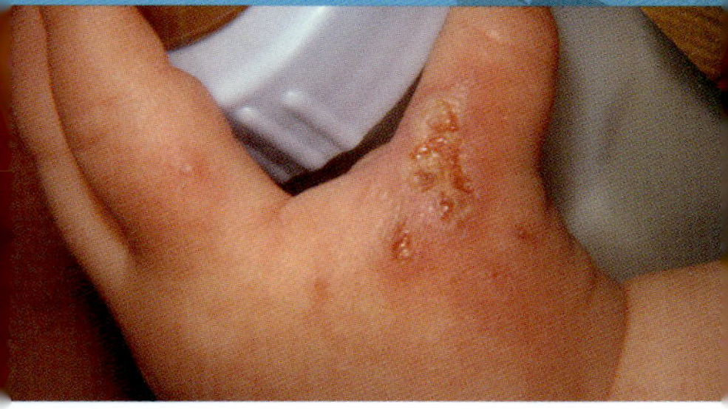

Herpetic whitlow. Grouped vesicles on red base at base of thumb in a thumbsucker.

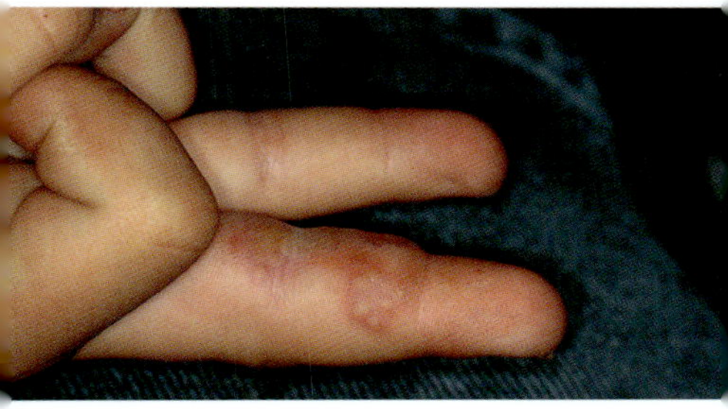

Herpetic whitlow. Grouped vesicles on middle finger of child.

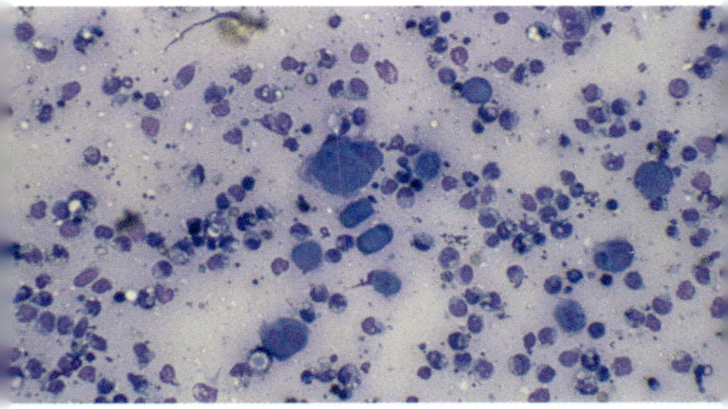

Photomicrograph of smear of blister contents showing transformed epidermal cells (giant cells) in herpes simplex infection.

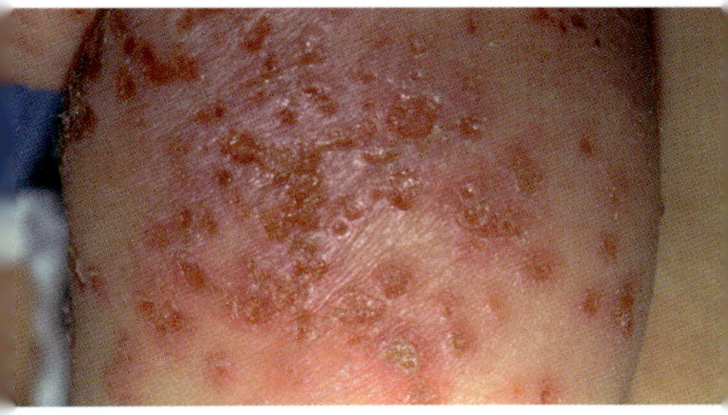

Eczema herpeticum. Numerous vesicles and erosions in child with atopic dermatitis and HSV 1 infection.

Herpetic whitlow Herpes finger and hand infections occur in 10% of infants and children. Because the stratum corneum is thicker in these areas, the vesicles appear deceptively deep.

Herpes progenitalis Teens and young adults may have prodromal pain followed by grouped vesicles on a red base on the genitalia. Severe infections may produce fever, lassitude, lymphadenopathy, and severe pain. HHV-2 is responsible for this recurrent sexually transmitted disease.

Herpes simplex in the immunosuppressed Atypical appearances of HSV occur in the immunosuppressed, genetic immune deficiencies, children with cancer, or the malnourished child. Grouped vesicles progress to giant bullae and erosions often with purpura or hemorrhage. After 24–48 hours, widespread lesions may appear. The red base may not be evident.

Eczema herpeticum (Kaposi's varicelliform eruption) Children with atopic dermatitis may develop superinfection with HHV-1 with multiple groups of vesicles and high fever. Rarely, herpes encephalitis or pneumonia may ensue if untreated.

TREATMENT

Neonatal HSV should be treated with high-dose intravenous acyclovir at 20–40 mg/kg per dose every 8 hours. Skin, eye, and mucous membrane disease is treated for 14 days; disseminated and CNS disease for 21 days. In addition, maintenance of fluid and electrolyte balance, and temperature regulation are necessary. The baby should be isolated.

Oral acyclovir, famciclovir, or valacyclovir These are effective in localized cutaneous infections. Topical therapy is ineffective. Treatment does not prevent recurrences and, if frequent recurrences develop, 6 months of acyclovir prophylaxis may be considered.

Herpes keratitis This can be treated with topical vidarabine 3% or 1–2% trifluridine ointment.

Varicella and herpes zoster

DDx ref 1 • 8 • 13

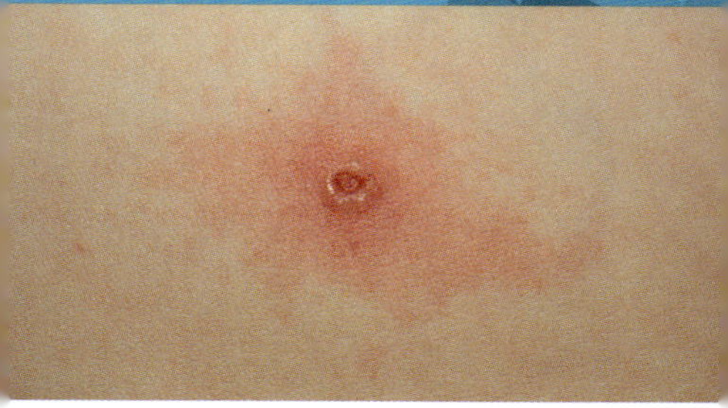

Varicella. Discrete umbilicated vesicle on a red base.

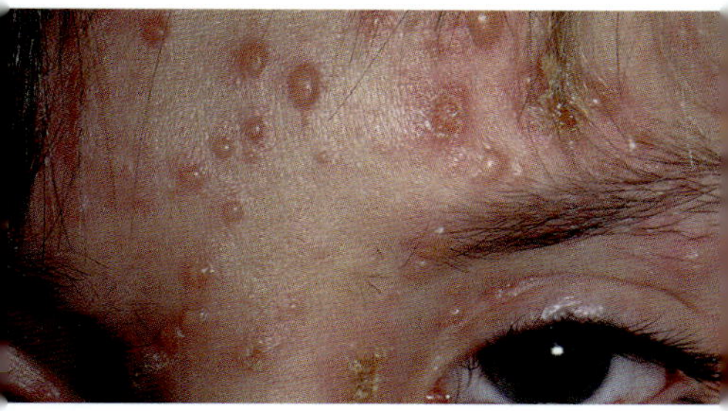

Varicella. Multiple discrete vesicles and crusted lesions on a child's face.

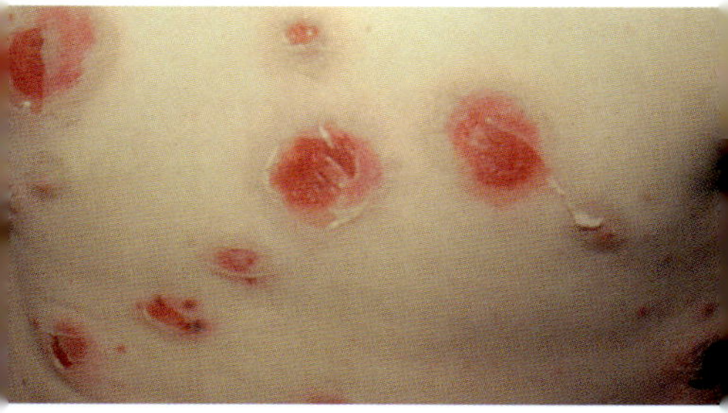

Varicella with bullous impetigo. Large erosions at sites of secondary infection of varicella vesicles.

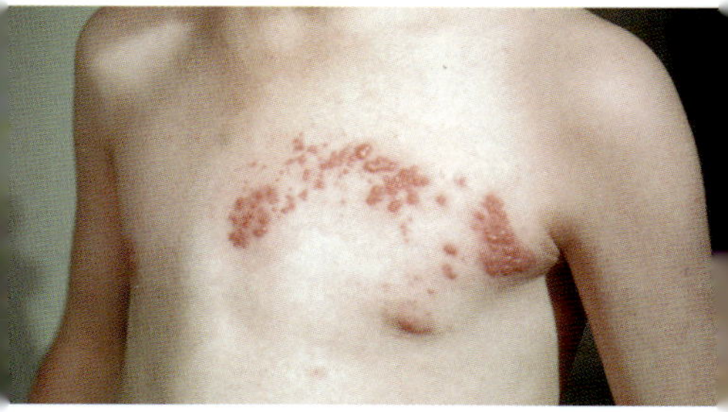

Herpes zoster. Several groups of vesicles over left thoracic dermatomes in a child with herpes zoster.

CLINICAL FEATURES

Varicella is characterized by the abrupt onset of crops of vesicles.

In newborns Crops of vesicles appear within the first 10 days after birth when maternal varicella occurred 2–3 weeks prior to birth. Lesions mimic neonatal herpes simplex infections. Rarely, premature infants are exposed to varicella after birth and may develop severe, widespread varicella with pneumonia. The congenital varicella syndrome follows intrauterine infection before 20 weeks' gestation and presents as vesicles and neuromuscular disease.

Childhood varicella begins as discrete red macules that evolve into vesicles within 24–48 hours. Moist crusts appear, dry, are shed, and shallow erosions develop. Successive crops of vesicles appear over the next 2–5 days, such that lesions in different stages are observed at the same time. Skin lesions may appear at sites of sun exposure or skin trauma. Mucosal lesions are common. A low-grade fever occurs and the illness is mild. Children within the same family vary considerably as to how many lesions they develop, from 10 in one child to hundreds in another. Varicella lasts 7–10 days. The disease is highly contagious from 1–2 days before skin lesions appear to 5–6 days afterward.

Secondary bacterial infection with staphylococcal or Group A streptococcus occurs in 2–3%. Rarely, pneumonia may complicate varicella in some otherwise healthy children, and in the immunosuppressed child severe pneumonia may ensue accompanied by high fever, encephalitis, hepatitis, and disseminated intravenous coagulation. Reye syndrome of encephalopathy and fatty infiltration of the liver may develop in children treated with aspirin.

Varicella vaccines are effective preventatives of varicella.

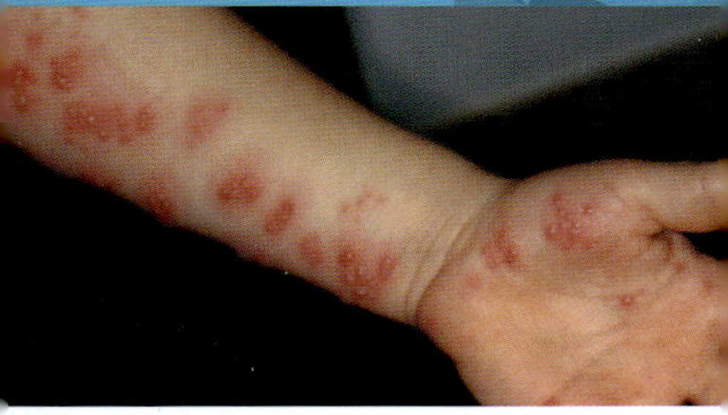

Herpes zoster involving the arm of a child with many groups of vesicles.

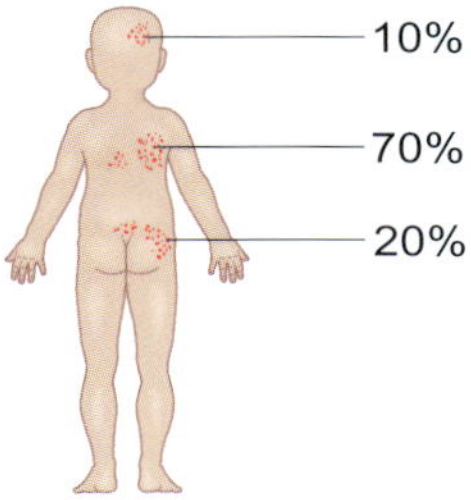

Distribution of herpes zoster in childhood.

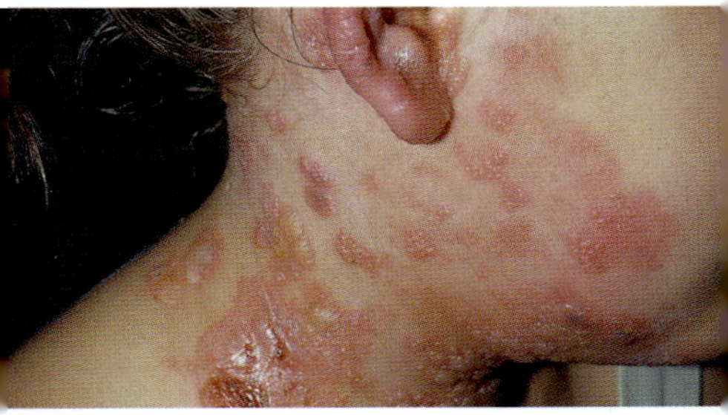

Ramsay Hunt syndrome. Grouped vesicles over the ear, cheek, and neck in a child with accompanying facial palsy.

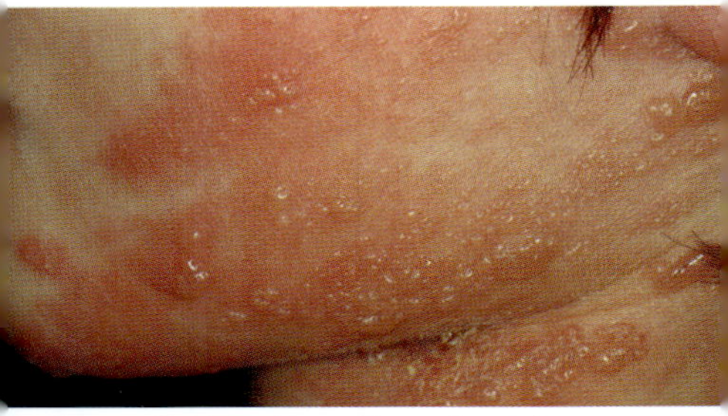

Ramsay Hunt syndrome. Grouped vesicles over the ear, cheek, and neck.

Herpes zoster represents reactivation of the varicella virus in several adjacent dermatomes on one side of the body lasting 7–10 days. Two to three groups of blisters on a red base are seen. The thoracic segments are most frequently involved (70%). Rarely, dermatomal pain may precede the cutaneous eruption, especially in head and eye involvement. Involvement of the ear and cheek may be accompanied by acute facial paralysis in children (Ramsay Hunt syndrome). It is rare for post-zoster neuralgia to occur in children.

Zoster may be the presenting symptom in childhood AIDS, but rarely in childhood cancer. In immunosuppressed children, dissemination may occur 1–5 days after the typical dermatomal pattern appears. This results in a varicella-like picture and can be accompanied by severe pneumonia and other organ involvement.

TREATMENT

In newborns and premature infants administration of zoster immune globulin may modify varicella. Intravenous high-dose acyclovir, valacyclovir, famciclovir, and foscarnet all have been successful in treating varicella.

In the healthy child varicella does not require specific therapy. Wet dressings and soothing baths, and oral antihistamines to relieve itching may be helpful. Salicylates should be avoided.

Secondary bullous impetigo Treatment is based on sensitivity and culture results. Acyclovir and similar antivirals should be considered only in children with immune suppression including steroid-dependent asthmatic children or other chronic pulmonary diseases, the Ramsay Hunt syndrome, or ophthalmic zoster with severe pain. Doses of 30 mg/kg in four daily doses is recommended for a total of 5 days of treatment. Varicella vaccine is efficacious if administered within 72 hours of exposure.

Post-varicella scarring always concerns parents. What appear to be purple-red scars return to normal skin in 6–12 months. Parents should be advised to wait for at least 12 months before considering treatment of scars.

3 DDx ref

BLISTERS (VESICLES AND BULLAE)

Hand, foot, and mouth disease

88 • 8 • 24

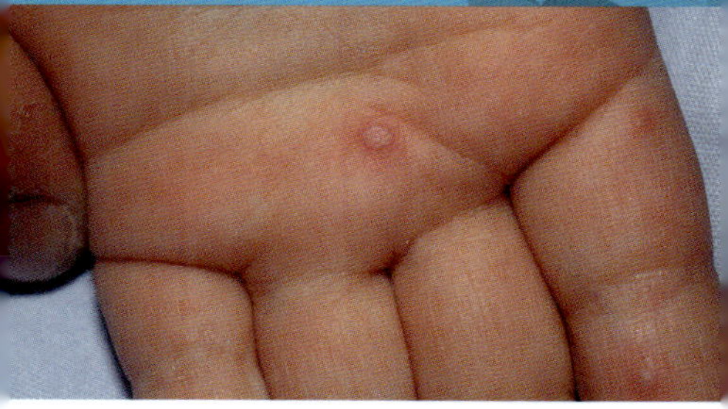

Hand, foot, and mouth disease. Oval blisters with a red base in child due to Coxsackie virus A16 infection and enterovirus 71.

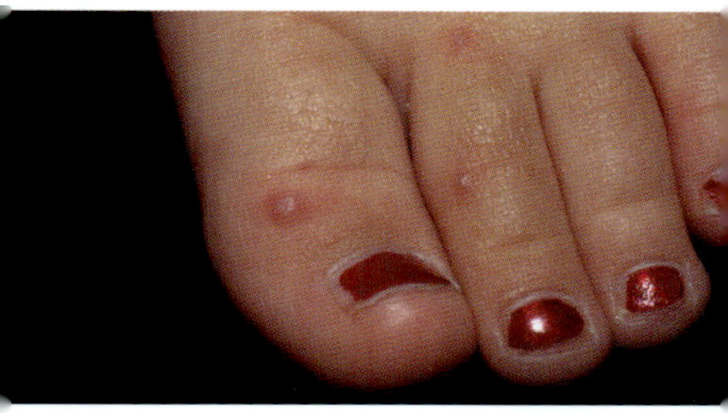

Tiny oval blisters on the feet of a girl with hand, foot, and mouth disease.

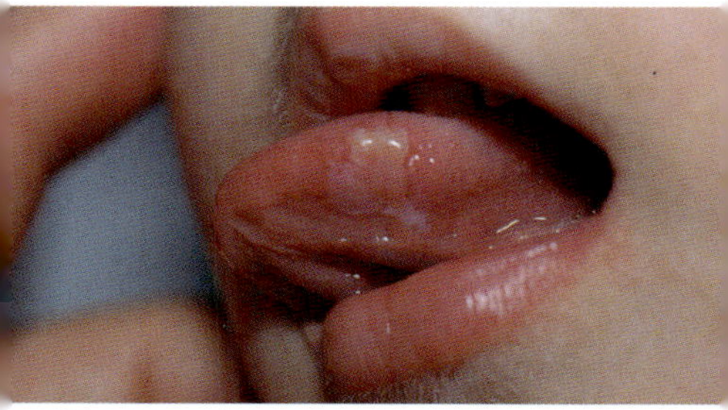

Discrete erosion on the tongue of a child with hand, foot, and mouth disease.

4 DDx ref

BLISTERS (VESICLES AND BULLAE)

Sucking blisters

15 • 10 • 11

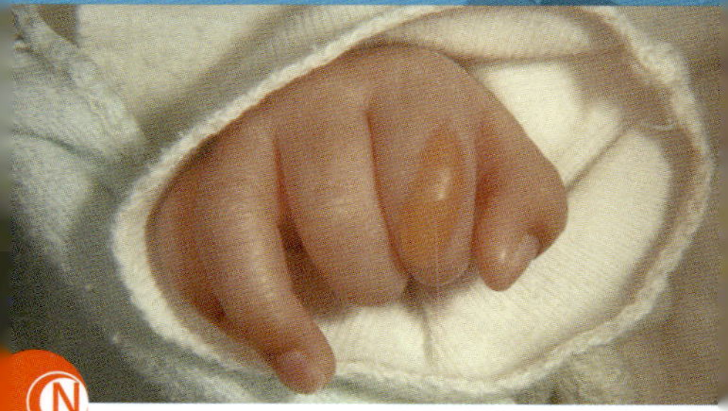

N Sucking blister. Oval noninflammatory blister on the finger of a newborn.

3

BLISTERS (VESICLES AND BULLAE)

Hand, foot, and mouth disease

DDx ref 88 • 8 • 24

CLINICAL FEATURES

This acral condition is seen as an abrupt onset of tiny 1–2-mm red papules that evolve within hours to the characteristic 1–3-mm oval or linear vesicles. Location on the palms and soles or the dorsum of the hands and feet is accompanied by discrete shallow oral erosions. Lesions are few in number but exceptionally, many lesions on the distal arms and legs have been described. The infection is due primarily to Coxsackievirus A16 and occurs in epidemics. Occasionally, Coxsackie viruses A2, A5, or A10 are responsible. It is a mild disease with little or no fever and lasts 4 or 5 days. The incubation period is 3–5 days and the child is contagious from 2 days before the onset of the eruption to 2 days after.

Atypical hand, foot, and mouth syndrome due to enterovirus 71 is a severe disease with more widespread blistering accompanied by high fever and lassitude. There is potential for dissemination in children with atopic dermatitis. Mortality has been reported. Shedding of the nails due to nail matrix arrest is seen following the illness.

TREATMENT

The more common mild forms of the disease require no specific treatment. In the severe enterovirus 71 infection, intravenous immunoglobulin or the newer antiviral agents have been used. Immunizations are being developed.

4

BLISTERS (VESICLES AND BULLAE)

Sucking blisters

DDx ref 15 • 10 • 11

CLINICAL FEATURES

Sucking blisters are usually solitary oval blisters or erosions present at delivery of the newborn. They occur on the dorsum of fingers, wrists, and forearm as the result of vigorous intrauterine sucking. They resolve within 2 or 3 days.

TREATMENT

No treatment is necessary.

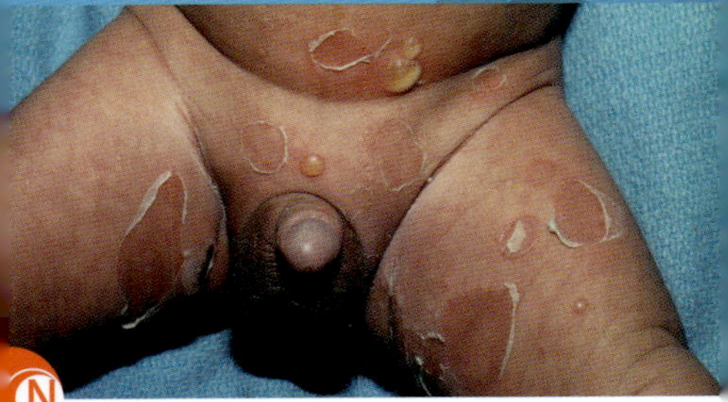

N Newborn with bullous impetigo. Flaccid, thin-roofed blisters and erosions involve the abdominal skin.

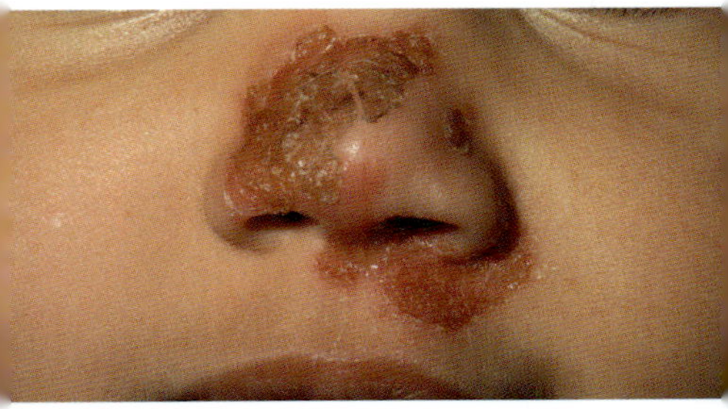

Impetigo in an infant. Crusts have spread from beneath the nose.

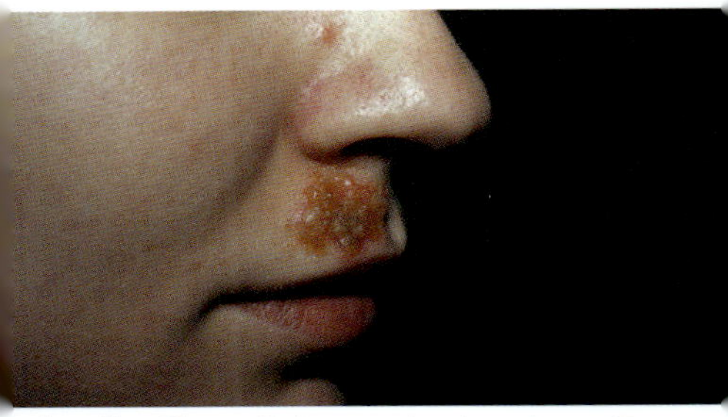

Impetigo. Diagnostic honey-colored crusts on skin above upper lip.

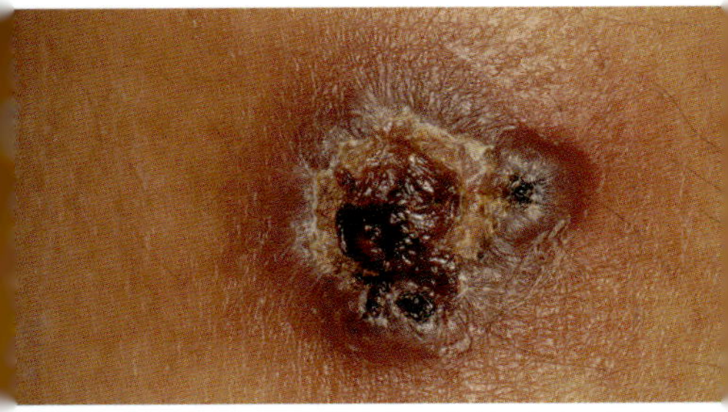

Ecthyma. Dry, firm crust surrounded by indurated border.

CLINICAL FEATURES

Moist, honey-colored crusts are considered diagnostic of impetigo. Impetigo begins as tiny 1–3-mm vesicles with thin fragile roofs that evolve into moist crusts. The face, nose, and extremities are the most frequent sites of involvement.

Bullous impetigo is the term used when large bullae surround a central moist crust or form shallow erosions with a thin remnant of blister roof as an outer zone. This form is the predominant presentation in newborns. Whether blisters are large or small, impetigo is the preferred term.

Staphylococcus aureus **and streptococcus** are responsible for the lesions of impetigo, with up to 50% of *S. aureus* due to MRSA in North America. Colonization of the skin occurs days to months before microscopic breaks in the skin permit the bacteria to invade. Poor hygienic habits such as nose-picking enhance the spread of impetigo. Nasal carriage of pathogenic bacteria is common. In a few children, nephritogenic strains of streptococcus have been responsible.

Ecthyma while due to the same bacteria, differs in clinical appearance from impetigo by the presence of indurated borders surrounding a firm, dry crust. Direct pressure on the crust produces purulent material to extrude from beneath the crust. Ecthyma represents involvement of the entire epidermis while impetigo involves only the upper epidermis.

TREATMENT

Topical antibiotics Topical mupirocin plus good hand washing are the preferred treatment strategies. If infected areas are large, culture and antimicrobial sensitivities help determine treatment. Cephalexin 40–50 mg/kg per day for 10 days is often effective when accompanied by daily hand washing with an antibacterial soap.

As MRSA remains a concern and antibiotic resistance increases, knowledge of effective MRSA treatment in your area is required and guided by sensitivity testing of bacterial cultures, including attempts to reduce nasal carriage. If nephritogenic strains are suspected, an active program of treatment for both affected children and contacts will reduce the risk of glomerulonephritis.

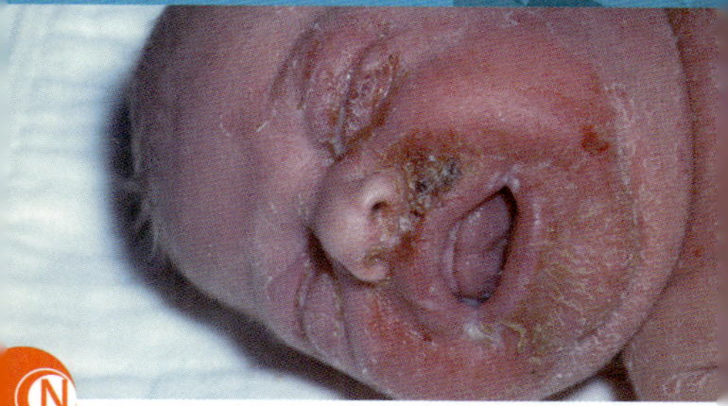

N Newborn with SSSS. Red, tender skin with perioral and periorbital crusting.

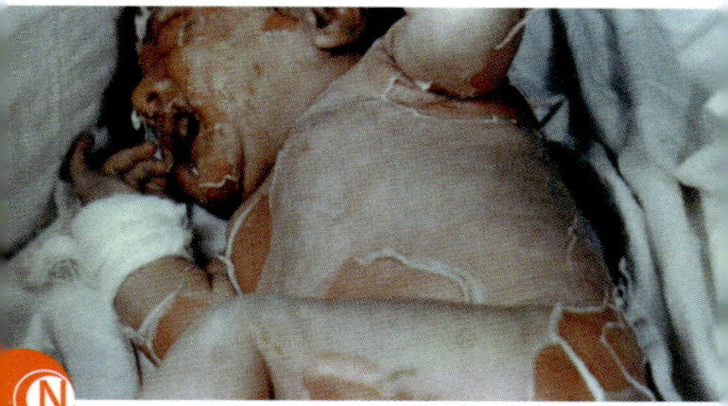

N Newborn with SSSS with widespread red, shiny erosions surrounded by thin peeling epidermis.

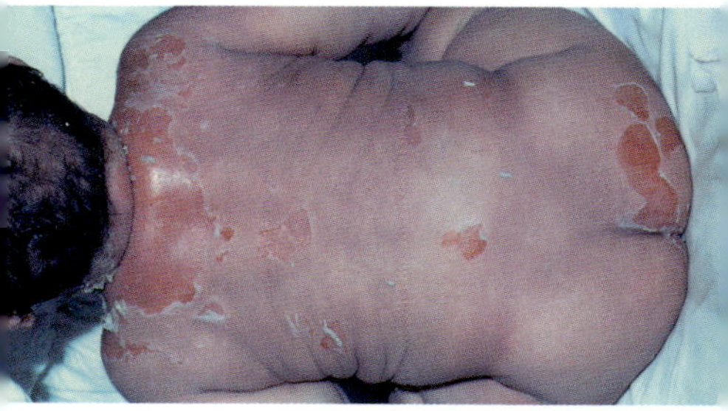

Infant with SSSS. Red, painful skin and red, shiny erosions with thin epidermal peeling.

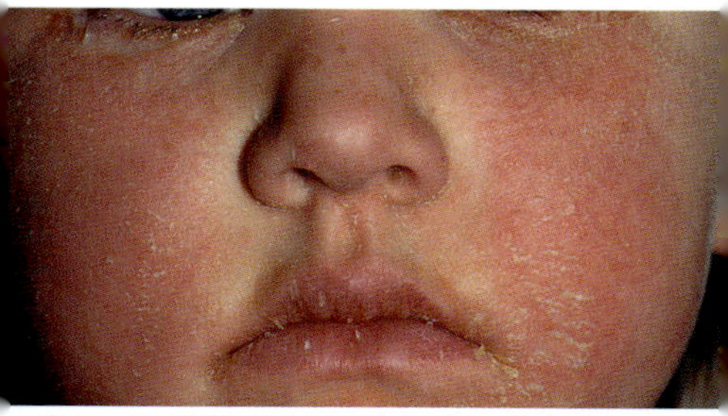

Child with SSSS. Painful red cheeks with initial perioral crusting.

CLINICAL FEATURES

The abrupt onset of red, exceedingly painful skin that separates with the slightest friction leaving red, shiny erosions with a border of thin peeling epidermis characterizes SSSS.

Newborns will have the entire cutaneous surface involved with an inability to maintain temperature control and will lose fluids and electrolytes. Mortality may be high as newborns do not readily make antitoxin. It may be introduced into the nursery by a staph carrier.

In infants and toddlers the involvement may be more localized to the upper body, and development of painful perioral, periorbital, and neck crusting is characteristic. Intact blisters are seldom seen. SSSS often occurs following a mild upper respiratory infection. The nares often harbor the responsible staphylococci. It is rarely seen over age 5 years. Infants and toddlers readily make neutralizing antitoxin, limiting the reaction to 1–3 days.

SSSS is the result of a bacterial toxin staph exfoliatin A, a serine protease that binds to desmoglein I and is produced by only certain strains of staphylococci (Phage group II). A tiny amount of staph produces enough toxin to exfoliate a human.

The toxin circulates to the skin from the infectious site and specifically injures the granular layer of the epidermis, producing a separation of the outer one third of the epidermis after the slightest friction to the skin.

TREATMENT

Newborns Should be hospitalized for 1–3 days and must have prompt administration of intravenous dicloxacillin and clindamycin or other antistaph drugs, and restoration of fluid and electrolytes. Temperature control is necessary. Minimal handling of the baby is imperative as friction to the skin induces more separation and pain. Screening cultures of nursery personnel and visitors and institution of sterile techniques is critical, as nursery epidemics with a high mortality rate have been described.

Infants and toddlers require minimal handling for the first 24 hours. Treatment with oral antibiotics such as dicloxacillin 15–50 mg/kg per day for 7–10 days is recommended. After the pain diminishes, a lubricating ointment may be applied twice daily to speed healing of desquamated sites.

7

BLISTERS (VESICLES AND BULLAE)

Miliaria

DDx ref 1 • 26 • 23

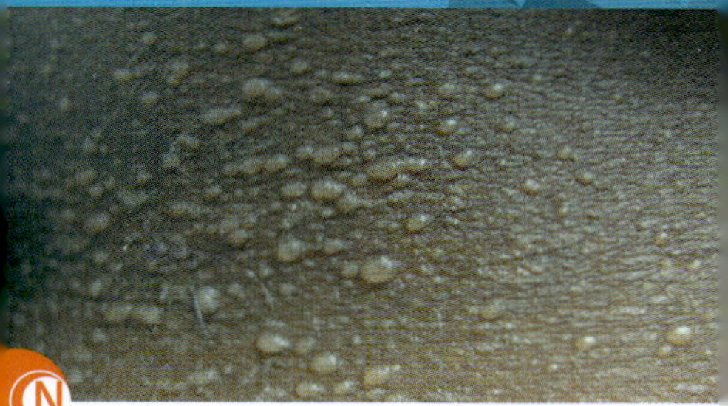

Miliaria cristallina. Multiple 1–2-mm vesicles in sweat pores of a newborn.

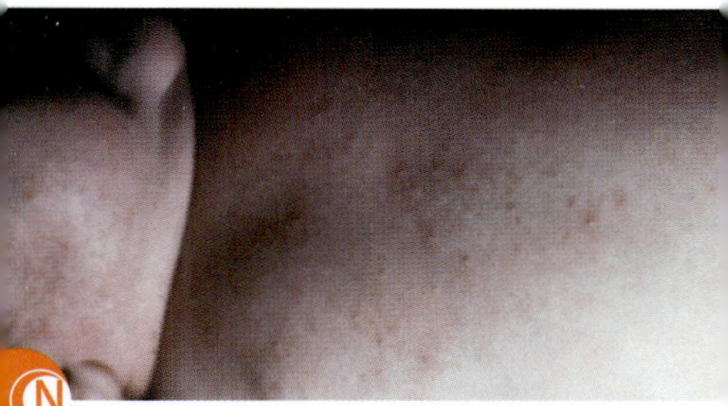

Miliaria rubra. Tiny red papules on the chest of an infant.

8

BLISTERS (VESICLES AND BULLAE)

Dermatitis herpetiformis

DDx ref 1 • 2 • 88

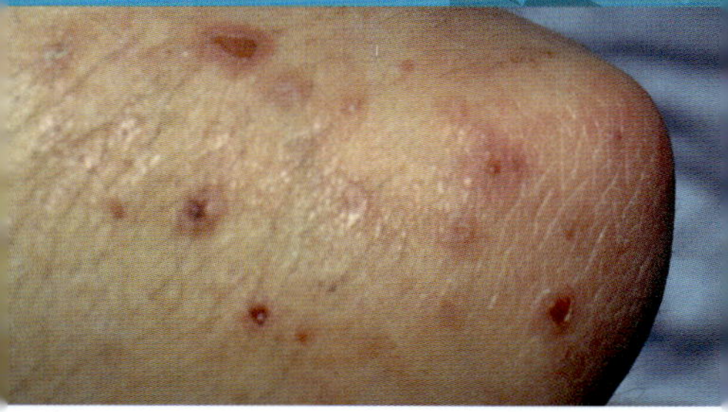

Grouped blisters and erosions around the elbow in a child with dermatitis herpetiformis (DH).

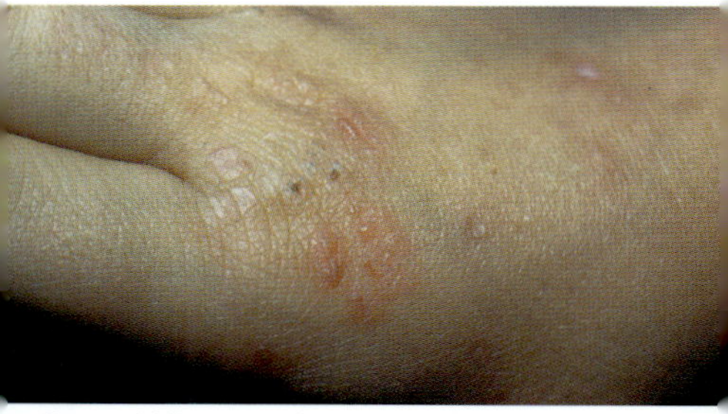

Grouped blisters on the dorsum of the hand in a child with DH.

7 DDx ref 1 • 26 • 23

BLISTERS (VESICLES AND BULLAE)

Miliaria

CLINICAL FEATURES

In newborns and especially premature infants, obstruction of the outer one third of the sweat duct presents as 1–2-mm discrete, clear vesicles without inflamed skin (miliaria cristallina). With cooling, the vesicles disappear in 24–48 hours leaving a tiny white scale.

It also occurs in older children in areas of sunburn. Infants may also develop miliaria rubra, characterized by tiny red papules or papulovesicles usually on flexural areas (neck, axillae, groin) and the trunk. This is due to deeper obstruction of the lower one-half of the sweat duct.

Both forms of miliaria are induced by heat retention on the skin or induced sweating, airtight clothing, or dressings. Immobilized children may develop miliaria from plastic bed-covers. Secondary infection with *S. aureus* may occur, producing pustules in the sweat pores (miliaria pustulosa). This is more prevalent in hot, humid conditions.

TREATMENT

Allowing the skin surface to dry and cool is the treatment of choice. Causes of overheating of the skin must be corrected. Cooling lotions will not be effective unless the overheating is corrected. Avoidance of overclothing the baby will be preventative.

8 DDx ref 1 • 2 • 88

BLISTERS (VESICLES AND BULLAE)

Dermatitis herpetiformis

CLINICAL FEATURES

In dermatitis herpetiformis (DH) IgA antibodies are directed at epidermal transglutaminase. All patients with DH have gluten-sensitive enteropathy, although it may be mild or asymptomatic. DH is characterized by severely pruritic grouped papules, vesicles, or urticarial lesions. Patients usually become symptomatic in the adolescent years.

Classic sites of predilection for DH are the elbows, knees, buttocks, and upper trunk, but lesions may occur anywhere, including the scalp.

Urticarial lesions are common and DH may initially be misdiagnosed as chronic urticaria. Pruritus is often so severe that intact vesicles are not seen and the patient presents with only excoriations.

Biopsy of perilesional skin with immunofluorescence evaluation reveals IgA in the dermal papillae. DH is most prevalent in Northern European populations and may be associated with the development of lymphoma in adult life.

TREATMENT

Patients respond within weeks to a few months to a gluten-free diet, although it is difficult for a child to follow rigorously.

Dapsone 0.5–2.0 mg/kg per day is an effective treatment, but it is associated with the risk of serious side-effects including methemoglobinemia, hemolysis, and hypersensitivity syndrome. Before starting dapsone, serum glucose 6 dehydrogenase, compete blood count, and liver function tests should be evaluated. Complete blood counts and liver function tests should be followed throughout therapy, which is lifelong.

Sunburn

DDx ref 6 • 31 • 52

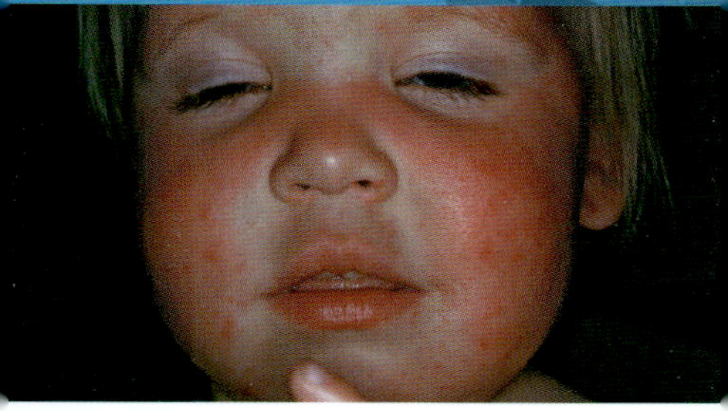

Acute sunburn on the face of a child.

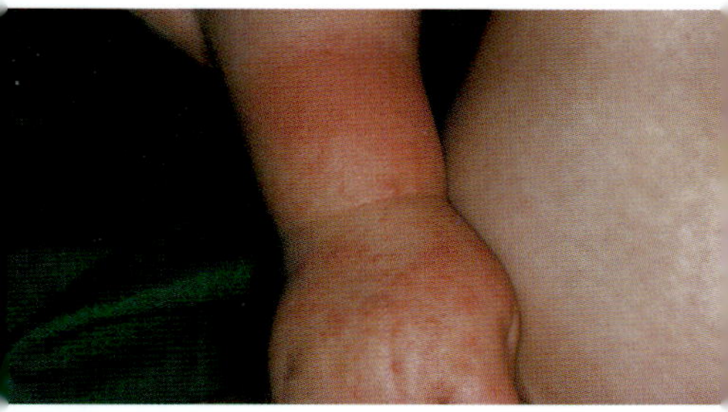

Acute sunburn on the arm of a child. Note the sharp demarcation due to protective clothing.

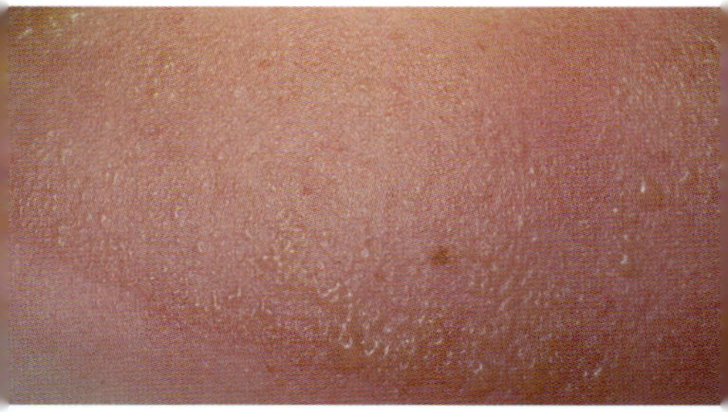

Sunburn with vesiculation on the neck of an adolescent.

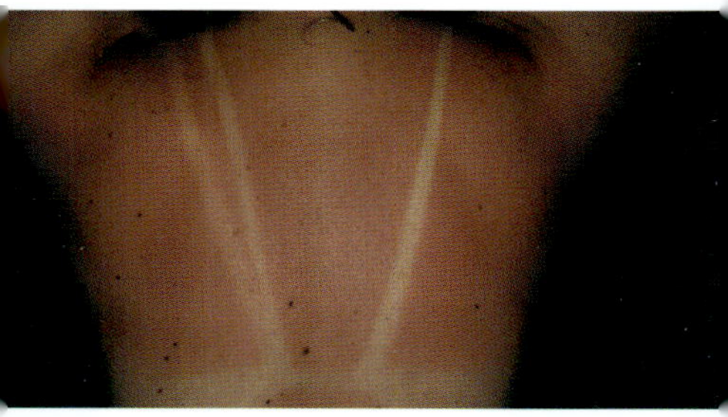

Sunburn on the back of an adolescent. Note uninvolved skin protected by clothing.

Sunburn

DDx ref 6 • 31 • 52

CLINICAL FEATURES

Sunburn occurs readily in fair-skinned children and correlates with the amount of melanin pigment in the epidermis.

Newborns and infants are very susceptible, as they have not created their normal amount of melanin pigment.

The first signs are red, tender skin in sun-exposed areas, such as the face, ears, and cheeks, the back of the neck, the V of the anterior neck, and the extensor surfaces of the arms and legs. Protective clothing will produce sharp demarcation of normal skin from sun exposed areas. The redness will begin quickly from 30 minutes to 4 hours after sun exposure.

Edema and blistering develop within 6–12 hours if the sun exposure is severe. In severe sun exposure in newborns and infants, their sweating rate is reduced and may contribute to collapse from heatstroke. The concomitant heating of the skin may also result in miliaria crystallina within areas of sunburn. Tenderness of the skin makes sleep difficult, and fever, headache, and fatigue are common. Some 2–7 days after sun exposure, the outer half of the epidermis is shed in white sheets of desquamation.

Investigation into exposure to medications that may accentuate sunburn, including sulfonamides, phenothiazines, ibuprofen, naproxen, tetracyclines, griseofulvin, and tretinoin should be instituted. It should be remembered that prolonged sunburn reactions occur in the rare types of xeroderma pigmentosum.

TREATMENT

The pain and redness of acute sunburn can be relieved by wet dressings or cool compresses. If given within 6 hours of exposure, indomethacin or aspirin may modify the sunburn. Topical steroids and anesthetics are not efficacious in sunburn.

Prevention Sunburn is 100% preventable and prevention is the key in children. Sun exposure between the hours of 10 a.m. and 3 p.m. should be minimized. Children should wear hats, sunglasses, and clothing and use a UVB and UVA protective sunscreen that is waterproof with a sun protective factor (SPF) of 30 or greater. It should be applied before sun exposure and reapplied every 1–2 hours. Water activities diminish the sun protection, even with the 'waterproof' sunscreens.

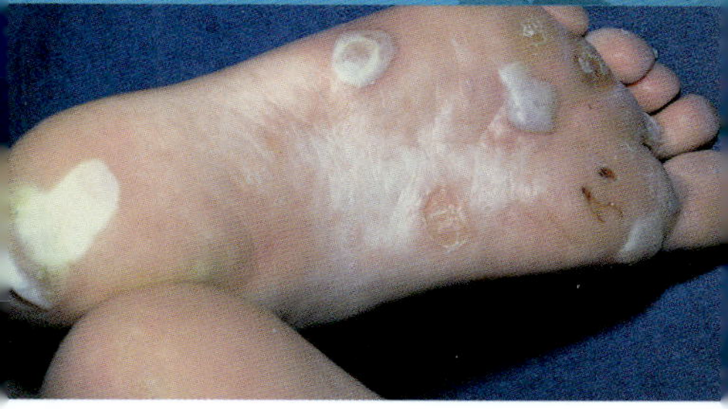

Epidermolysis bullosa simplex, localized.

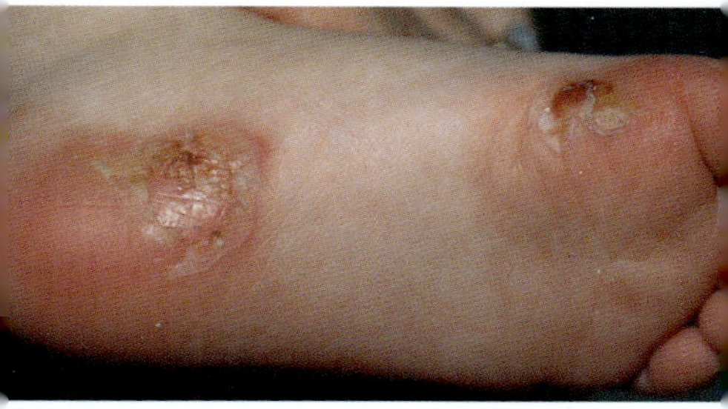

Epidermolysis bullosa simplex, generalized discrete blisters on a toddler's foot.

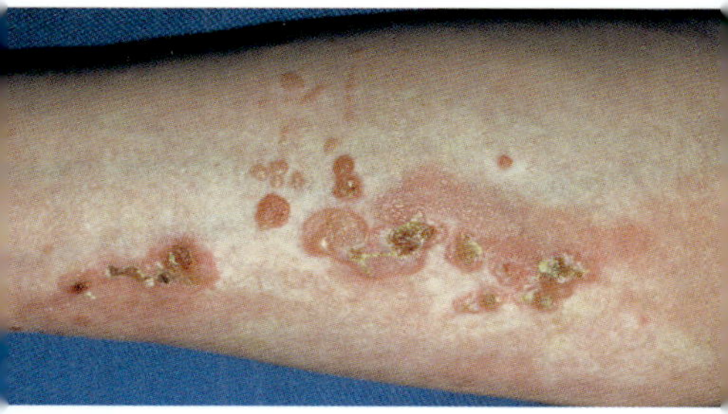

Epidermolysis bullosa simplex, generalized. Grouped blisters on the leg of a child.

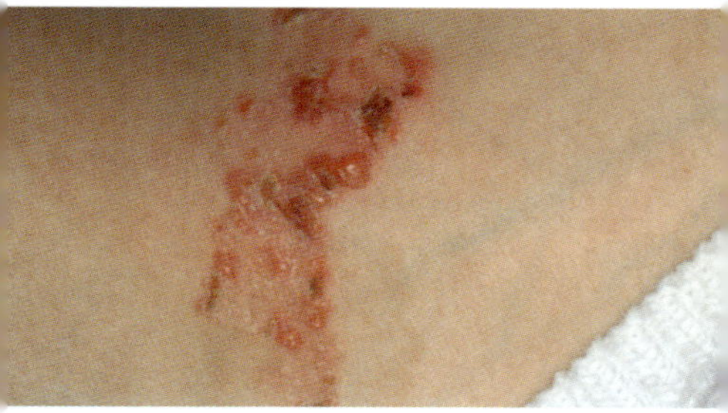

Epidermolysis bullosa simplex, generalized. Grouped blisters on the arm of a child.

CLINICAL FEATURES

Epidermolysis bullosa simplex (EBS) is characterized by blister formation within the epidermis, most commonly in the basal layer, and in rarer forms, in the suprabasilar layer. There are mutations in six different genes that cause EBS. These are keratin 5, keratin 14, plectin, $\alpha6\beta4$ integrin, plakophilin, and desmoplakin. A new form of EBS caused by mutations in the dystonin gene has been described. The defects in the most common types of EBS are in keratins 5 or 14. There are multiple other rare variants.

The most common form of EBS is localized to the hands and feet (EBS-localized). It was formerly named EBS-Weber–Cockayne. In EBS-localized, blisters usually are not present at birth and first occur in late childhood or early adolescence. Blisters of the hands and feet develop after minor frictional trauma. Frequent superinfection of blisters on the feet occurs. Focal palmar and plantar hyperkeratosis may be seen. It often has its onset and is most symptomatic in warm weather.

EBS may also be generalized There are two major forms of generalized EBS. These are EBS-generalized other (formerly EBS-Koebner) and EBS-Dowling–Meara. In EBS-generalized, blisters often present at birth or in the neonatal period. The lesions are more numerous on the distal extremities, but may also be seen on the elbows and knees. In EBS-generalized, other the lesions are discrete.

EBS-generalized Dowling–Meara is characterized by grouped blisters resembling herpes simplex. Onset is usually at birth. Severity of blisters varies greatly, both within and among families. Widespread areas of grouped blisters are typical, and hemorrhagic blisters are found. Mucosal involvement may interfere with feeding. During infancy, blistering may be severe and extensive, may involve mucous membranes, and may result in shedding of nails and formation of milia. Both hyper- and hypopigmentation develop. Improvement may occur during mid–late childhood.

TREATMENT

Treatment is symptomatic and supportive. Drain blisters with a sterile needle or blade. Do not remove the blister roof. If the blister roof is gone, apply Vaseline and a non-stick bandage. Secure the bandage with Kerlix and netting. Avoid strenuous activity in warm weather. Antibiotics may be necessary if the blisters become infected.

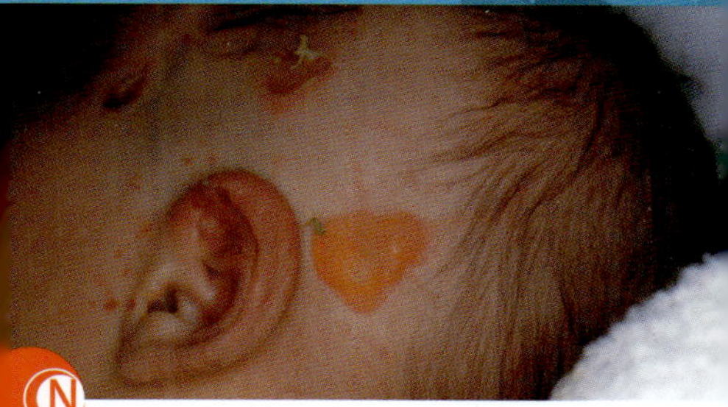

Junctional epidermolysis bullosa. Newborn with a few scattered blisters.

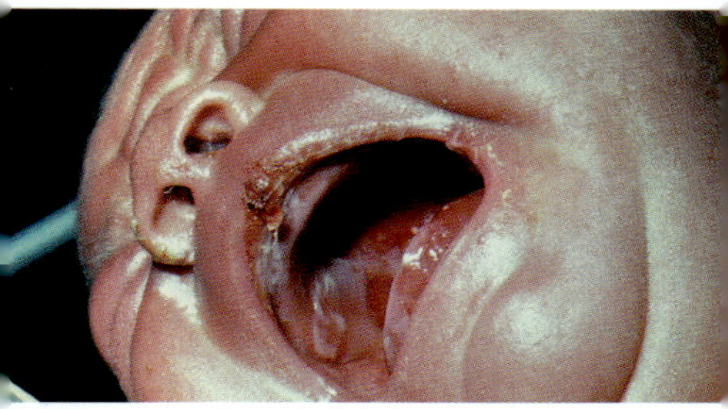

Junctional epidermolysis bullosa. Severe oral erosions in an infant.

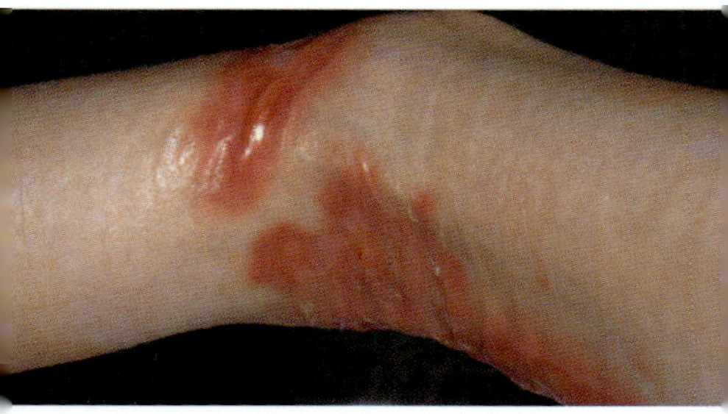

Scarring (dystrophic) epidermolysis bullosa. Hemorrhagic bulla.

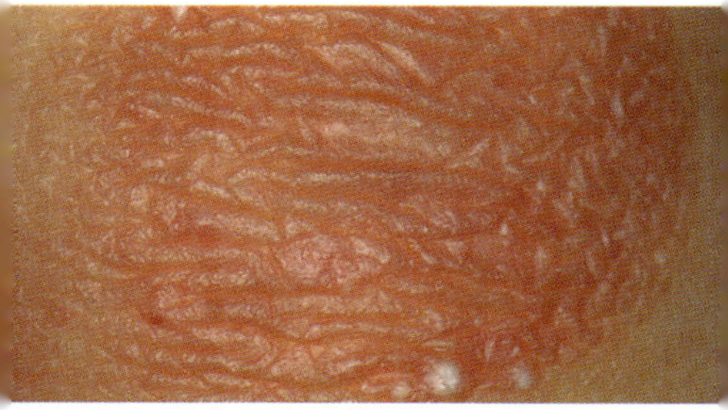

Recessive dystrophic epidermolysis bullosa. Multiple white milia at border of scar.

CLINICAL FEATURES

Junctional epidermolysis bullosa (JEB) may be divided into two subtypes. These are JEB-Herlitz (JEB-H) and JEB-other. JEB-H is a life-threatening autosomal recessive disease caused by mutations in laminin-332 (formerly laminin-5). Blisters may be present at birth and continue to develop throughout the neonatal period. Oral mucosa becomes severely affected and interferes with eating, often resulting in failure to thrive. Non-healing granulation tissue may develop over bony prominences such as the spine, ear, or mid-face. Healing is delayed and these large erosive plaques may provide a portal of entry for bacterial infection, and septicemia is often the cause of death. Most patients die within 3 years. JEB-other is a heterogeneous group of disorders.

Mutations have been found in laminin-332, type XVII collagen, and $\alpha 6\beta 4$ integrin. Blisters may be severe early in life, making distinction between JEB-Herlitz difficult but in general, these conditions are much milder. Mucous membrane lesions and non-healing granulomas are rarely, if ever, seen. The $\alpha 6\beta 4$ integrin subtype is associated with pyloric stenosis.

Dystrophic epidermolysis bullosa (DEB) consists of dominant dystrophic epidermolysis bullosa (DDEB) and recessive dystrophic epidermolysis bullosa-severe generalized (RDEB-sev gen), formerly known as RDEB-Hallopeau–Siemens. All forms of DEB are caused by mutations in type VII collagen. In DDEB, blisters may be seen at birth and are limited in number and characteristically form over acral prominences. Lesions heal with soft, wrinkled scars, milia, and pigmentary alteration. Nails are frequently lost and replaced by scars. Mucous membrane disease is minimal and, when present, quite mild. Blistering continues throughout life and in many cases is mild, causing little restriction of activity. Anemia and failure to thrive are rarely seen.

RDEB-sev gen is the most debilitating form of EB, although the clinical spectrum is wide. In severe cases, blistering is present at birth and heals with scarring. Milia formation within the scars is common. Nails are lost and scarring of the digits leads to fusion into a club-like appearance. Scarring alopecia of the scalp is common and severe scarring of the eyelids may occur. Blisters and erosions of the oral mucosa result in limitation of eating, immobilization of the tongue, and esophageal stricture. Laryngeal bullae may cause respiratory stridor. The teeth may be malformed. Anemia, malnutrition, and failure to thrive are common. Secondary bacterial and candidal infection is frequent. Squamous cell carcinoma arising in the chronically scarred areas is a leading cause of death.

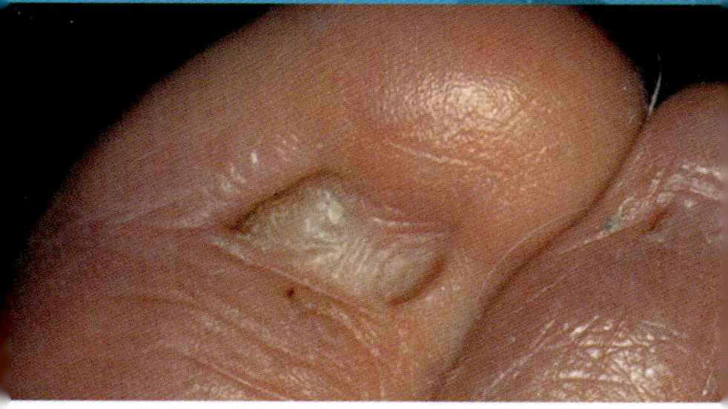

Recessive dystrophic epidermolysis bullosa. Missing toenails and scarring.

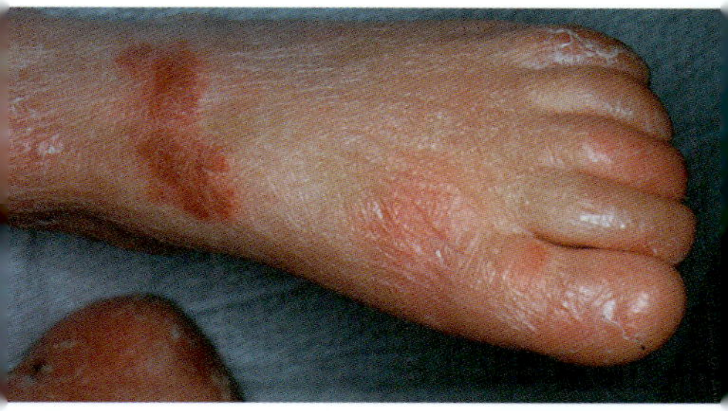

Recessive dystrophic epidermolysis bullosa. Loss of toenails, and pseudowebbing of digits.

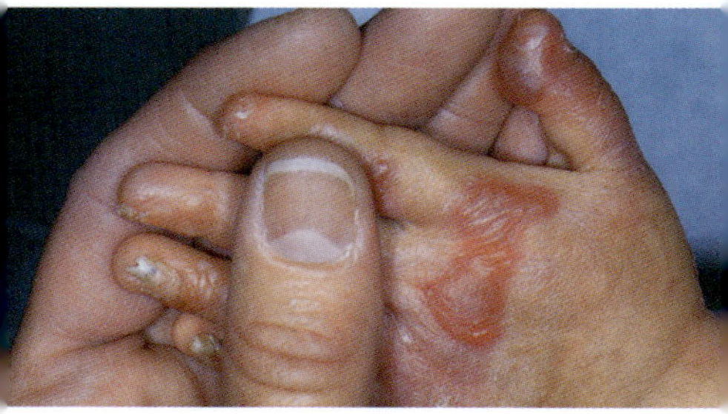

Dominant dystrophic epidermolysis bullosa. Blister, scar formation, milia, and loss of a fingernail in infant.

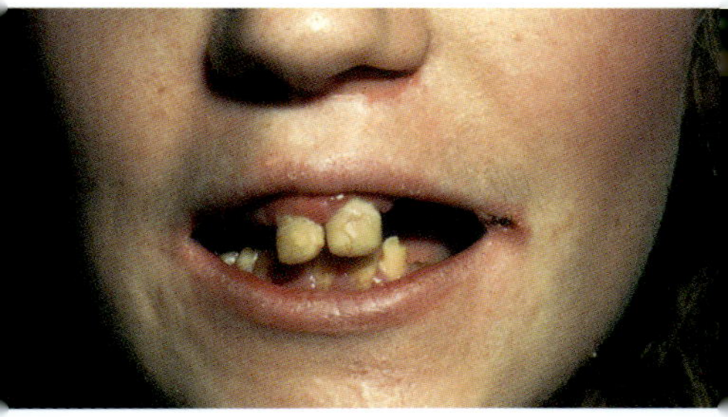

Recessive dystrophic epidermolysis bullosa. Loss of teeth and restriction of mouth opening in child.

TREATMENT

Treatment for the scarring forms of EB is symptomatic and supportive, but much more intensive than for the non-scarring forms. Treatment at a specialized EB center is optimal. Skilled nursing techniques and general healthcare are required. Saltwater baths for dressing changes help reduce the pain. Stem cell treatments are an active area of research.

Blisters should be drained and bandaged as with the non-scarring forms. Tissue engineered skin grafts may be used on large non-healing ulcers.

Neonates should be fed multiple small feedings with a soft nipple.

Gentle handling, soft, loose fitting clothing, and a sheepskin for sleeping are required. Adequate nutrition must be maintained and nutritional supplements and gastrostomy are often required. Esophageal dilatation and stricture excision with colonic interposition may be needed. Iron supplementation and transfusions are necessary to treat chronic anemia.

A multidisciplinary approach is required to deal with general well-being, esophageal strictures, dental abnormalities, extremity fusion, laryngeal disorders, urethral meatal stenosis, conjunctival scarring, and psychosocial issues. Any verrucous growths should be biopsied to evaluate for squamous cell carcinoma.

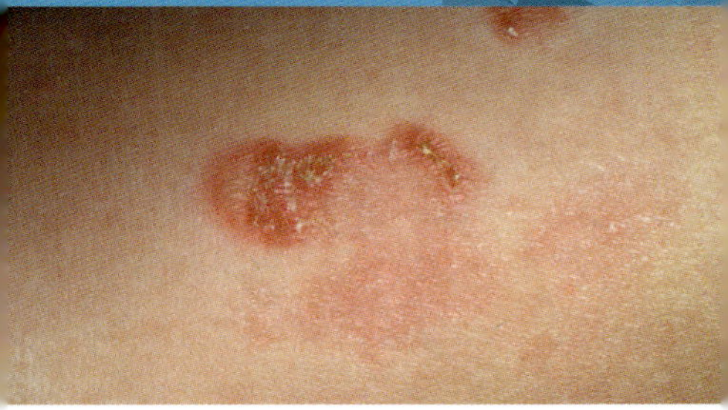

Crusted lesions on the arm of a child with pemphigus foliaceous.

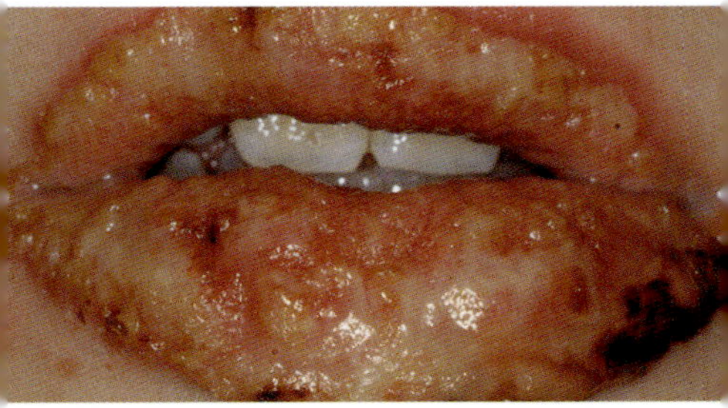

Completely eroded lips in an adolescent with pemphigus vulgaris. His mouth was also severely eroded.

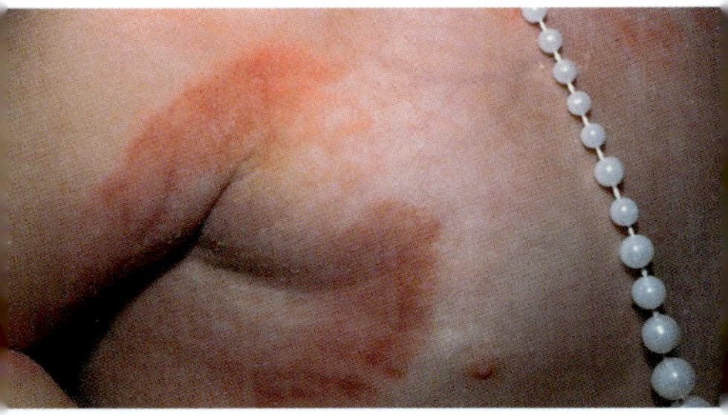

Trauma-induced erosions in an infant with pemphigus vulgaris.

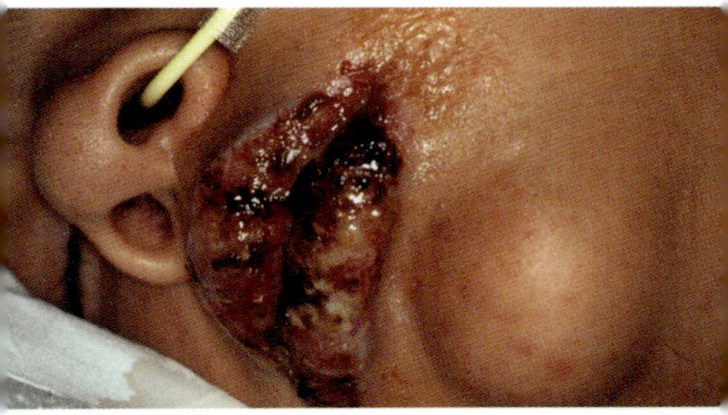

Hemorrhagic crusts on lips and eroded conjunctiva in a boy with PNP and Castleman's tumor.

CLINICAL FEATURES

There are three forms of pemphigus.

Pemphigus foliaceous (PF) is caused by circulating antibodies to the 50-kDa portion of the 160-kDa desmoglomal protein, desmoglein 1. PF patients develop superficial blisters, which rupture quickly, leaving erosions surrounded by erythema. They heal with crusting and scaling. Lesions are most common on the scalp, face, neck, and upper trunk. Once lesions appear they tend to be persistent. Mucous membrane lesions are minimal or absent. The patient may complain of pruritus or a stinging pain. An endemic form is seen in Brazil (fogo selvagem). PF tends to be less severe than pemphigus vulgaris (PV).

Pemphigus vulgaris (PV) is caused by circulating antibodies to desmoglein 3. In PV, oral lesions usually present for months before the development of skin lesions. The oral lesions are seen as painful erosions of the lips, tongue, and buccal mucosa. The pain from the oral lesions may limit eating and drinking, leading to malnutrition. Other mucosal sites may be involved. After a few months, flaccid blisters and crusted lesions may appear anywhere on the body. In a variant of PV, pemphigus vegetans, verrucous, malodorous lesions develop in the groin and axilla.

Paraneoplastic pemphigus (PNP) is usually associated in children with Castleman's tumor, a thoracic B lymphocyte hyperplasia. Antibodies against desmoplakin 1, desmoplakin 2, envoplakin, periplakin, and desmoglein 3 are found. PNP begins with severe, widespread oral disease. Target-like lesions on the skin, and severe cuticle involvement may be seen. Oral lesions interfere with nutrition, and weight loss is seen. Severe pulmonary involvement and sloughing of airway mucosa (bronchiolitis obliterans) occurs.

TREATMENT

Localized PF may be treated with super-potent topical steroids. More widespread disease requires oral methylprednisolone 1 mg/kg per day. Long-term remission is usually achieved.

PV treatment often requires methylprednisolone 1–2 mg/kg per day and mycophenolate mofetil 500–1000 mg twice a day. Rituximab may lead to long-term remission and should begin as soon as possible. After the first course of Rituximab, the child begins weaning off steroids.

Treatment of PNP is similar to therapy of PV. Removal of the Castleman's tumor may be beneficial. Mortality is high.

13 DDx ref 1 • 2 • 14

BLISTERS (VESICLES AND BULLAE)

Linear IgA dermatosis

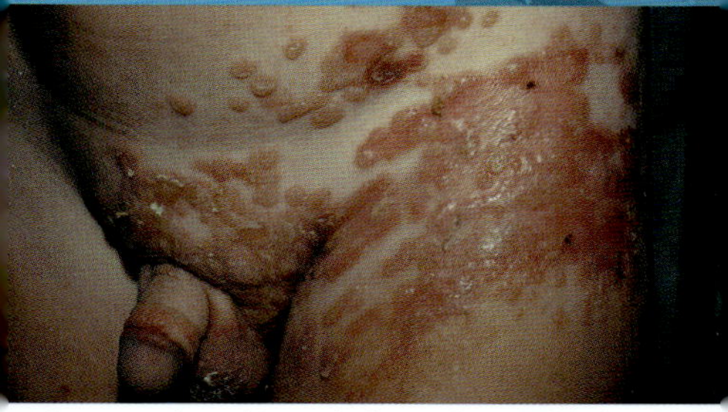

Sausage-shaped tense bullae and crusted lesions in a toddler with linear IgA dermatosis.

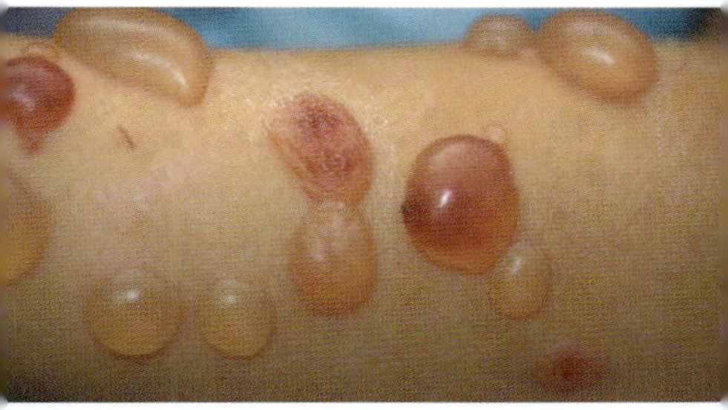

Tense blisters on the arm of a child with linear IgA dermatosis.

14 DDx ref 13 • 12 • 11

BLISTERS (VESICLES AND BULLAE)

Pemphigoid

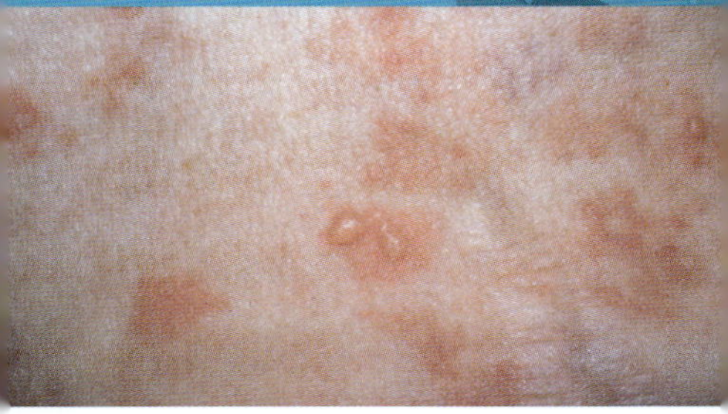

Tense blisters on the leg in childhood bullous pemphigoid.

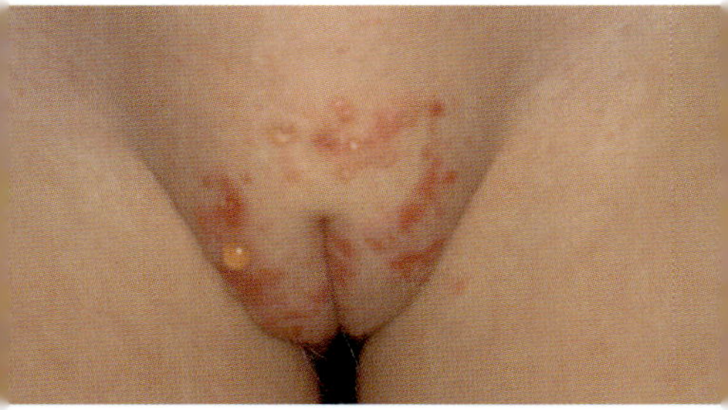

Vulvar blisters, erosions and early scarring in a preschool child with localized vulvar pemphigoid.

13 BLISTERS (VESICLES AND BULLAE)

Linear IgA dermatosis

DDx ref 1 • 2 • 14

CLINICAL FEATURES

Linear IgA dermatosis is a heterogeneous autoimmune disorder with antibodies targeting multiple antigens. The most common antigens are LABD97 and LAD-1, which are degradation products of BP 180 (type 17 collagen). It may also be drug-induced, usually by vancomycin. Biopsy of perilesional skin with immunofluorescence evaluation reveals linear IgA deposition at the basement membrane. The blisters of linear IgA dermatosis are characteristically sausage-shaped, grouped in an annular or rosette-like fashion around a central crust, and occur most commonly in the inguinal area. Multiple tense blisters, some with hemorrhage, may be seen. Toddlers are usually affected. Pruritus may be absent or very intense.

TREATMENT

Linear IgA usually responds promptly to dapsone 0.5–2.0 mg/day. Oral methylprednisone, mycophenolate mofetil, and erythromycin may be used in cases unresponsive to dapsone. Improvement with dapsone is usually seen within a few weeks. Once clear, linear IgA dermatosis is unlikely to recur. The usual course is 2–4 years.

14 BLISTERS (VESICLES AND BULLAE)

Pemphigoid

DDx ref 13 • 12 • 11

CLINICAL FEATURES

Bullous pemphigoid (BP) is caused by circulating antibodies to either the 180-kDa or 230-kDa BP antigen (type 17 collagen). Immunofluorescence findings include linear deposition of IgG and/or C3 at the dermoepidermal junction. The infantile form of BP usually presents with blisters on the palms, soles and scalp, whereas the childhood form is more likely to present with vulvar lesions, and a subset of girls with BP will have only vulvar lesions. Individual lesions vary greatly in size, are tense, and filled with serous fluid that may become hemorrhagic. Lesions may be pruritic or painful and may heal with scarring. Mucosal lesions are seen less commonly than in pemphigus vulgaris. Rarer variants include those associated with lichen planus and solid organ transplant rejection.

TREATMENT

Infants and children with localized disease may be treated with super-potent topical steroids. Those with more generalized disease will require treatment with methylprednisolone (1–2 mg/kg per day). Remission is usually achieved in several weeks to a few months and relapses are very rare. There is no difference in response to treatment for any of the types of BP.

15 DDx ref

BLISTERS (VESICLES AND BULLAE)

Incontinentia pigmenti

1 • 127 • 92

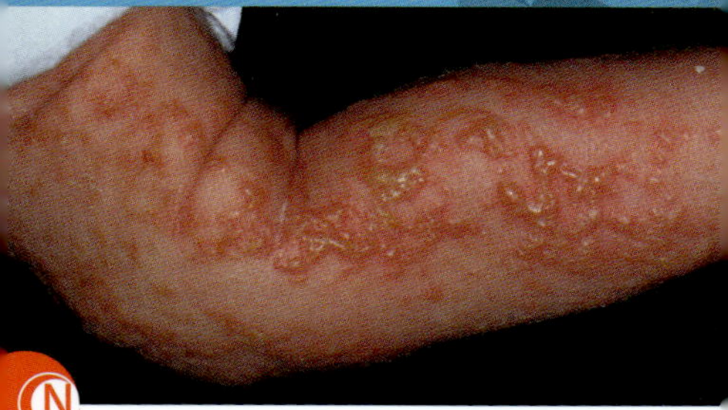

Incontinentia pigmenti. Linear vesicles and crusts in an affected newborn girl.

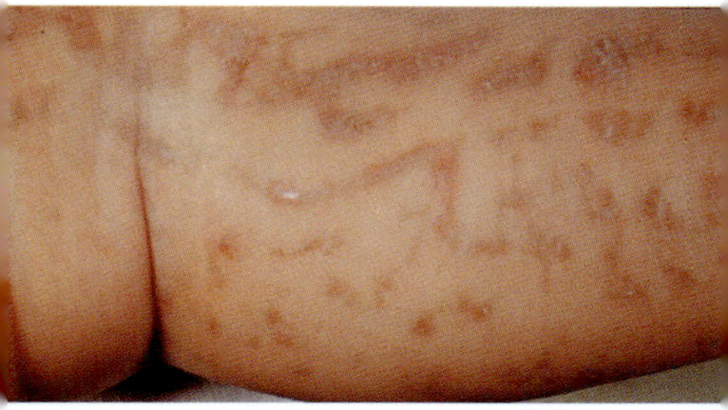

Incontinentia pigmenti. Whorled pigmentation of an extremity in sites of previous blisters.

16 DDx ref

BLISTERS (VESICLES AND BULLAE)

Epidermolytic hyperkeratosis

5 • 6 • 70

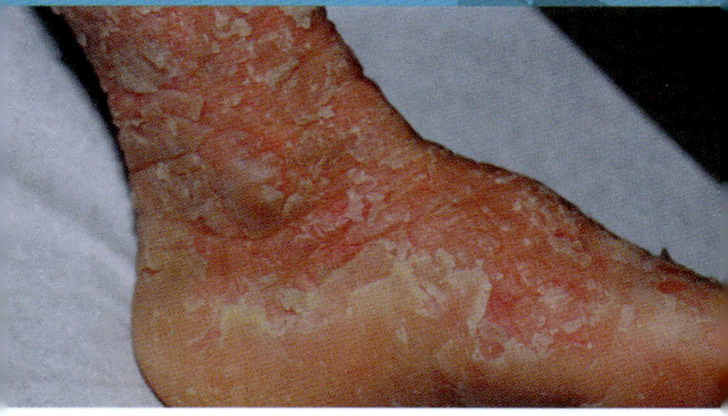

Epidermolytic hyperkeratosis. Thickened, malodorous skin on legs and ankles.

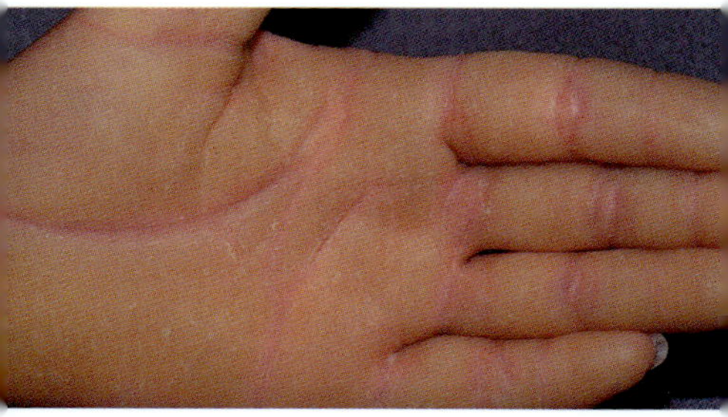

Epidermolytic hyperkeratosis. Hyperkeratosis of the palms and deep fissures of the creases.

15 DDx ref 1 • 127 • 92

BLISTERS (VESICLES AND BULLAE)

Incontinentia pigmenti

CLINICAL FEATURES

Incontinentia pigmenti is an X-linked disorder, lethal in males except in mosaic form, caused by mutations in the gene encoding NF-κb essential modifier (NEMO). Four distinct clinical types of skin lesions are seen.

Initial lesions are curvilinear vesicles following the lines of Blaschko occurring in the first week of life. This is followed by a warty verrucous phase that may last until 1 year.

The third phase is curvilinear macular hyperpigmentation that may occur at areas not initially affected. The hyperpigmentation fades and in adulthood is replaced by hypopigmented, slightly atrophic scarred areas. There may be some overlap of the phases.

Blood eosinophilia may be seen early in life. Dental abnormalities are common, including oligodontia, hypodontia, and peg-shaped teeth. Retinal vascular proliferation leading to retinal detachment and loss of vision may occur.

CNS disease is reported to occur in up to 20% of children and may present as mental retardation, seizures, and spasticity. Rarely, limb abnormalities may also occur.

TREATMENT

No treatment is required for the skin disease. Ophthalmologic examination should be performed on all patients. Referral to dentistry, neurology, and orthopedics is dependent on degree of involvement.

16 DDx ref 5 • 6 • 70

BLISTERS (VESICLES AND BULLAE)

Epidermolytic hyperkeratosis

CLINICAL FEATURES

Epidermolytic hyperkeratosis is caused by mutations in the genes encoding for keratins K1 and K10.

Newborns have generalized erythroderma with widespread blisters and erosions. With time, blistering ceases and erythema decreases and is replaced by a generalized hyperkeratosis. Thick, warty, dirty-yellow scales develop on the acral areas. Palmoplantar keratoderma is associated with K1 defects. *Staphylococcus aureus* infection is common during the neonatal period and infancy. Malodor due to bacterial colonization of the skin is a major social problem. Hair, nails, mucosa, and sweat glands are normal.

TREATMENT

In the newborn period fluid and electrolyte balance must be controlled and signs of bacterial sepsis should be evaluated and treated urgently.

Antibacterial cleansers and intermittent courses of systemic antibiotics are generally necessary. Keratolytic agents are often poorly tolerated and there is a risk for systemic absorption due to the large surface area treated and the abnormal skin barrier. Oral retinoids are effective, but must be used cautiously due to side-effects. Treatment may begin at 1 mg/kg per day, but then titrated to the lowest effective dose.

17 DDx ref

BLISTERS (VESICLES AND BULLAE)

Diffuse cutaneous mastocytosis

6 • 48 • 16

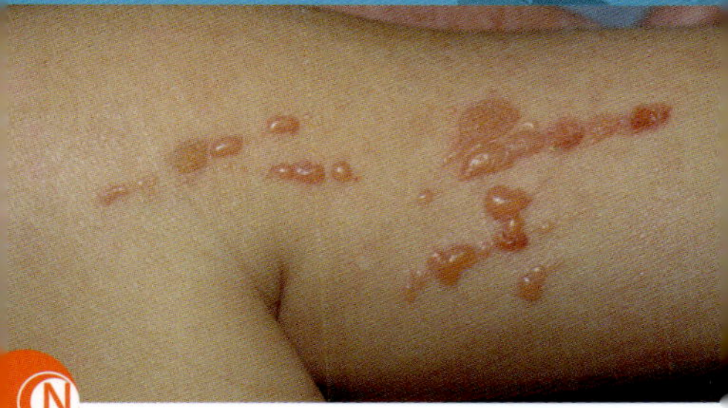

Diffuse cutaneous mastocytosis. Linear blisters from stroking the infant's skin.

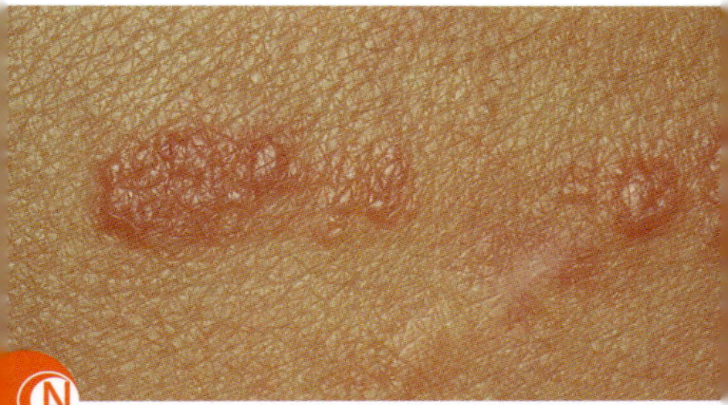

Diffuse cutaneous mastocytosis with thickened, leathery, yellowish skin.

18 DDx ref

BLISTERS (VESICLES AND BULLAE)

Bullous drug reactions

14 • 13 • 65

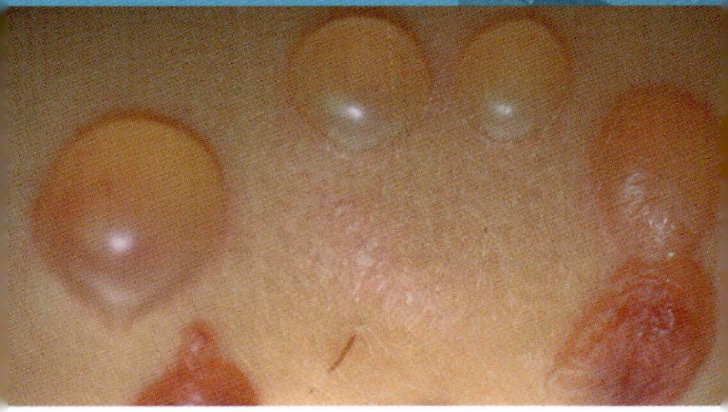

Tense bullae in child treated with vancomycin.

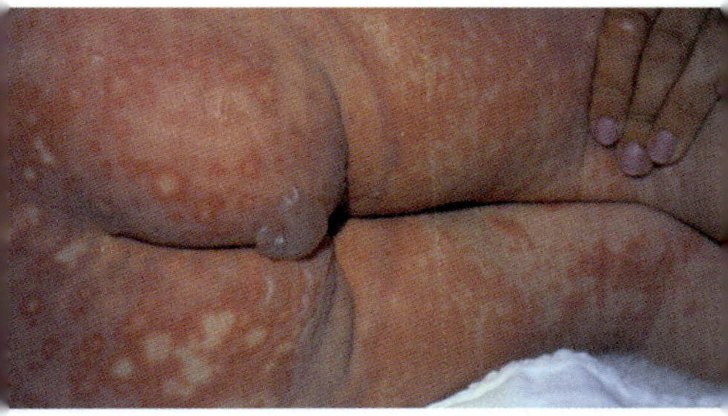

Bullous macules with islands of uninvolved skin in Stevens–Johnson syndrome.

17 DDx ref

BLISTERS (VESICLES AND BULLAE)

Diffuse cutaneous mastocytosis

6 • 48 • 16

CLINICAL FEATURES

Diffuse cutaneous mastocytosis presents as blistering in the neonatal period. Involvement is generalized and discrete hyperpigmented macules and papules as in urticaria pigmentosa are not seen. The blisters are often large and leave large denuded erosions. After a severe blistering episode, 5–10 days may be required to regranulate mast cells. Marked dermographism is present. With time, the skin becomes thickened, pink to yellow, with a doughy feel and a texture resembling orange peel. Recurrent bullae, intractable pruritus, and flushing attacks are common. Severe syncopal episodes and death from prolonged hypotension have been reported.

Gastrointestinal symptoms are seen as the child becomes older, including chronic diarrhea and recurrent episodes of vomiting associated with abdominal pain. Gastrointestinal stromal tumors may appear in adults.

TREATMENT

Oral H1 antihistamines are the first line of therapy. Cetirizine 2.5–10 mg given every morning with hydroxyzine 1 mg/kg at bedtime is an excellent initial therapy. Alternatively, hydroxyzine 1 mg/kg may be given every 6 hours. H2 antihistamines and oral cromolyn sodium may be valuable in infants with gastrointestinal symptoms. Phototherapy with narrow band UVB or psoralens plus UVA (PUVA) twice a week will minimize symptoms.

18 DDx ref

BLISTERS (VESICLES AND BULLAE)

Bullous drug reactions

14 • 13 • 65

CLINICAL FEATURES

In bullous drug reactions, tense bullae develop, usually on the extremities but often may be widespread. They usually begin within 2 weeks of starting the drug. Vancomycin is the most common cause of these eruptions and is associated with linear IgA deposition at the dermal–epidermal junctions (see DDx ref 13 Linear IgA Dermatosis). Bullae may also be seen in fixed drug eruptions (see DDx ref 53 Fixed Drug Eruptions), erythema multiforme (see DDx ref 35 Erythema Multiforme) and in Stevens–Johnson syndrome (SJS) and toxic epidermal necrolysis (TEN) (see DDx ref 20 Stevens–Johnson Syndrome (SJS) and Toxic Epidermal Necrolysis (TEN)).

TREATMENT

Begins with removal of the offending drug. Other supportive care depends upon clinical features and is reported in topics 13, 20, 35, and 53.

MUCOSAL EROSIONS (BLISTER BASES)

Aphthous ulcers

1 • 35 • 3

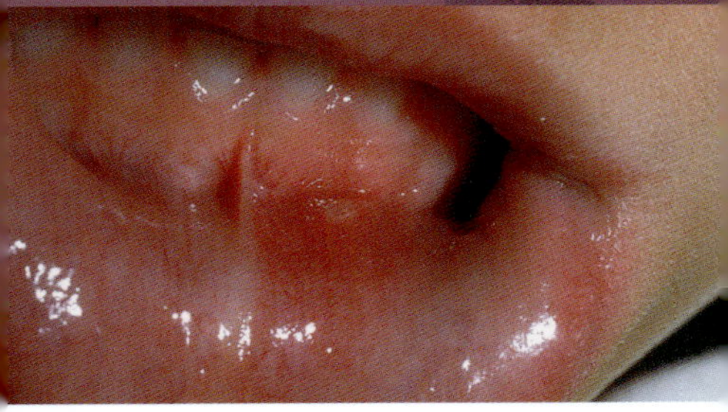

Minor aphthous ulcer with red border in a child's mouth.

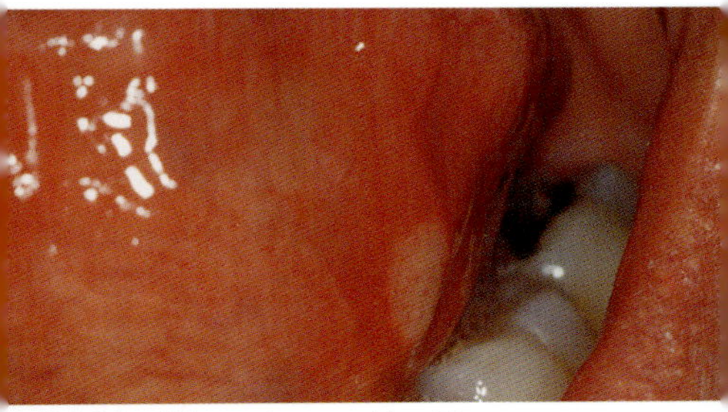

Painful aphthous ulcer on side of tongue.

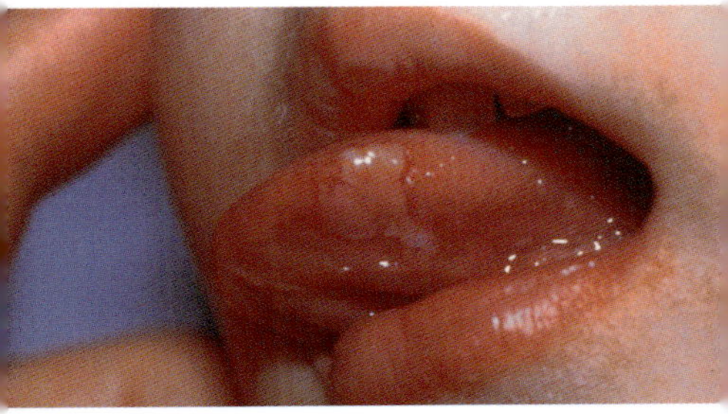

Large painful ulcer on side of tongue in a child with complex aphthosis and vaginal lesions.

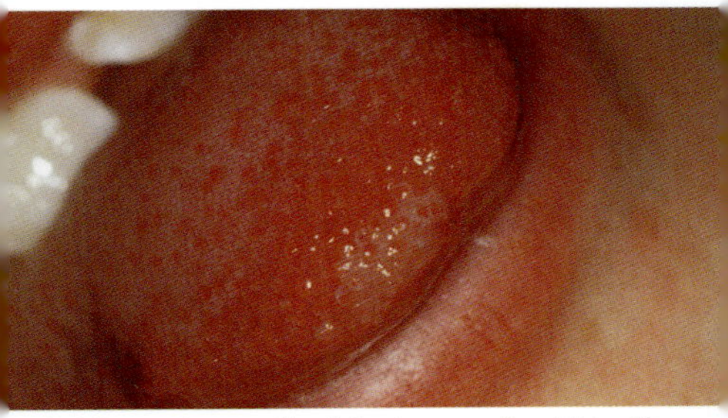

Aphthous ulcer on tip of the tongue of a child with periodic fever (FAPA) syndrome.

Aphthous ulcers

DDx ref 1 • 35 • 3

CLINICAL FEATURES

Aphthae are recurrent, tender, shallow 1–10-mm erosions of the oral mucosa and lips, including gums, tongue, palate, and buccal mucosa. They have a yellow-gray base surrounded by a red zone. Healing occurs in 7–10 days without scarring.

Recurrences are irregular, several months apart, and consist of 2–4 lesions. The uncommon severe forms are characterized by large ulcers greater than 10 mm, and almost continuous disease (major aphthae). This often impairs eating and provides continuous discomfort for the child.

Large ulcers may, in addition to the oral cavity, occur on the genitalia in complex aphthosis. A few children with associated systemic features should be investigated for the possibility of FAPA (fever, aphthous ulcers, pharyngitis, adenitis) syndrome and related periodic fever syndromes, and Behçet's disease (oral and genital aphthae, arthritis, uveitis, vasculitis), cyclic neutropenia, or inflammatory bowel disease. Although there may be abnormalities of the immunoregulatory process in aphthae and related syndromes, the cause is unknown.

TREATMENT

Mild attacks may be treated with liquid antacids to coat the erosions, oral cyanoacrylate dental adhesives, or daily rinsing of the oral cavity with an enzyme solution containing amyloglucosidase and glucose oxidase. Silver nitrate cautery will reduce pain without altering healing time.

Topical steroids in an adhesive base may be used for severe lesions. Oral prednisone 1–2 mg/kg per day for 3–5 days may be necessary for severe involvement that impairs eating. In FAPA and related periodic fever syndromes, prednisone for 1 or 2 days may abort an attack.

For major aphthae colchicine has been effective.

Stevens–Johnson syndrome (SJS) and toxic epidermal necrolysis (TEN)

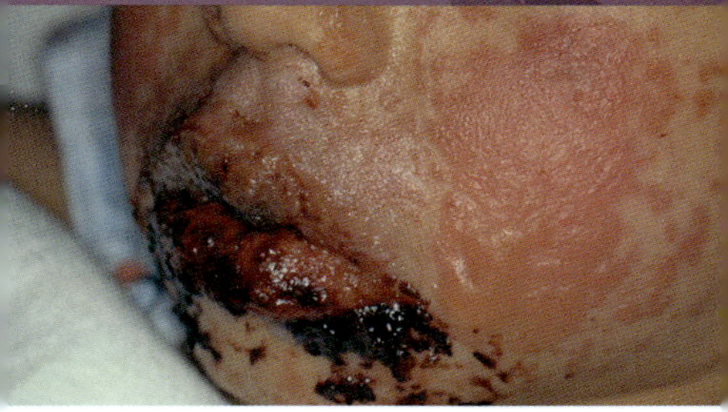

Severe oral and skin involvement in SJS.

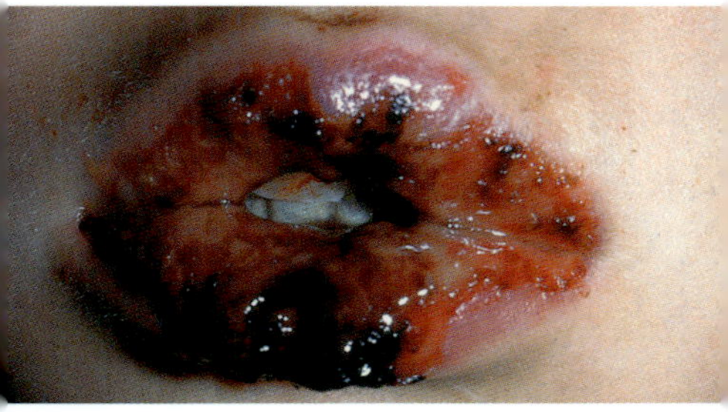

Classic hemorrhagic crusts of lips in a child with SJS.

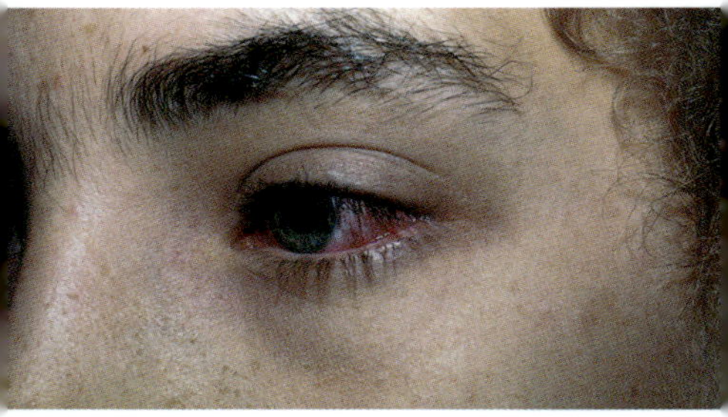

Early conjunctival involvement in SJS with red eyes.

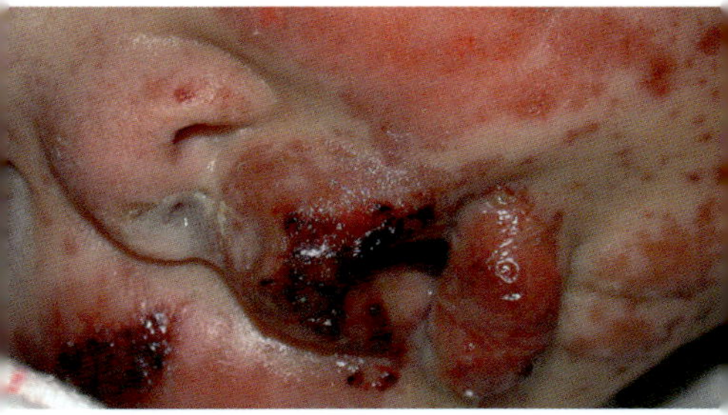

Child with hemorrhagic crusts of lips plus necrosis of skin of cheeks in overlap between SJS and TEN.

20

Stevens–Johnson syndrome (SJS) and toxic epidermal necrolysis (TEN)

DDx ref 65 • 12 • 18

CLINICAL FEATURES

Both SJS and TEN can have overlapping mucocutaneous lesions, but SJS is predominantly a mucosal disease and TEN predominantly has skin involvement. SJS is uncommon but life-threatening in childhood. TEN is rare in childhood. They both occur mostly in children aged 2–10.

SJS begins after a prodrome of fever, headache, and sore throat followed by severe oral mucosal necrosis and often conjunctival redness, then necrosis. At least two mucosal surfaces are involved and may include genital mucosa, respiratory mucosa, and gastrointestinal mucosa. Rarely, only oral mucosa has been involved. Skin lesions are less common but large areas of bulla formation and necrosis of skin may occur. Hemorrhagic crusts on the lips are characteristic. Mycoplasma infection has been associated and may be predominantly mucosal.

TEN demonstrates widespread sheets of epidermal necrosis with large areas of denuded skin and often no mucosal involvement. The course of both conditions may be prolonged for several weeks and accompanied by an inability to eat or drink, dehydration, fever, lymphadenopathy, and cough. Both are characterized by toxic injury to epithelium. Complications of SJS include mucosal scarring with the ocular complications the most concerning. Loss of skin pigment and shedding of nails may occur. TEN may have burn-like scarring of skin and permanent pigment loss.

Reported mortality rates vary because of the differences in severity and the lack of a uniform classification. Generally, it is 1% for SJS and 30% for TEN. Almost all cases of SJS or TEN are drug related, with nonsteroidal anti-inflammatory agents, sulfonamides, and anticonvulsants the most often implicated. Mycoplasma infection is commonly associated.

TREATMENT

Admission to a burn unit or pediatric intensive care unit is recommended. The suspected offending drug must be discontinued. Support of fluids and electrolytes, respiratory toilet, fever control, and prevention of infection of denuded skin are needed. It is not clear whether the commonly used anti-inflammatory drugs alter the course of the disease, but intravenous prednisone 2 mg/kg per day for 4–5 days or intravenous immunoglobulin therapy 1.5–2.0 g/kg per day for 4 days may shorten the disease more than supportive care alone. There is no consensus on any treatment modality.

Ophthalmologic care is best instituted early to prevent conjunctival scarring. Amniotic membrane has been promising in conjunctival scar prevention.

21 DDx ref

MUCOSAL EROSIONS (BLISTER BASES)

Geographic tongue

12 • 19 • 83

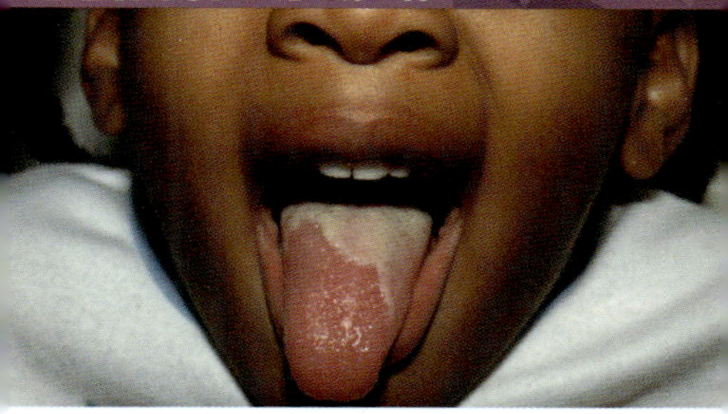

Smooth, pink area surrounded by inflamed gray area in child with geographic tongue.

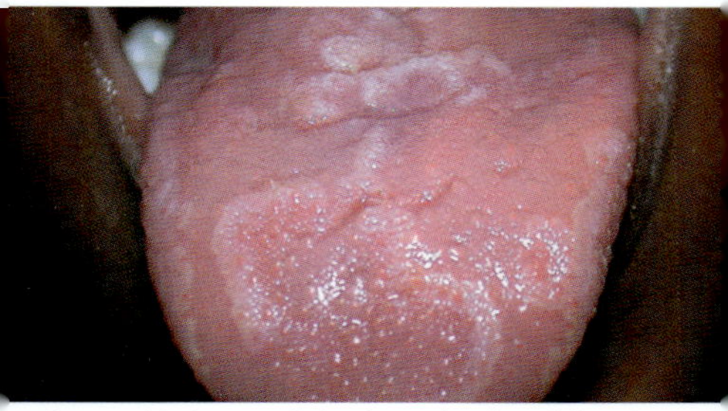

Geographic tongue. Raised gray borders delineate smooth pink areas of a child's tongue.

22 DDx ref

MUCOSAL EROSIONS (BLISTER BASES)

Mucosal erosions in immunobullous and hereditary bullous diseases

20 • 19 • 18

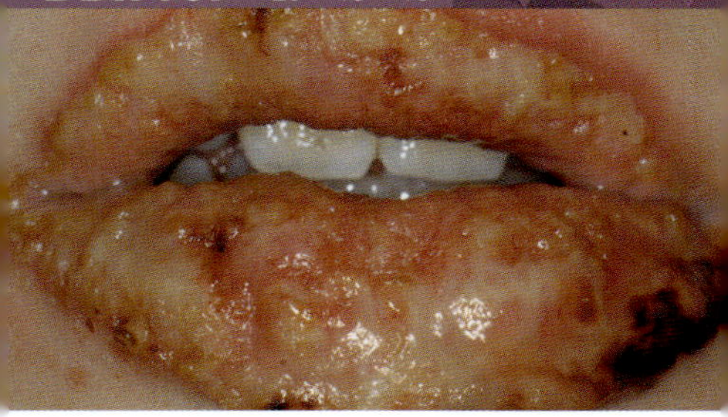

Childhood pemphigus vulgaris with severe erosions in oral mucosa and on the lips.

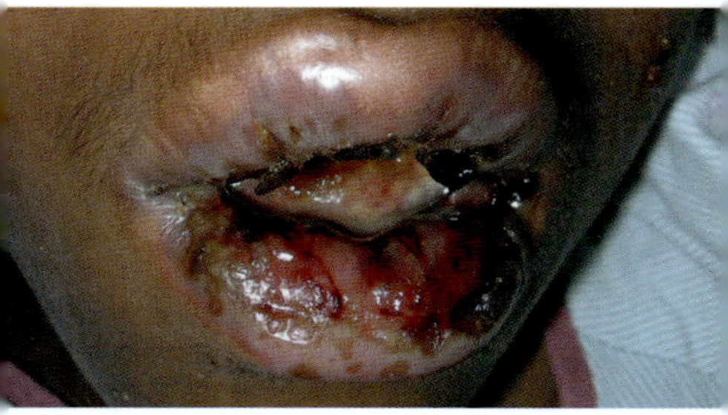

Lip and mucosal erosions in child with pemphigus vulgaris.

MUCOSAL EROSIONS (BLISTER BASES)

21 Geographic tongue

DDx ref 12 • 19 • 83

CLINICAL FEATURES

The annular smooth patches on the tongue mimic erosions, the smooth areas represent villous atrophy, and the raised areas show inflammation similar to that found in psoriasis. Geographic tongue is usually asymptomatic in the child, but uncommonly, is painful. The areas change from day to day, adding to the difficulty in diagnosis. Spontaneous remissions occur.

TREATMENT

No treatment is necessary unless symptomatic. Liquid antacids will soothe the discomfort.

MUCOSAL EROSIONS (BLISTER BASES)

22 Mucosal erosions in immunobullous and hereditary bullous diseases

DDx ref 20 • 19 • 18

CLINICAL FEATURES

Oral erosions are also seen in immunobullous diseases and are particularly characteristic of pemphigus vulgaris and paraneoplastic pemphigus. They are rarely seen in dermatitis herpetiformis and not at all in children with linear IgA disease, bullous pemphigoid, or pemphigus foliaceous.

Of the hereditary mechanobullous diseases, mucosal erosions are prominent in the oral cavity of newborns with recessive dystrophic epidermolysis bullosa, and with junctional epidermolysis bullosa. In those two conditions, mucosal lesions, particularly oral lesions, become progressively worse. In most forms of epidermolysis bullosa simplex, newborns do not have mucosal involvement except in the EBS-generalized and Dowling–Meara type. Oral involvement in EB simplex improves with age.

23 DDx ref

PUSTULAR LESIONS

Folliculitis

25 • 7 • 24

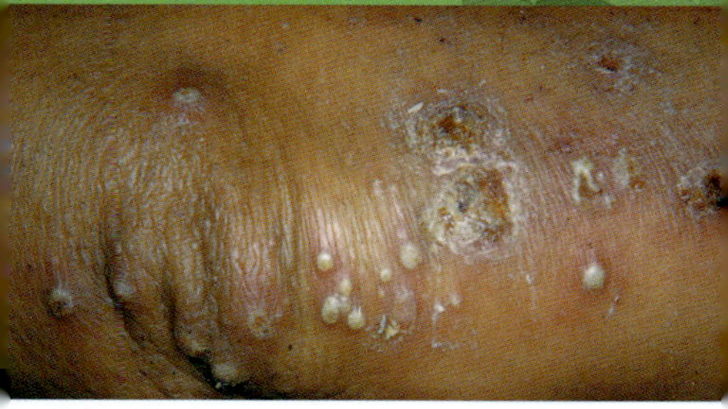

Folliculitis: Staphylococcal superficial folliculitis and ecthyma.

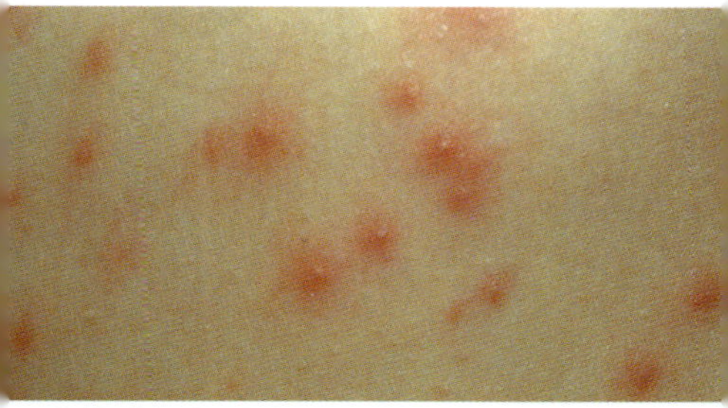

Folliculitis: Staphylococcal superficial folliculitis. Multiple pustules on a red base.

24 DDx ref

PUSTULAR LESIONS

Infantile acropustulosis

88 • 23 • 34

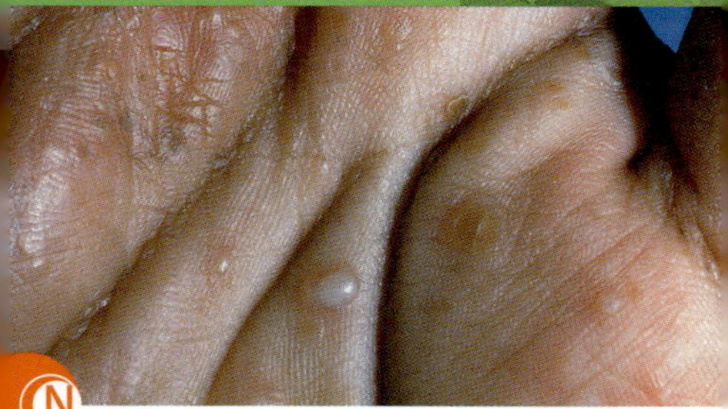

Infantile acropustulosis. Vesicles and pustules on the palm of an infant.

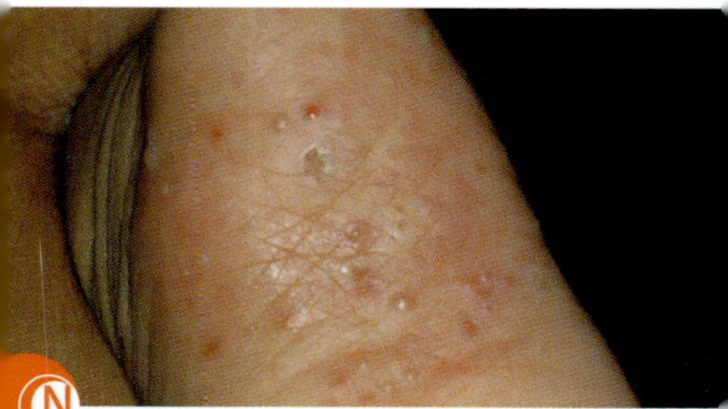

Infantile acropustulosis. Vesicles and pustules on an infant's heel.

23 PUSTULAR LESIONS

Folliculitis

DDx ref 25 • 7 • 24

CLINICAL FEATURES

Folliculitis is seen as 1–2-mm discrete pustules restricted to follicular openings. In a few children with folliculitis, impetigo or ecthyma may also be seen. Most folliculitis is bacterial in origin and *Staphylococcus aureus* the most frequent pathogen. Occasionally, *Pseudomonas aeruginosa* or other Gram-negative bacteria will produce folliculitis in special circumstances, such as 'hot tub' folliculitis.

Poor hygiene and warm moist conditions are predisposing factors as is air-tight skin occlusion and prolonged immersion in water. Ask about other family members or close contacts who may be affected. Bacterial cultures are not routinely done.

TREATMENT

Topical antibiotics and good skin hygiene are the mainstays of therapy. Topical mupirocin, erythromycin, clindamycin, retapamulin 1%, or benzoyl peroxide 5% gel preparations should be used twice daily for 7–10 days.

Thorough hand washing with antibacterial soaps daily for the affected child, family members, and close contacts. In recurrent or persistent cases, nasal carriage of *S. aureus* may be eliminated with mupirocin 1% nasal ointment daily for 5 days. For recurrent cases, bleach baths one to two times a week may help. For bleach baths, add 1/4 cup of sodium hypochlorite [Clorox] in 40 gallons of lukewarm water for 5–10 minutes.

Oral anti-staph antibiotics such as dicloxacillin 15–50 mg/kg per day or cephalexin 40–50 mg/kg per day may be considered in severe infections or when impetigo or ecthyma is also present. In Gram-negative infections, proper chlorination of hot tubs or spas should be emphasized.

24 PUSTULAR LESIONS

Infantile acropustulosis

DDx ref 88 • 23 • 34

CLINICAL FEATURES

Recurrent crops of pruritic pustules and vesicles on the palms and soles characterize infantile acropustulosis. Onset may be at birth or any age up to 3 years. Pruritus is expressed as irritability and fretfulness in infants without the coordination to scratch effectively. Vesicles resolve with scale and, sometimes, lichenification. The itchy lesions mimic scabies.

TREATMENT

Mid- to strong-potency topical steroid ointments or creams applied twice daily will relieve symptoms, but not influence the recurrences. Occasionally, oral antihistamines such as hydroxyzine 2 mg/kg per day may be required to control pruritus.

PUSTULAR LESIONS

Acne and steroid rosacea

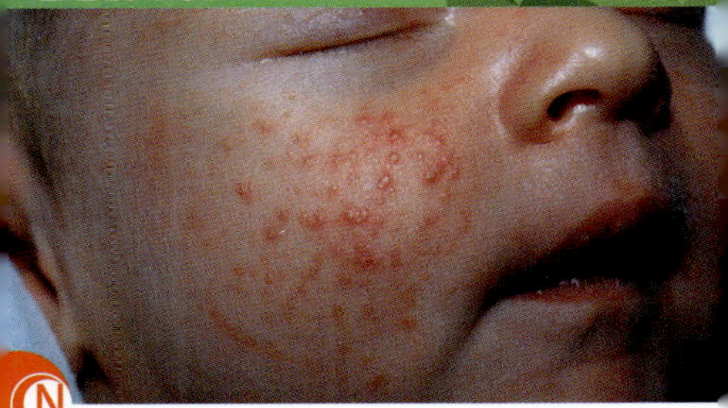

Neonatal acne. Papules and pustules on the cheek of a 3-week-old infant.

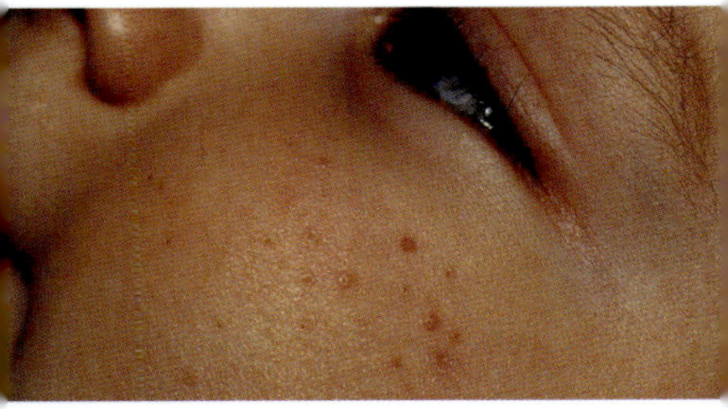

Resolving neonatal acne on the cheeks of a 3-month-old infant.

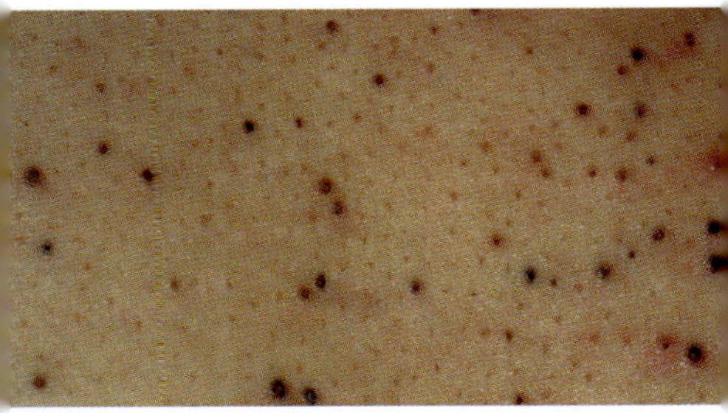

Acne vulgaris. Open comedones (blackheads).

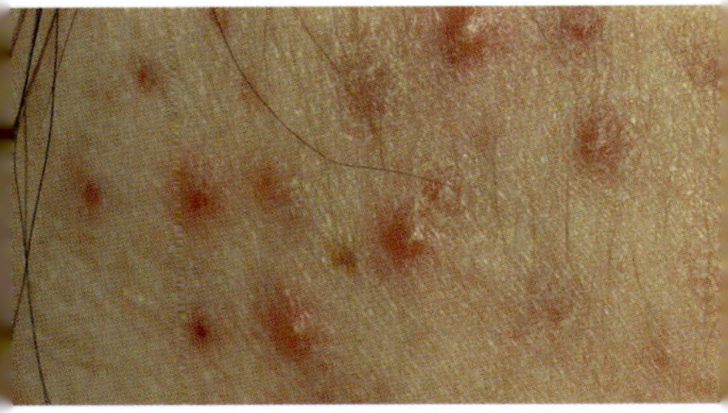

Acne vulgaris. Teen with red papules and pustules on face.

Acne and steroid rosacea

CLINICAL FEATURES

Acne is a disorder of sebaceous follicles that are found on the head, chest, and back. It is androgen dependent as sebaceous follicles convert circulating androgens to DHT, resulting in plugging of the follicles with cells, increased sebum production, overgrowth of the bacteria *P. acnes*, and subsequent inflammation. Lesions begin with small white papules (closed comedones) or blackheads (open comedones) that progress to red papules and pustules. Deep lesions of red nodules, cysts, and scars may develop.

Neonatal acne starts at 4 weeks of age with red papules and pustules on the cheeks, upper chest, and back. Comedones are uncommon. It is related to maternal androgens and clears by 6 months as the androgen effects decline.

Infantile acne starts at 6–16 months of age with red papules, pustules, and nodules on the cheeks. It requires 18 months to 3 years to clear.

Acne vulgaris starts at 7–10 years of age with closed and open comedones on the face, chest, and back. During teen years, red papules, pustules, and nodules appear. Some 85% of teens will have some acne, and acne lasts into the mid-20s for most.

Teenage boys are five times more likely than girls to develop the deep nodules, cysts, and scars characteristic of nodulocystic acne. About 1% of teenage boys will suffer from nodulocystic acne. Some of the scars are keloidal.

Acne conglobata appears as an abrupt onset of nodulocystic acne without systemic symptoms. It often accompanies hidradenitis suppurativa and dissecting cellulitis of the scalp.

Acne fulminans is sudden-onset hemorrhagic and ulcerative acne with joint and bone pain. It may be part of the SAPHO syndrome (synovitis-acne-pustulosis-hyperostosis-osteitis).

Girls with acne may rarely present with signs of hirsutism, premature pubarche, irregular menses, or male pattern alopecia. They should have laboratory screening for hyperandrogenism. This includes total testosterone, free testosterone, luteinizing hormone/follicle stimulating hormone ratio, prolactin, dehydroepiandrosterone, and 17-hydroxyprogesterone.

Steroid rosacea (perioral dermatitis) is an acne variant with pustules and red papules on the perinasal, perioral, and lower eyelid skin. It is seen mostly in toddlers and preschool children. Often, a history of an affected family member and a history of topical steroid use may be obtained.

TREATMENT

Treatment of acne is based upon the severity and natural history.

PUSTULAR LESIONS

Acne and steroid rosacea

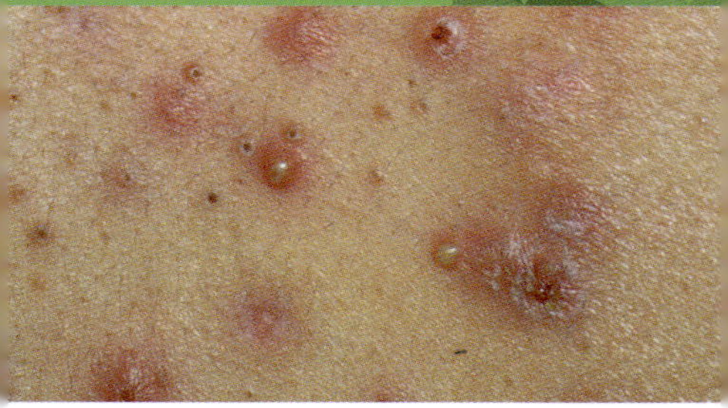

Acne vulgaris. Pustules, red papules, open and closed comedones demonstrating lesions in different stages at one time.

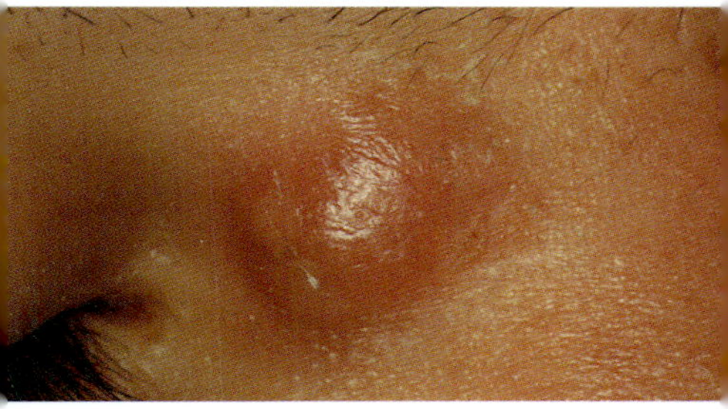

Nodulocystic acne. Red cyst on face of adolescent.

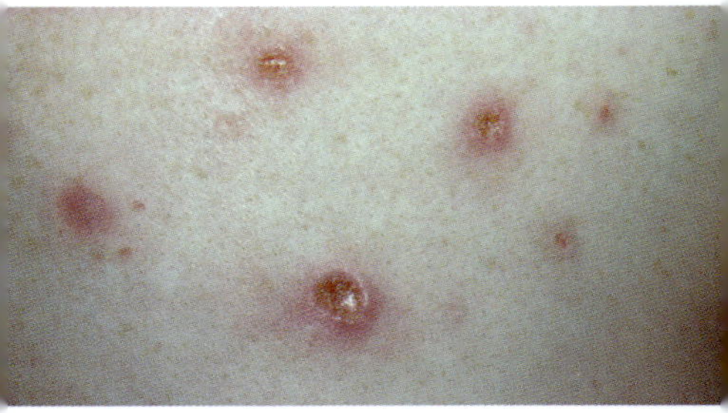

Excoriated acne vulgaris. Atrophic scars eventuate from excoriations.

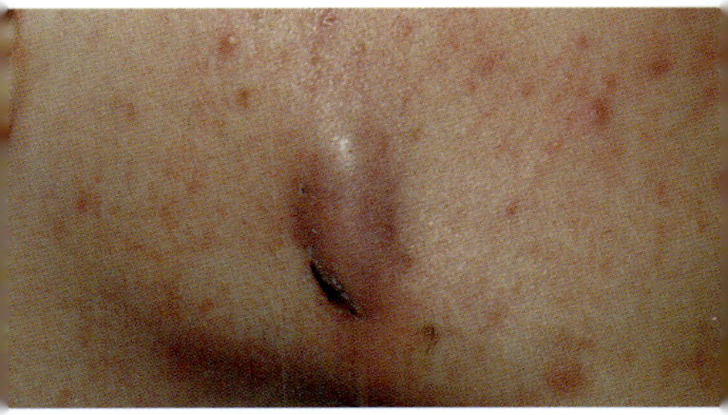

Hypertrophic scar in nodulocystic acne.

Neonatal acne usually requires no treatment as it will clear without sequelae by 6 months.

The remainder of acne types including infantile acne are treated based on the clinical appearance. If comedones only, daily topical retinoid can be used as monotherapy. With red papules and a few pustules, a daily retinoid and benzoyl peroxide gel are used. If poor response, a topical antibiotic can be added. With many red papules and pustules, an oral antibiotic can be added to the regimen. All treatment regimens require about 3 months for significant improvement. All children with acne, who have many inflammatory lesions, should begin on combination therapy such as a topical retinoid plus benzoyl peroxide and an oral antibiotic (see table below). Those treated with oral antibiotics should be also treated with topical 5% benzoyl peroxide gel or wash to minimize antibiotic resistance.

Selected Acne Treatment Products

Product	Form	Size
TOPICAL KERATOLYTICS (apply once daily)		
Retinoids		
Tretinoin	0.05% solution	28 mL
	0.025% cream	20 g, 45 g
	0.05% cream	20 g, 45 g
	0.1% cream	20 g, 45 g
	0.01% gel	15 g, 45 g
	0.025% gel	15 g, 45 g
	0.1% micro gel	20 g, 45 g
	0.04% micro gel	20 g, 45 g
Adapalene	0.1% lotion	30 mL
	0.1% gel	15 g, 45 g
	0.1% gel with 2.5% BPO	
Tazarotene	0.05% gel	30 g, 100 g
	0.1% gel	30 g, 100 g
	0.1% cream	30 g
TOPICAL ANTIBIOTICS (apply once or twice daily)		
Benzoyl peroxide	2.5%, 3%, 4%, 5%, 6%	30 g, 45 g, 60 g
	8%, 10% gel	90 g
	2.5%, 4%, 5%, 8%, 10% lotion	30 mL, 150 mL
Clindamycin phosphate	1% solution	30 mL, 60 mL
	1% gel	30 g, 42.77 g, 60 g
	1% pledgets	60
Clindamycin/BPO	1% gel/5% gel	25 g, 45 g, 50 g
Azelaic acid	20% cream	30 g
SYSTEMIC ANTIBIOTICS (one or two capsules twice daily)		
Tetracycline hydrochloride		250- and 500-mg capsule
Erythromycin		250- and 500-mg capsule
Minocycline		50- and 100-mg capsule
Doxycycline		50- and 100-mg capsule
ORAL RETINOIDS (40-mg capsule twice daily for 16–20 weeks)		
Isotretinoin		10-, 20-, 30-, and 40-mg capsules

25

PUSTULAR LESIONS

Acne and steroid rosacea

DDx ref 23 • 7 • 40

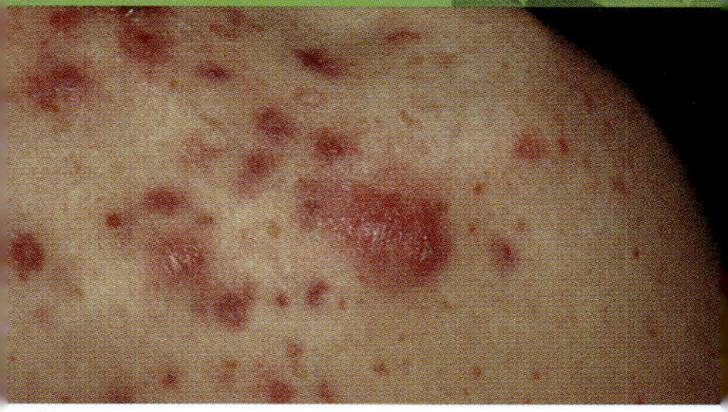

Nodulocystic acne with red nodules, cysts, papule, and pustules on a teenage boy's back and shoulder.

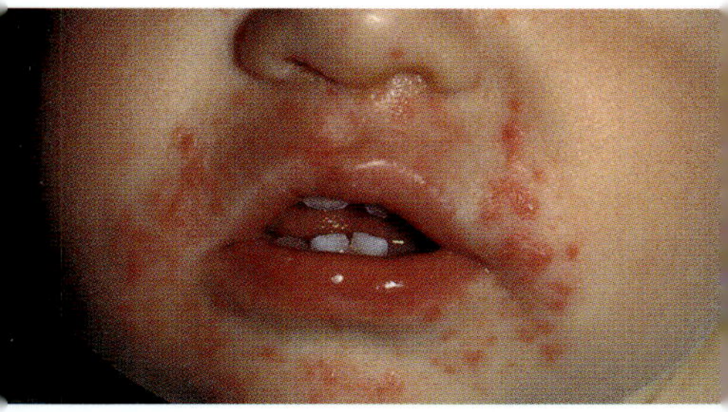

Steroid rosacea. Perioral involvement with red papules and pustules.

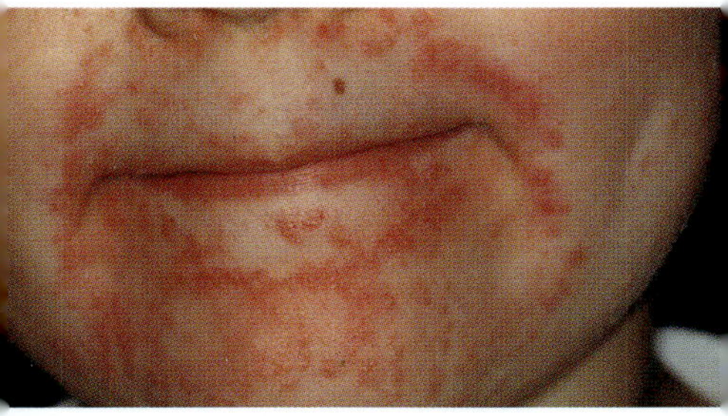

Steroid rosacea. Perioral and perinasal red papules in a 6-year-old boy.

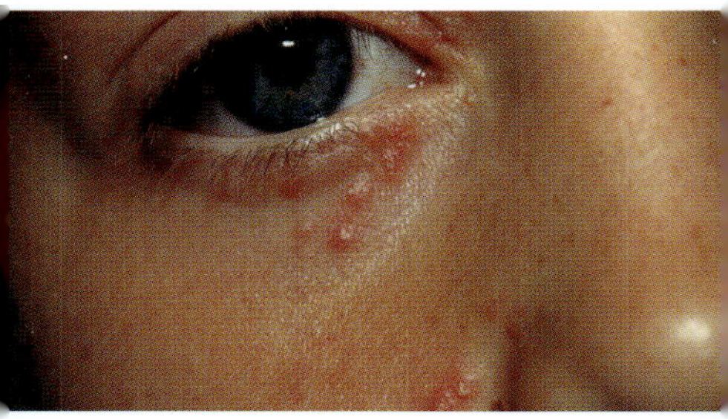

Steroid rosacea. Perinasal and lower eyelid pustules.

Factors that aggravate acne may interfere with the therapeutic response. This includes use of oil- or propylene glycol-based cosmetics, hairstyling mousse, face creams, and hair sprays. The use of noncomedogenic products may help.

Some girls will benefit from oral contraceptive therapy with improvement after 3 or 4 months. Girls with confirmed hyperadrenalism should be managed by an endocrinologist.

Severe acne unresponsive to combination therapy and teens that suffer from nodulocystic acne or acne conglobata will require treatment with oral isotretinoin. Isotretinoin (13 cis retinoic acid) is started at 0.5–1.0 mg/kg per day and treatment continued to total dose of 120–150 mg/kg. Doses lower than 0.5 mg/kg per day result in a high rate of relapse.

Side-effects of therapy include dry skin, lips, eyes, and nose. Elevated levels of liver enzymes and blood lipids may occur and baseline liver function tests and blood lipids should be obtained and monitored monthly for first 2 months.

For girls teratogenicity is a major limiting factor of retinoid use. Of pregnancies while on isotretinoin, 25% will result in fetuses with severe CNS malformations. Strict adherence to contraceptive recommendations and pregnancy testing guidelines is vital. In the USA, isotretinoin is restricted to those that register in the government 'iPLEDGE' program. Treatment longer than 6 months is not recommended to reduce the likelihood of bony side-effects. Of those treated, 40% will require no further treatment, 45% will need re-institution of standard combination therapy, and 15%, after a 4–6-month period, will require a second course of isotretinoin.

Acne fulminans requires the use of a systemic anti-inflammatory such as glucocorticoids or anti-TNF agents in combination with isotretinoin.

Steroid rosacea will initially worsen when topical steroids are withdrawn. Children treated 4–6 weeks with either a topical antibiotic (clindamycin, erythromycin twice daily) or oral antibiotics such as erythromycin under age 8, or doxycyline if older, will clear completely. Metronidazole 0.75% gel daily has also been effective.

26 DDx ref

PUSTULAR LESIONS

Transient neonatal pustular melanosis

1 • 7 • 24

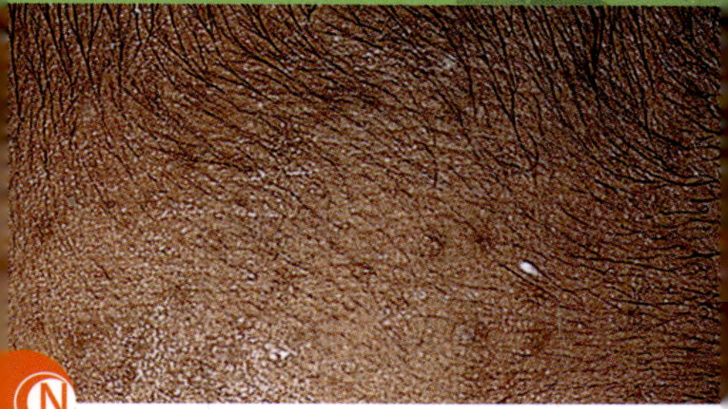

N Transient neonatal pustular melanosis. Multiple macules at sites of previous pustules on a 10-day-old infant.

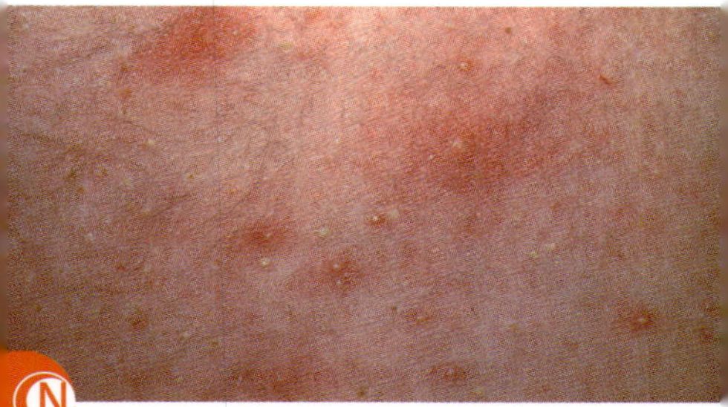

N Transient neonatal pustular melanosis. Red macules, papules, and pustules in a newborn.

27 DDx ref

PUSTULAR LESIONS

Pyoderma gangrenosum

1 • 29 • 34

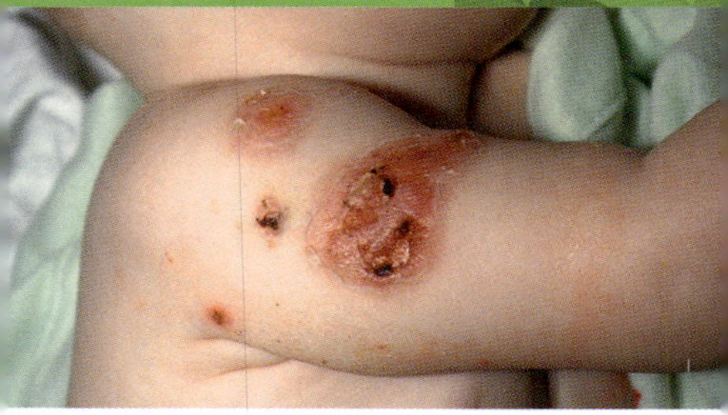

Multiple ulcerated lesions following attempted surgical debridement of pyoderma gangrenosum lesion (pathergy).

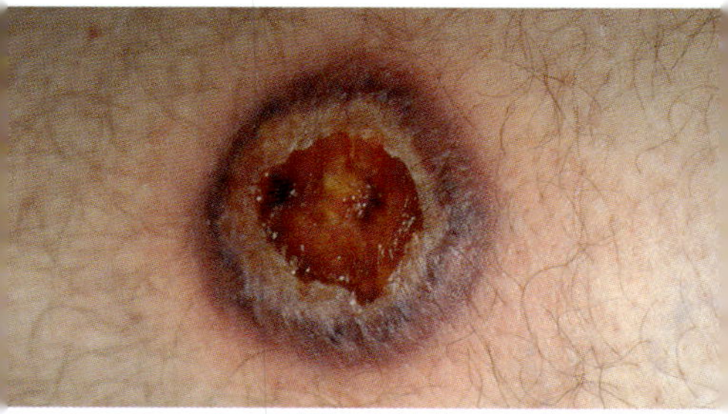

Pyoderma gangrenosum. Ulceration with characteristic loosely attached epidermis and purple border.

26 DDx ref 1 • 7 • 24

PUSTULAR LESIONS

Transient neonatal pustular melanosis

CLINICAL FEATURES

At birth, vesicles and/or pustules are seen on the face and trunk. Ruptured vesicles or pustules will have a fine collarette of white scale. Brown pigmented macules appear at the sites of involvement as lesions heal. Vesicles and pustules disappear by 5–7 days of age, but brown macules may take 3 months to clear. The course and distribution are similar to erythema toxicum, but in the vesicles, neutrophils rather than eosinophils are seen. Predominantly, black infants have transient neonatal pustular melanosis.

TREATMENT

No treatment is necessary.

27 DDx ref 1 • 29 • 34

PUSTULAR LESIONS

Pyoderma gangrenosum

CLINICAL FEATURES

Pyoderma gangrenosum begins as a 3–8-mm red papule that progresses within hours to a pustule, then ulcerates with a surrounding loosely attached epidermis and an outer lilac-colored border. The ulcer relentlessly enlarges to 2 cm or more.

Skin lesions may appear at sites of trauma (pathergy). Skin lesions are solitary in half the children with lesions primarily on the arms and legs. Sheets of activated neutrophils undermine the skin.

Surgical debridement results in expansion of lesions because of pathergy and should not be done.

Associated diseases such as inflammatory bowel disease, rheumatoid arthritis, or a myelodysplastic disorder may be found. Endoscopy for inflammatory bowel disease, a bone marrow for myelodysplastic disorders, and rheumatic consultation should be obtained. Untreated, childhood pyoderma gangrenosum has a mortality of 10%.

TREATMENT

Immunosuppressive drugs, such as oral cyclosporine or tacrolimus are the most effective at controlling the disease. Since their initial effects are slow, high-dose oral glucocorticoids may be required to initiate a remission.

Long-term (years) immunosuppressive therapy is required and adjunctive therapy such as dapsone or colchicine or topical tacrolimus may help maintain improvement. Infliximab has shown encouraging results in children unresponsive to usual therapy.

RED PAPULES AND NODULES

Furunculosis and cellulitis

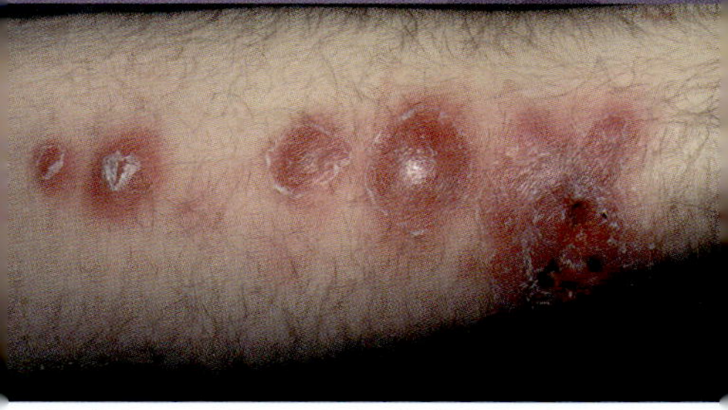

Staphylococcal furunculosis. Multiple tender red nodules on a teen's arm.

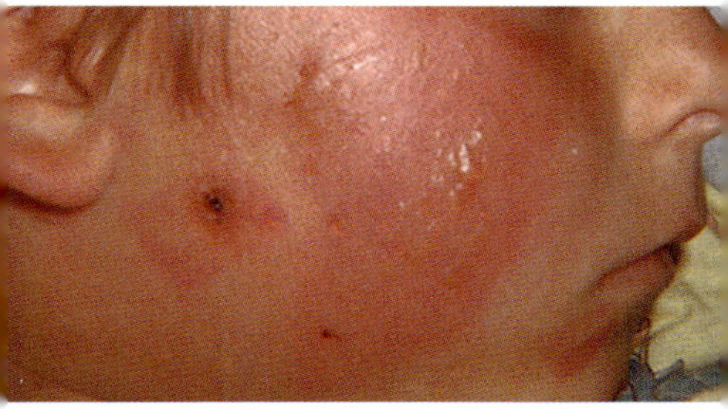

Cellulitis of the cheek of a child, with red, tender skin surrounding a puncture wound.

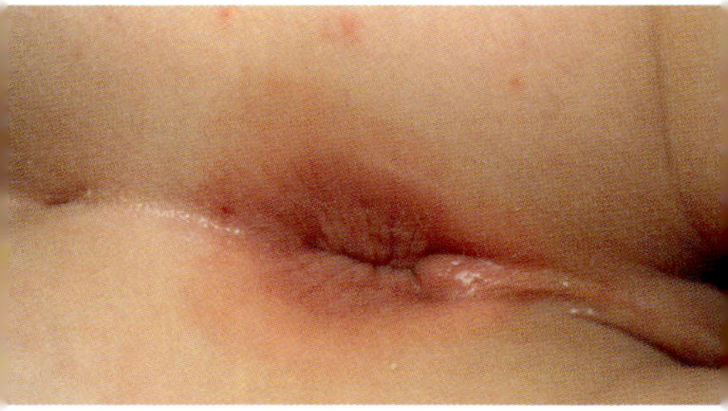

Streptococcal perianal cellulitis. Infant with tender red perianal skin.

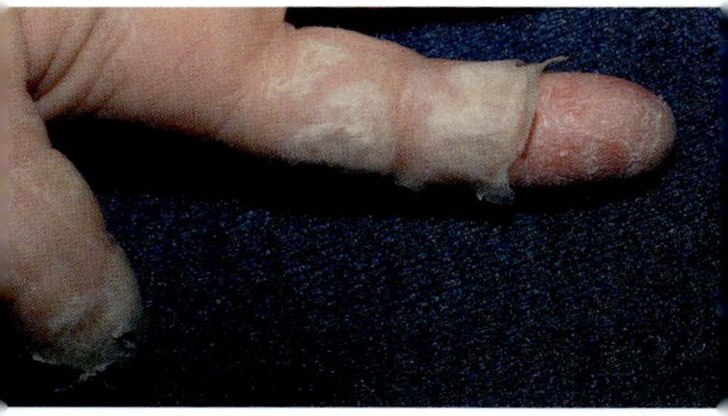

Blistering distal dactylitis. Red, tender fingertips and peeling skin in a preschool boy.

CLINICAL FEATURES

Furunculosis appears as tender red nodules and confluence of several adjacent furuncles produces a skin abscess. *S. aureus* is most commonly responsible for childhood furunculosis, but Gram-negative organisms such as *Pseudomonas* are occasionally responsible.

Cellulitis appears as tender, warm, red plaques with ill-defined borders. Regional adenopathy and fever are seen with cellulitis. In infants and toddlers, cellulitis may be seen over joints such as hip, shoulder, or knee. Extension into the joint cavity creating a septic arthritis is a concern.

Streptococcus is usually responsible and sepsis may result. Staphylococcal cellulitis can also occur but extends more slowly than streptococcal cellulitis.

Hemophilus influenza cellulitis is far less common since immunization with hemophilus B vaccine has been more widely used in infants.

Perianal cellulitis is seen in infants and toddlers as perirectal redness and tender skin. Pain upon defecation is common. Perivaginal extension may be seen.

Cellulitis of the fingertips in infants is called 'blistering distal dactylitis'.

Blood cultures may be more reliable than local cultures in identifying the responsible bacteria in febrile children that require hospitalization.

TREATMENT

The treatment of choice for furunculosis or abscesses is surgical incision and drainage. This may be difficult in toddlers with multiple lesions.

More severe cases may require systemic antistaphylococcal antibiotics such as dicloxacillin 15–50 mg/kg per day or cephalexin 40–50 mg/kg per day for 7–10 days.

Cellulitis including perianal cellulitis and blistering distal dactylitis should be treated with antibiotics that target *Streptococcus* pyogenes. If staphylococcal infection is suspected, then antistaphylococcal antibiotics such as those for furunculosis should be used.

29 DDx ref

RED PAPULES AND NODULES

Necrotizing fasciitis

27 • 28 • 61

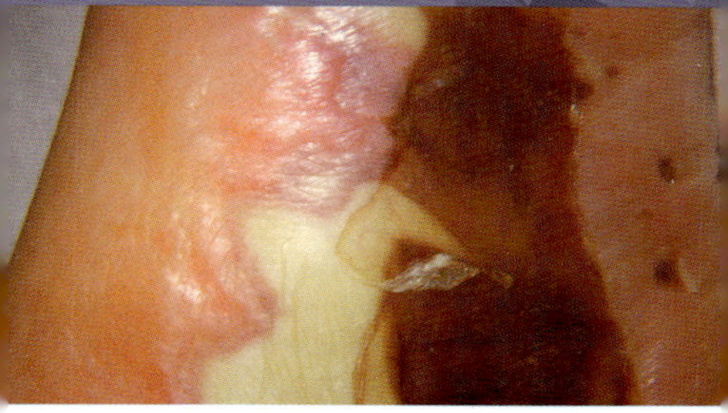

Necrotizing fasciitis. Central black, painless area with surrounding red swollen skin.

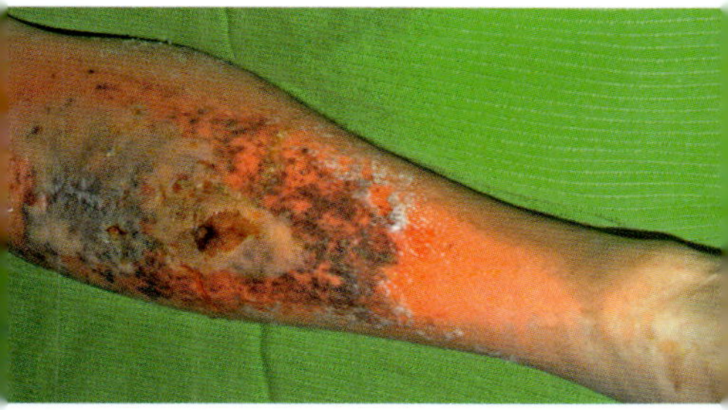

Necrotizing fasciitis. Painful red swollen leg with black necrotic areas.

30 DDx ref

RED PAPULES AND NODULES

Mycobacterial infections

28 • 89 • 99

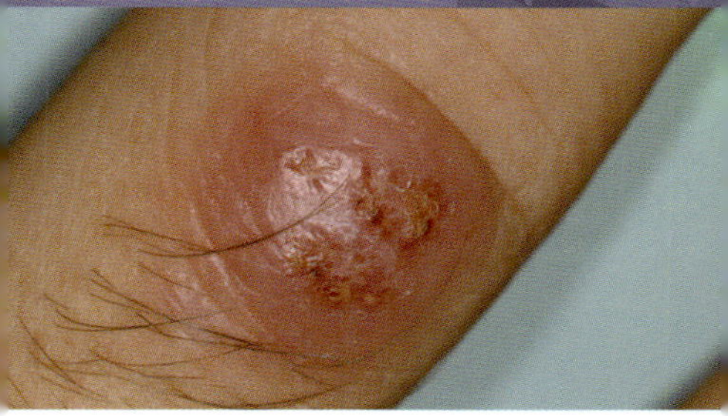

M. marinum infection. Red nodule from the finger of a teen from a fish aquarium.

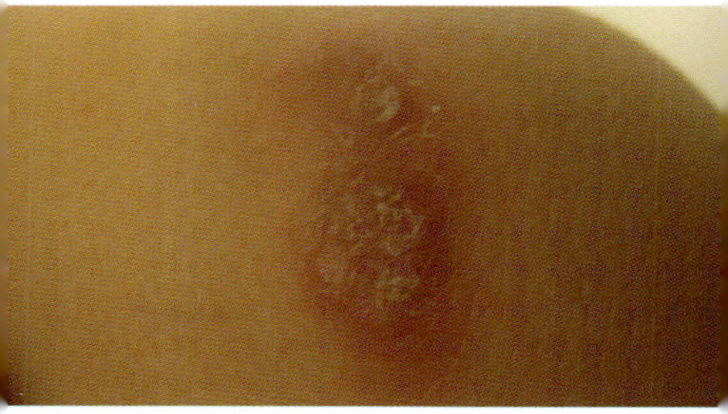

M. marinum infection. Red nodules on a child's leg from a swimming pool abrasion and infection.

29 RED PAPULES AND NODULES

Necrotizing fasciitis

DDx ref 27 • 28 • 61

CLINICAL FEATURES

Lesions begin as red, tender, swollen skin that mimics cellulitis, but within a few hours central bullae appear accompanied by severe pain. The bulla collapses and a central purulent area develops as the red swollen skin area enlarges. Pain subsides when a black center ensues, correlating with the destruction of cutaneous nerves. Shock may then develop. Over the next 2 days, frank gangrene appears.

Necrotizing fasciitis represents deep bacterial infection within the subcutaneous fat, underlying fascia and muscle compartments. Strep pyogenes infections are most common but 30% may have polymicrobial infections. Blood flow deep in the skin is compromised and infarction occurs.

Immunosuppressed or uncontrolled diabetic children are the most susceptible and a leg or arm is usually involved.

Rarely, newborns develop necrotizing fasciitis on the abdominal wall. An MRI will delineate the depth of involvement.

TREATMENT

Necrotizing fasciitis is a surgical emergency and requires surgical exposure of the fascia and underlying compartments to relieve pressure on the blood vessels and nerves.

Fluid management to ensure adequate venous return combined with intravenous high-dose broad spectrum antibiotics and a bacterial protein synthesis inhibitor such as clindamycin.

Even with prompt surgical intervention, loss of limb and mortality is high.

Correction of diabetic ketoacidosis, if present, can be most useful.

30 RED PAPULES AND NODULES

Mycobacterial infections

DDx ref 28 • 89 • 99

CLINICAL FEATURES

With the decrease in tuberculosis of skin, nontuberculous mycobacterial infections are more likely to be seen. These uncommon infections present as persistent red nodules or ulcerated nodules. The most frequent is *M. marinum* obtained from fish aquariums or swimming pools. Others reported include *M. fortuitum*, *M. kansasii*, *M. buruli*, and *M. chelonae*. All require a wound to enter the skin. Some will infect bone and lung as well. Otherwise healthy children can be infected but immunosuppressed children or the child with cancer will be especially susceptible.

Skin biopsy of infected areas for special mycobacterial culture and pathology is diagnostic.

In mild infections spontaneous clearing in 4 months may be expected.

Large or ulcerated lesions require systemic antimicrobial agents.

TREATMENT

Antituberculous drugs such as the combination of ethambutol 15 mg/kg per day in children over 5 years of age plus rifampin may be effective. In vitro sensitivity testing may not correlate with the clinical response.

Clarithromycin plus rifampin has been successful and fluoroquinolones have been also useful in some.

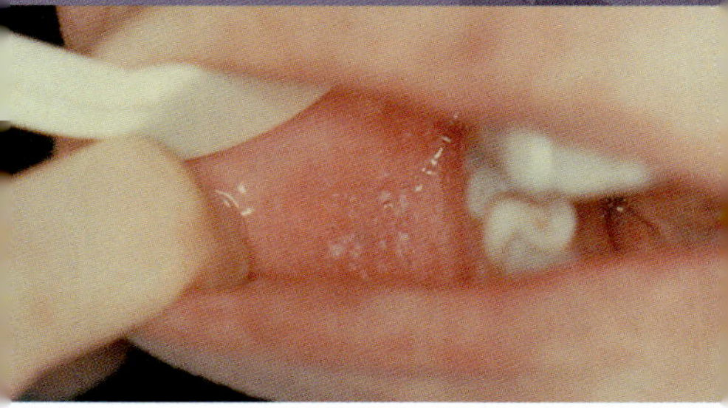

Koplik's spots. Red buccal mucosa with 1 mm white macules in a child with measles.

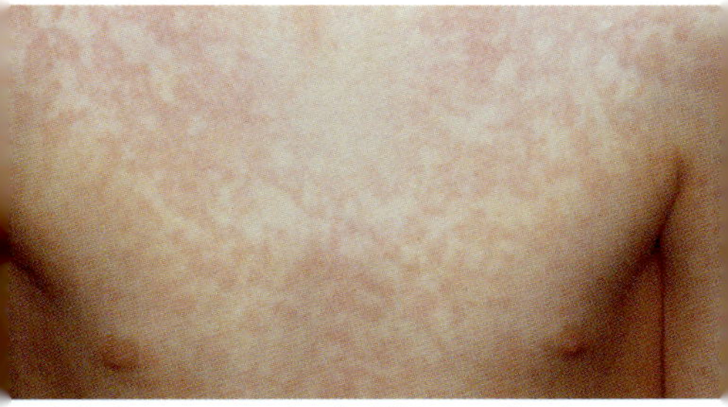

Infectious mononucleosis. Widespread red papules over the chest of a preteen.

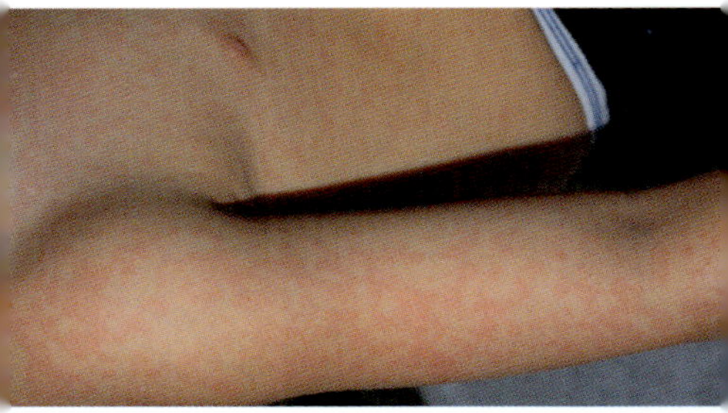

Erythema infectiosum. Lacy rash on right arm and trunk following red cheeks.

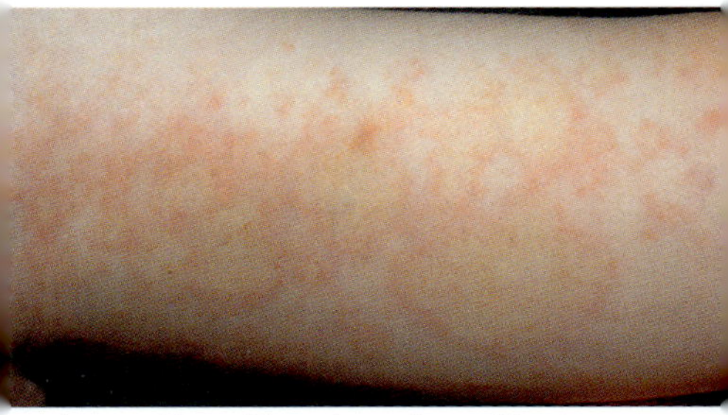

Asymmetric periflexural exanthem with a lacy rash on one inner arm.

CLINICAL FEATURES

Viral exanthems are quite common in childhood. Two major patterns are discrete red papules and macules (measles-like or morbilliform) and a lacy red macular pattern.

Morbilliform eruptions are seen in rubeola, rubella, roseola, enterovirus infections, and infectious mononucleosis. The child with rubeola (measles) has a prodrome of high fever, barking cough, rhinitis, and conjunctivitis lasting 3–5 days, followed by red oral mucosa with 1–2-mm white macules (Koplik's spots). A generalized morbilliform eruption follows, accompanied by cervical lymphadenopathy. Bacterial otitis media, pneumonia, or encephalitis may complicate.

Rubella is a mild illness with a 3-day morbilliform rash and mild lymphadenopathy. Monoarticular arthritis can occur. Pregnant women exposed to rubella during the first trimester are at risk for congenital rubella, with heart, ear, eye, and CNS defects.

Roseola (HHV-6 infection) presents in toddlers with high fever yet appearing well. Rarely, convulsions at the onset of fever are described. After 2 or 3 days of fever, a transient morbilliform rash occurs.

Infectious mononucleosis (HHV-4, -5, -6, & -7 infections) is characterized by fever, generalized lymphadenopathy, fatigue, sore throat with exudative tonsillitis, headache, and splenomegaly. The morbilliform eruption lasts 1–5 days; fatigue can last up to 3 months. Serology for EBV IgM is positive and the most reliable diagnostic test. Liver function tests are often abnormal. In some, arthritis can occur and persist for several months. Drug eruptions mimic exanthems.

Lace-like eruptions are seen in erythema infectiosum (parvovirus B19 infection) and the asymmetric periflexural exanthem.

Erythema infectiosum has a distinct pattern of confluent red cheeks and a lacy red pattern on extremities and trunk that lasts 3–5 days but will recur upon sun exposure or overheating of the skin. A transient arthritis may develop.

Parvovirus B19 replicates within red blood cells and causes disruption of red cell production. In children with chronic hemolytic anemias, an aplastic crisis can occur. Pregnant women exposed to parvovirus B19 can have a fetus with hydrops fetalis.

Asymmetric periflexural exanthema shows a lacy eruption on one side of the body lasting 1–3 days in an otherwise well child. Some may generalize after initial unilateral presentation.

TREATMENT

Supplements of vitamin A in measles have reduced pulmonary disease. Measles immune globulin administered within 6 days may modify the disease. Measles and rubella can be prevented with vaccines.

Roseola and rubella usually require no treatment.

Infectious mononucleosis splenomegaly may be improved with systemic steroids reducing the risk of splenic rupture.

Erythema infectiosum and the asymmetric exanthema require no intervention. In suspected rubella or erythema infectiosum, avoidance of pregnant women is advised.

32

DDx ref

RED PAPULES AND NODULES

Syphilis

66 • 31 • 54

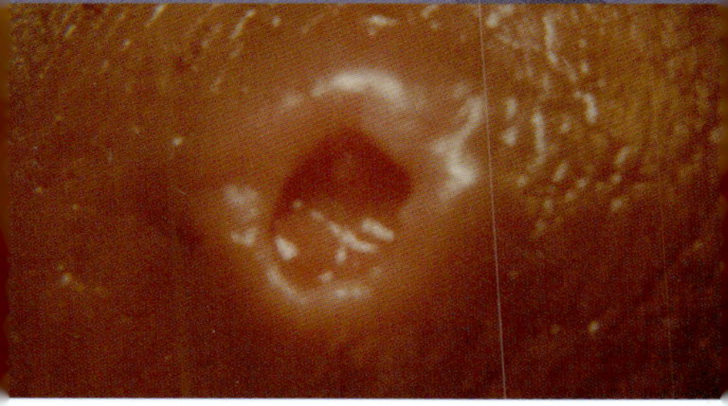

Syphilitic chancre in an 11-year-old boy, 3 weeks after exposure.

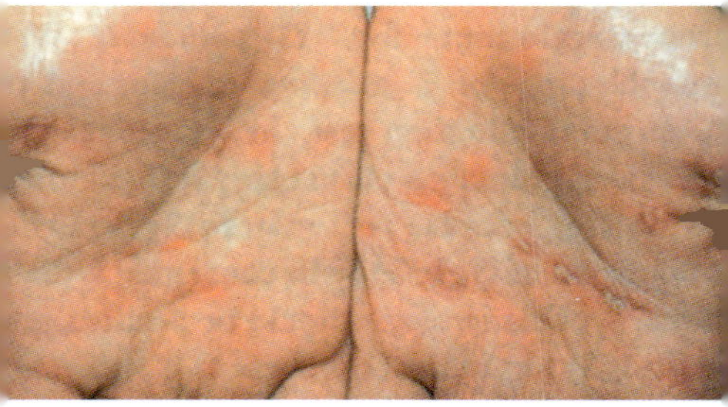

Secondary syphilis. Pink macules on the palms of a teen.

33

DDx ref

RED PAPULES AND NODULES

Cutaneous larva migrans

88 • 80 • 68

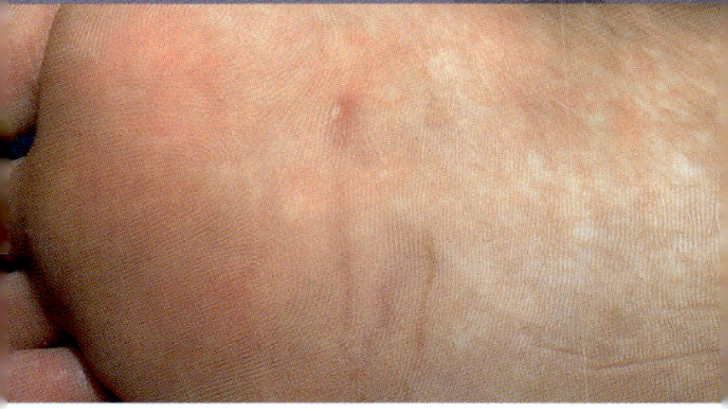

Creeping eruption. Serpiginous red track on the plantar forefoot in a child.

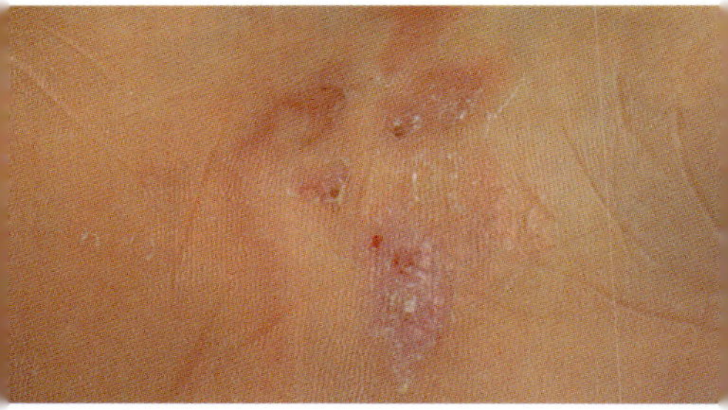

Serpiginous red track with excoriations on the foot of a child infested by larva of *A. brasiliensis*.

32 RED PAPULES AND NODULES
Syphilis

DDx ref 66 • 31 • 54

CLINICAL FEATURES

Secondary acquired syphilis is seen as widespread pink to red papules (morbilliform eruption) with pink macules on the palms and soles accompanied by fatigue, headache, and lymphadenopathy. Weeping erosive areas may be seen on oral or genital mucosa.

The secondary stage follows 6 weeks to 6 months with the appearance of a shallow ulcer with a red indurated border (primary chancre) due to *T. pallidum* infection. The eruption lasts weeks and is accompanied by low-grade fever and lassitude.

Newborns with congenital syphilis are often asymptomatic and the morbilliform rash as seen in secondary syphilis is transient and easily overlooked. Serologic tests for syphilis on the mother are critical for early diagnosis. If congenital syphilis is missed in the newborn, then late stage findings are not seen until 6 years of age.

Late congenital syphilis includes cloudy corneas, bilateral nerve deafness, notching of undersized central and lateral incisors, painless knee swelling, nasal septum perforation, saber tibia, and radial perioral scarring.

TREATMENT

Benzathine penicillin given IM at 50 000 units/kg per dose up to 2.4 million units.

If penicillin allergic, doxycycline 100 mg twice daily for 2 weeks is recommended.

Late syphilis signs cannot be reversed if treatment is delayed until they appear.

33 RED PAPULES AND NODULES
Cutaneous larva migrans

DDx ref 88 • 80 • 68

CLINICAL FEATURES

Itchy red, serpiginous areas that appear to pulsate is the pattern in cutaneous larva migrans (creeping eruption). Lesions are mostly on the foot and advance at 1 cm/day. A history of play along beaches in the southeast USA or Caribbean islands may be found. Use of footwear on the beach can be preventive.

A second pattern involves the perianal skin, thighs, or buttocks and advances at 5 cm/hour.

Children with foot lesions are infested with the dog and cat hookworm larvae, *Ancylostoma brasiliensis*. The perianal pattern is due to *Strongyloides stercoralis*.

TREATMENT

Topical 15% thiabendazole cream applied three times a day for 5–7 days often cures the foot lesions.

For perianal involvement oral thiabendazole 25 mg/kg twice a day for 2 days; albendazole 700 mg/day for 7 days or ivermectin 200 mg/kg in a single oral dose, are all effective.

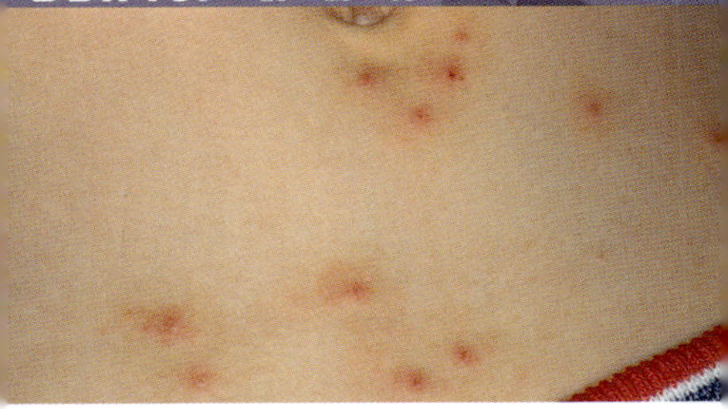

Papular urticaria. Clusters of red papules surrounded by an urticarial flare due to cat fleas.

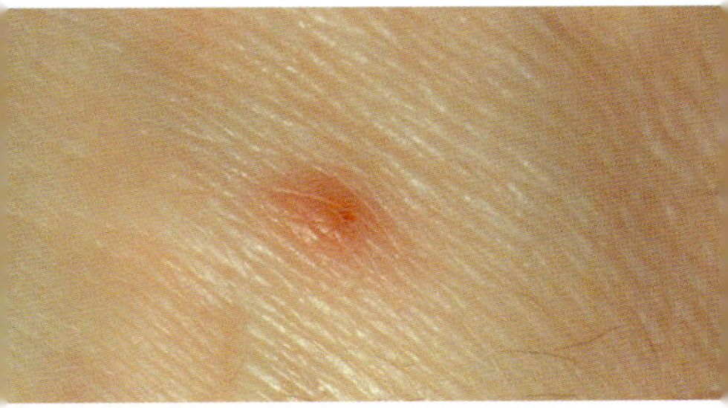

Papular urticaria. Characteristic red papule with central puncta.

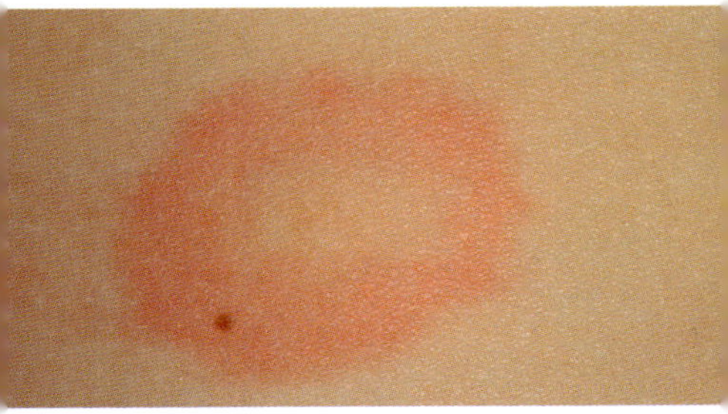

Papular urticaria. Giant red flare following insect exposure.

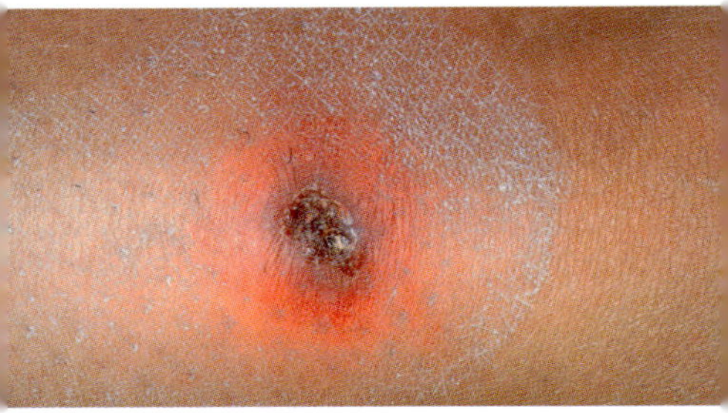

Venomous spider bite. Central necrosis and indurated red border in brown recluse spider bite.

CLINICAL FEATURES

Intensely itchy clustered red papules, some with an urticarial flare, are the most common form of insect bite reactions. A tiny central punctum is present. Children 18 months to 7 years are susceptible as they are hypersensitive, but older children and adults similarly exposed are not. Parents may have difficulty understanding why other household members are not affected. Typically, the recurrent crops lasting 2–10 days first develop in the spring and summer and last 3–9 months.

Cat fleas are the most common offender, followed by dog fleas, mosquitoes, lice, scabies, grain mites, grass mites or fowl mites, or non-venomous spiders. In the very sensitive child, giant urticarial flares are seen and the central papule becomes a vesicle or large bulla.

Venomous spiders such as the brown recluse, induce a red indurated plaque with central necrosis that is painful and sometimes hemorrhagic. Rapidly spreading tissue damage may occur within hours and produce a toxic appearance in the child with fever, nausea, vomiting, and syncope.

Widow spiders induce a painful red papule with a central punctum with sweating and piloerection of the surrounding skin. Abdominal cramps may ensue and lack of coordination followed by paralysis develop. Symptoms subside within 3 days.

TREATMENT

Papular urticaria requires insect avoidance and symptomatic treatment. Pets should be treated by a veterinarian and household fumigation may be necessary. Protective clothing with long sleeves is helpful.

The use of insect repellant such as a bite blocker or 6% DEET to make the child less attractive to the insect will help.

Prophylactic use of an oral antihistamine such as cetirizine once daily, and a moderate-strength topical steroid twice daily will relieve symptoms.

Venomous brown recluse spider bites require prompt intervention. In some, surgical excision of the bite site to remove the venom is helpful, and toxic-appearing children require hospitalization with fluid and electrolyte support.

Widow spider bites may be improved with widow antisera administered within hours of the bite.

Erythema multiforme

DDx ref 48 • 99 • 34

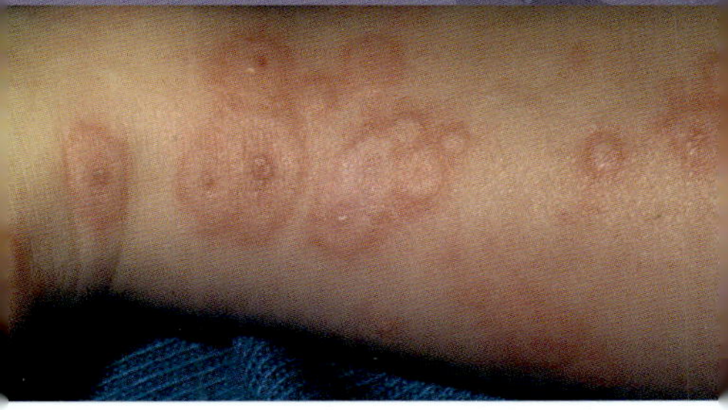

Early target lesions with a central dusky and an outer edematous zone.

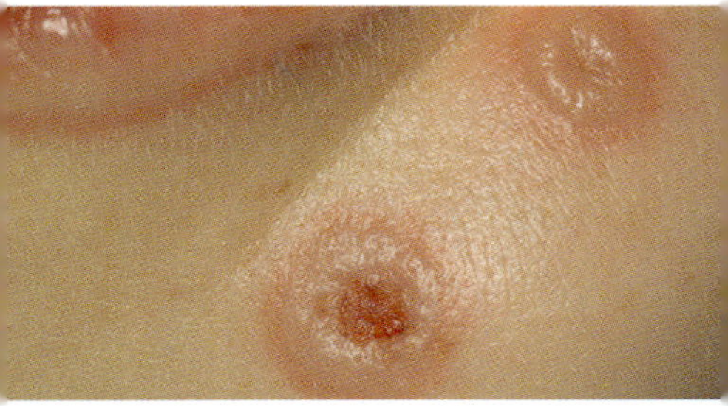

Fully developed target lesions with central necrotic crusted zone, edematous zone, and outer red zone.

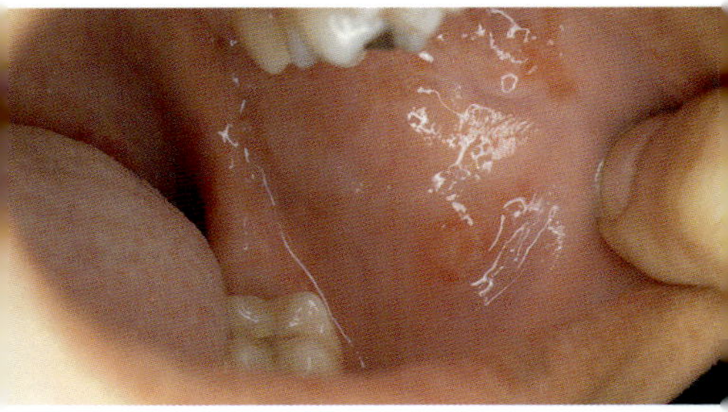

Oral shallow ulcers with a red base on buccal mucosa.

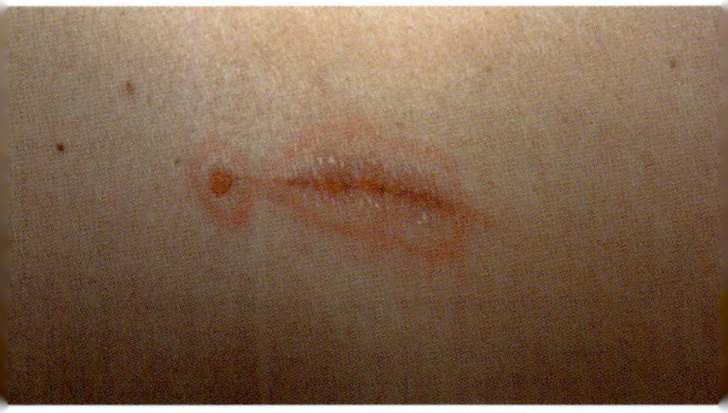

Isomorphic phenomenon (Koebner) at the site of an antecedent scratch on the arm of a teen with EM.

CLINICAL FEATURES

The abrupt onset of symmetrical red papules that evolve into diagnostic target lesions characterizes EM.

Target lesions are oval to round, fixed lesions that have three distinct zones: a central zone of epidermal damage seen as blister or crust formation, an edematous middle zone, and a red outer zone. Target lesions must display epidermal damage. Giant urticaria with a clear center is often mislabeled as target lesions.

EM skin lesions are fixed; that is, once they appear, they stay at the same site for 7–21 days, whereas urticaria lesions move to different skin sites within hours. Target lesions may itch or be painful. Herpes labialis may precede the onset of EM, but most often a prodrome is absent. The dorsum of the hands, palms and soles, and extensor extremities are the sites most often involved.

Sites of skin trauma that preceded the onset of lesions may develop target lesions in the configuration of the injury (Koebner phenomenon).

Oral mucosa is involved and in half of the children, a few shallow oral lesions will be seen.

EM is uncommon is recurrent, and predominantly seen in older children and teens. Recurrences are usually 1 or 2 each year.

The majority of children with EM will have HSV-1 or -2 associated disease and have detectable virus within their skin lesions even without a definite history of a preceding HSV infection. They may have delayed clearing of HSV from their skin. In a few, EBV or CMV infections may be precipitating agents.

TREATMENT

Symptomatic treatment with wet compresses and oral antihistamines will help with itching or pain.

Antiviral treatment even at the onset of symptoms is ineffective, as the skin injury has already been initiated.

Six months of daily prophylaxis with oral acyclovir at 20 mg/kg per day will often abort EM episodes and is reserved for children who suffer frequent recurrences.

Good sun protection can be useful in preventing the antecedent recurrent HSV.

Systemic steroids should be avoided, as their use may result in more frequent recurrences and prolonged, almost continuous episodes.

Erythema nodosum

DDx ref 37 • 47 • 30

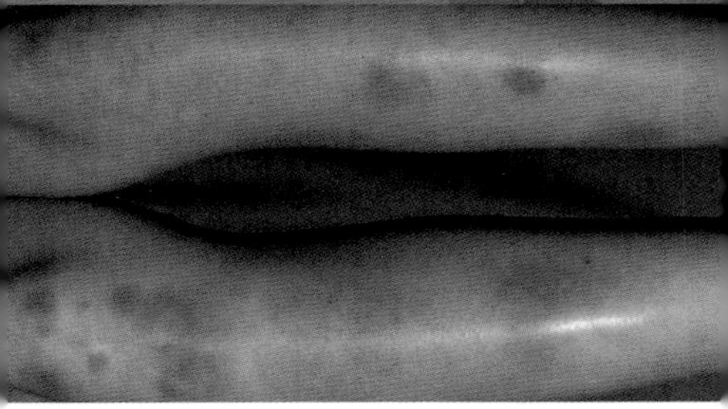

Painful red nodules on the anterior lower legs of an adolescent female.

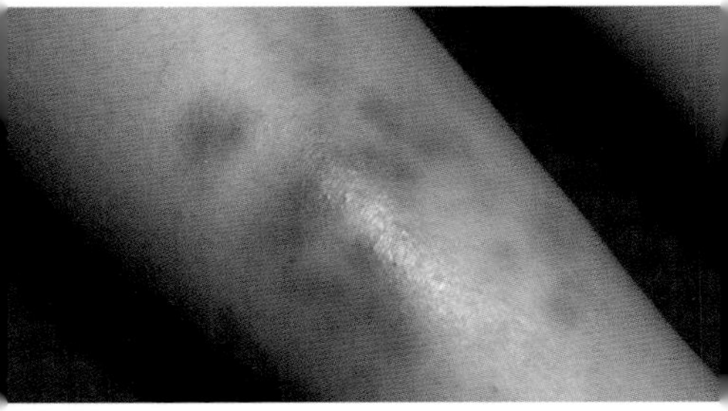

EN on the extensor lower leg of a teen.

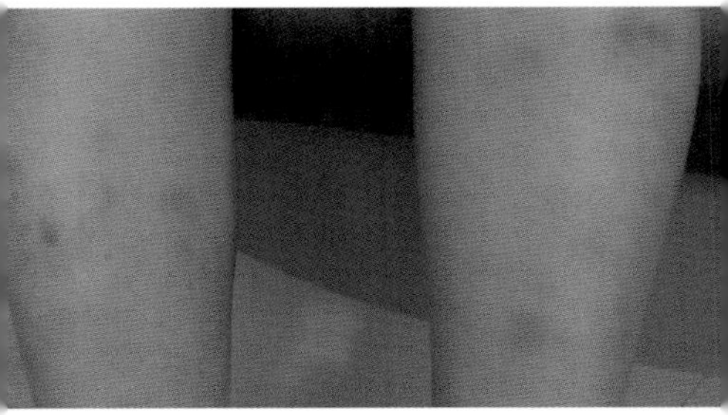

Evolving purple lesions in a 3-year-old child.

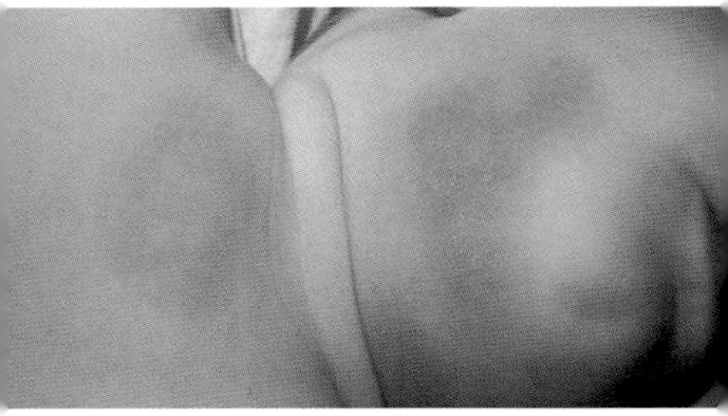

Atypical EN of the chin and chest of a toddler.

Erythema nodosum

DDx ref 37 • 47 • 30

CLINICAL FEATURES

The abrupt onset of symmetric, painful red nodules with indistinct borders on the extensor lower legs characterizes erythema nodosum. The child or teen will limp because of the pain. Girls are more likely than boys to have EN.

In preschool children EN is more likely to be asymmetrical and appear in non-characteristic sites such as soles, eyelids, neck, hands, or trunk. In 25% of children with EN, a prodrome of cough, sore throat, and fever will antecede the nodules. Nodules last 2–6 weeks and evolve like a bruise, with color change to purple, then yellow-brown.

Recurrences develop in 4%. EN is a chronic injury to blood vessels of the lower dermis and subcutaneous fat but fat cell destruction does not occur. Circulating immune complexes are implicated in the pathogenesis.

There are many infectious associations including streptococcus (30%), tuberculosis, sarcoidosis, histoplasmosis, tularemia, *Giardia*, EBV, hepatitis B, *Yersinia*, and coccidioidomycosis.

Other associated factors include inflammatory bowel disease, Behçet's syndrome, hereditary periodic fever syndromes, and Hodgkin's disease. Oral contraceptives also have been implicated.

TREATMENT

Symptomatic treatment with aspirin, indomethacin, or antihistamines suffice in many children as the condition resolves within 3 weeks. Some relief can be obtained with oral prednisone but its chronic use results in many undesirable side-effects.

Thalidomide has been helpful in severe EN.

RED PAPULES AND NODULES

Panniculitis

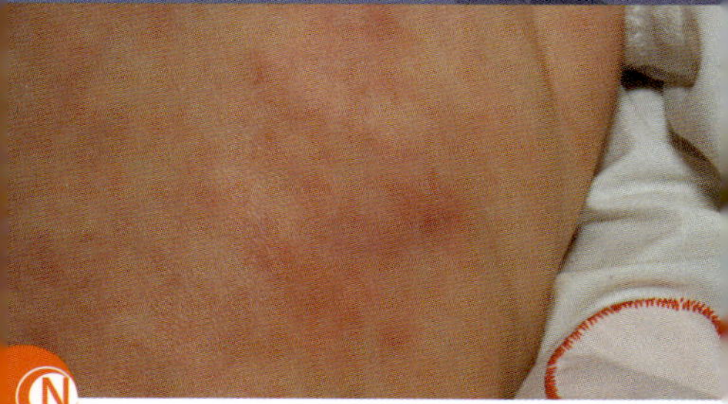

N Neonatal subcutaneous fat necrosis. Red nodules of immobile skin on the back of a 2-day-old infant.

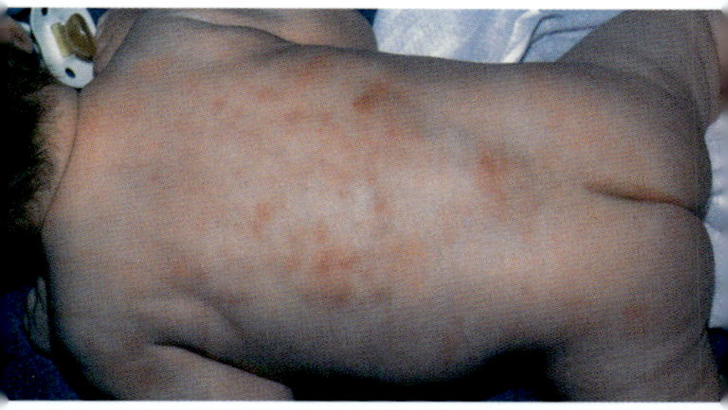

Subcutaneous fat necrosis. Multiple firm red nodules on the back of a 1-month-old infant.

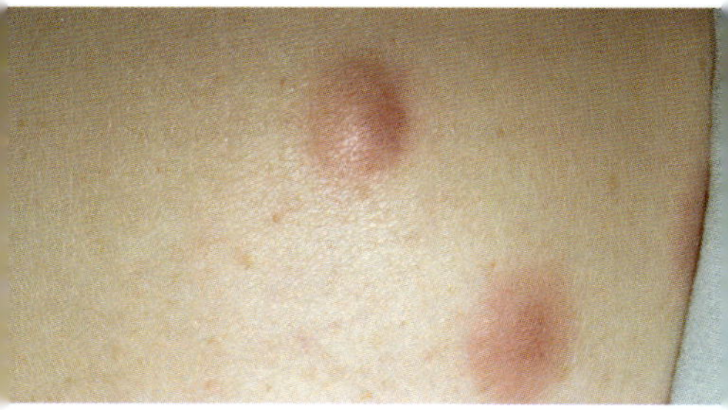

Lupus panniculitis. Red-purple nodules on the upper arm of a girl with lupus profundus.

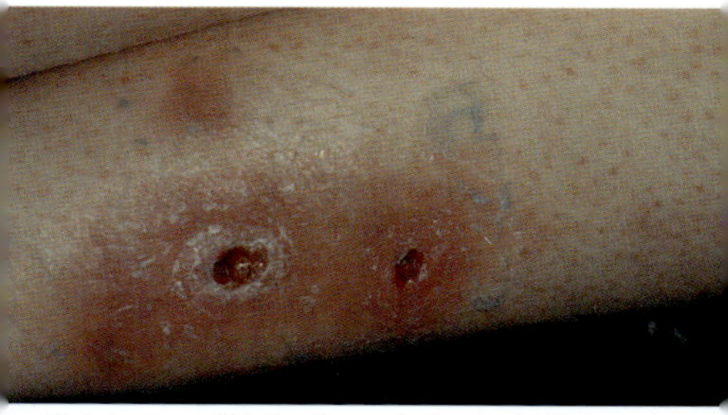

Nodular vasculitis (erythema induratum). Ulcerated red nodules on the calf of a teenage girl.

CLINICAL FEATURES

Panniculitis is characterized by red to red-purple nodules on the skin associated with fat cell destruction.

In the newborn panniculitis is called 'subcutaneous fat necrosis' and red nodules appear over the cheeks, buttocks, back, arms, and thighs. A major precipitating factor is cooling of the skin, including therapeutic neuroprotective cooling. Skin lesions begin in the first 14 days and resolve slowly over the next few months. The skin in the involved areas is initially immobile. Eventually, a skin depression may result. In a few newborns, extensive fat necrosis may be associated with hypercalcemia, with irritability, vomiting, and weight loss. Serum calcium levels should be monitored in babies with associated symptoms or widespread skin involvement.

Panniculitis in older children and teens is seen as red-purple nodules associated with lupus erythematosus or other connective tissue disease, or nodules that ulcerate, as seen in nodular vasculitis (erythema induratum).

Nodular vasculitis is associated primarily with tuberculosis and occasionally hepatitis C.

It is very rare in childhood to have the panniculitis seen with pancreatic disease, lipophagic panniculitis or alpha$_1$-antitrypsin deficiency. T-cell lymphoma may mimic panniculitis.

TREATMENT

No treatment is necessary in subcutaneous fat necrosis of newborns.

In infants with hypercalcemia, in addition to strategies to lower calcium levels and increase renal excretion of calcium, systemic steroids may be useful.

For the child with lupus panniculitis, systemic immune suppressants may be required, depending upon associated problems.

For nodular vasculitis there are no reliable studies on treatment. If tuberculosis is found, multidrug antituberculosis therapy is indicated. Systemic steroids or immunosuppressives have been traditionally used to improve symptoms.

38

RED PAPULES AND NODULES

Dermatofibromas

DDx ref 39 • 44 • 131

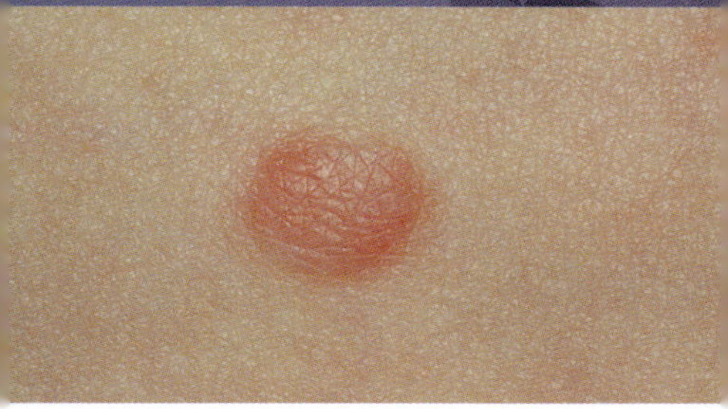

Early dermatofibroma. Pinkish-red nodule on the arm of a 2-year-old child.

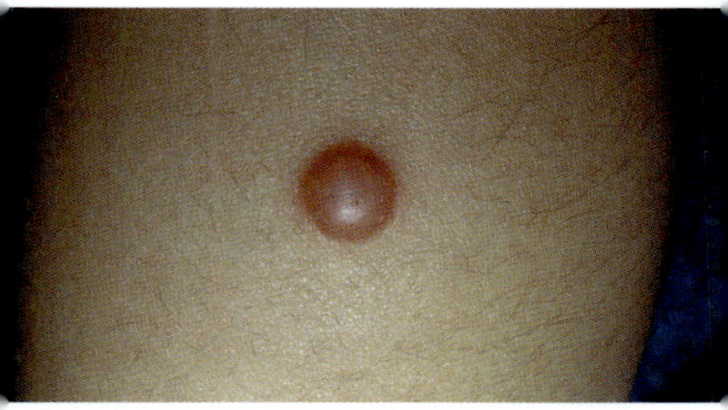

Late dermatofibroma. Brownish-red nodule on the leg of a teenager.

39

RED PAPULES AND NODULES

Keloids and hypertrophic scars

DDx ref 38 • 98 • 102

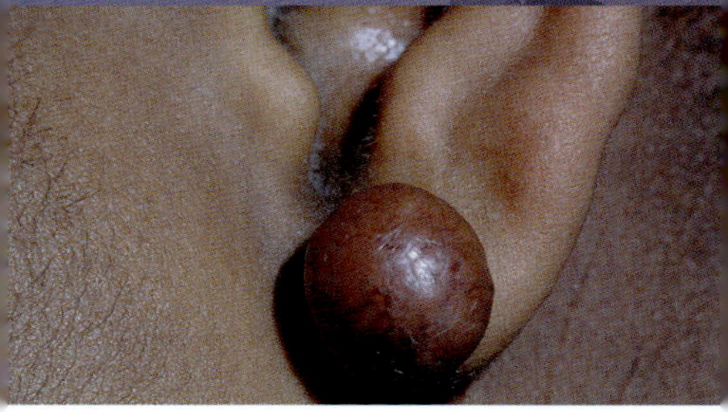

Keloid nodule on the earlobe from ear piercing.

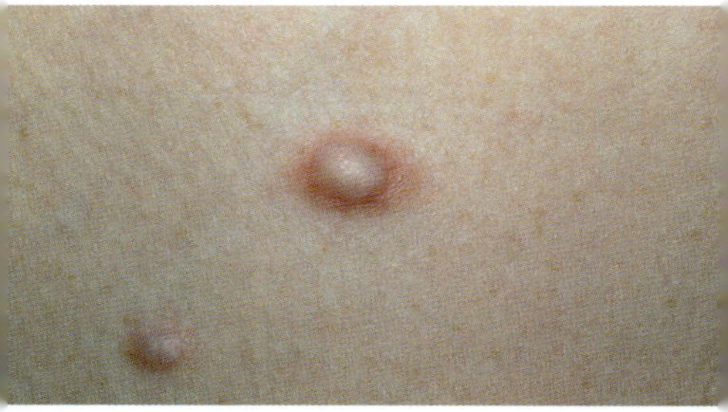

Hypertrophic scars at the site of a varicella lesion. They subsequently resolved.

38

RED PAPULES AND NODULES

Dermatofibromas

DDx ref 39 • 44 • 131

CLINICAL FEATURES

Small, firm nodules that are red at first, and later brown, are seen in dermatofibromas. Lateral pressure on the dermatofibroma will produce dimpling of the overlying surface.

They are frequently on the legs or trunk but may appear anywhere on skin. They are more common in the older child or teenager. Often, multiple lesions are present.

A prior history of trauma can sometimes be obtained. They may grow up to 1–2 cm. Once present, dermatofibromas persist. Rarely, they are painful.

TREATMENT

Usually no intervention is required. If painful, then surgical excision is recommended.

39

RED PAPULES AND NODULES

Keloids and hypertrophic scars

DDx ref 38 • 98 • 102

CLINICAL FEATURES

Keloids are firm, progressively enlarging nodules with a shiny, hairless surface, which begin at sites of skin trauma such as acne, surgical incision sites, burns, or varicella lesions. They may be painful or itch. They are most often on the earlobes following ear piercing but occasionally appear on the trunk or extremities. Stellate shapes develop as the keloid grows beyond the boundaries of the initial skin injury. Multiple genetic susceptibility loci for keloid development have been described and a few families have a dominant pattern of inheritance.

Progressive enlargement over 20–40 years is common resulting in lobulated or pedunculated masses.

Simple surgical excision often results in regrowth larger than the original keloid. Post-excision radiotherapy may successfully treat large symptomatic keloids.

Hypertrophic scars are raised, hairless, shiny nodules that appear at sites of skin injury. Unlike keloids, they do not spread beyond the original scar site and stop growth after a few months, and then slowly regress.

TREATMENT

Intralesional injections of glucocorticosteroids will soften and flatten the keloid. Surgery followed by intralesional injections of glucocorticosteroids weekly over 1 month may be effective for large keloids, particularly those around the ear.

The corticosteroid injections may result in hypopigmentation in the area.

No treatment for hypertrophic scars is usually necessary as regression is expected.

RED PAPULES AND NODULES

Angiofibromas

DDx ref 25 • 59 • 57

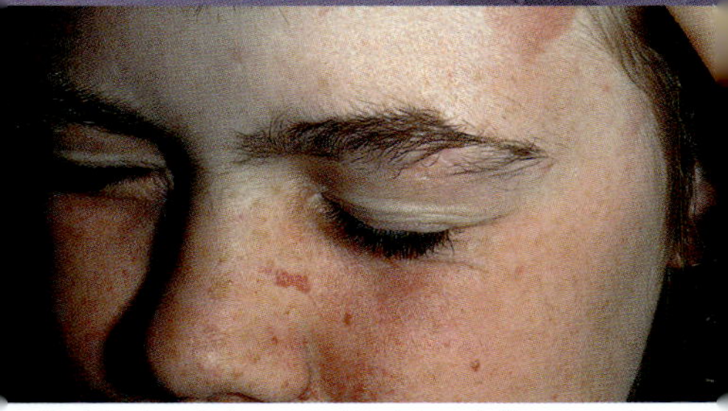

Red forehead plaque and facial angiofibromas of tuberous sclerosis.

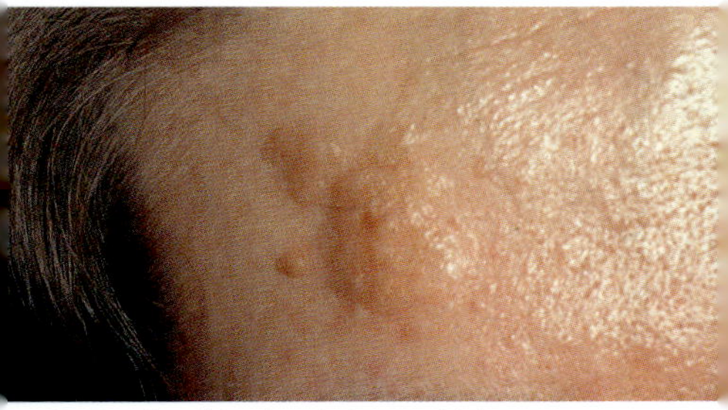

Flesh-colored forehead plaque of tuberous sclerosis.

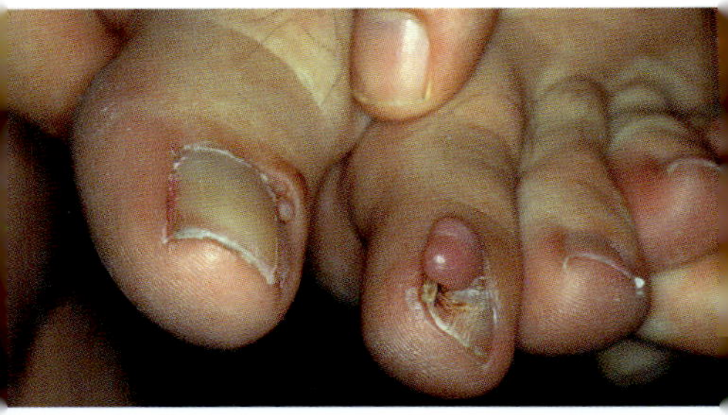

Periungual fibrous nodules (Koenen's tumors) on the toes of an adolescent with tuberous sclerosis.

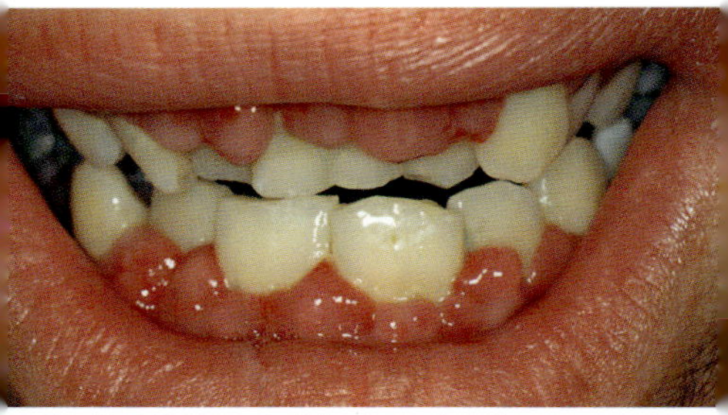

Gingival fibromas in tuberous sclerosis.

CLINICAL FEATURES

Angiofibromas are flesh- to red-colored papules or plaques. They are most commonly seen in the tuberous sclerosis complex.

Tuberous sclerosis complex (TSC) is an autosomal dominant genetic disease caused by mutations in the genes encoding for the proteins hamartin (TSC1) and tuberin (TSC2). There are major and minor criteria for the diagnosis of the TSC. Four types of skin disease are major criteria. These are facial angiofibromas or fibrous forehead plaques, non-traumatic ungual or periungual fibromas, hypomelanotic macules (≥3), and the shagreen patch. Gingival fibromas and confetti type white patches are minor criteria.

Multiple types of angiofibromas are seen in TSC. The first type to be noted is the facial angiofibromas. They are seen beginning at age 2 years, predominantly on the nose, cheeks, upper lip, and chin. They grow progressively throughout life. They may eventually cover the entire central face and bleeding with irritation may be a severe problem. When small in number and beginning after the age of 8 years, they have been confused with inflammatory papular acne. The other types of angiofibromas seen are the fibrous forehead plaque, periungual fibromas (Koenen's tumors), and gingival fibromas.

Periungual and gingival fibromas begin developing with adolescence. Periungual fibromas may be painful, destroy the nail, and bleed with trauma.

TREATMENT

If treatment is begun early in life facial angiofibromas respond well to vascular pulsed dye laser treatment. More established lesions may be treated with the carbon dioxide laser. Treatment of facial angiofibromas with topical rapamycin reduces their size.

Rapamycin inhibits mTOR activation and decreases the growth of the angiofibromas.

Hamartin and tuberin suppress mTOR activation. In TSC, mutation of hamartin or tuberin allows for unsuppressed activity of mTOR, leading to the unregulated growth of the facial angiofibromas.

Periungual fibromas may be treated with curettage and electrocautery of the base.

RED PAPULES AND NODULES

Tufted angiomas

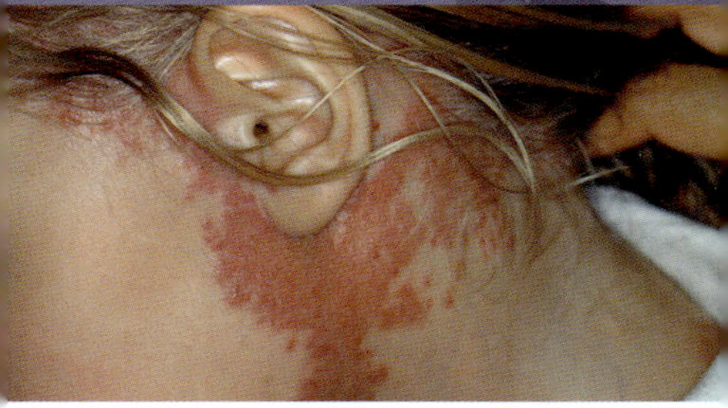

Plaque-type tufted angioma on the neck of a 4-year-old girl.

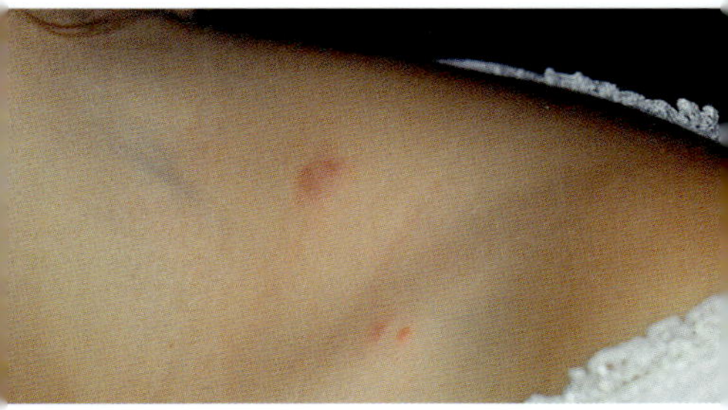

Satellite lesions of tufted angioma on the neck of the same girl as the previous image.

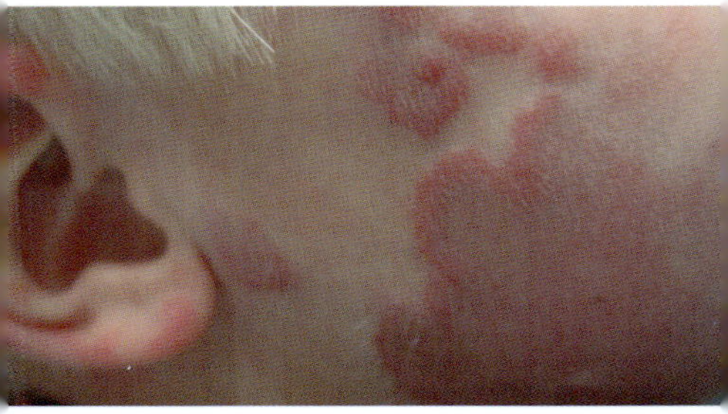

Plaque-type tufted angioma of the face.

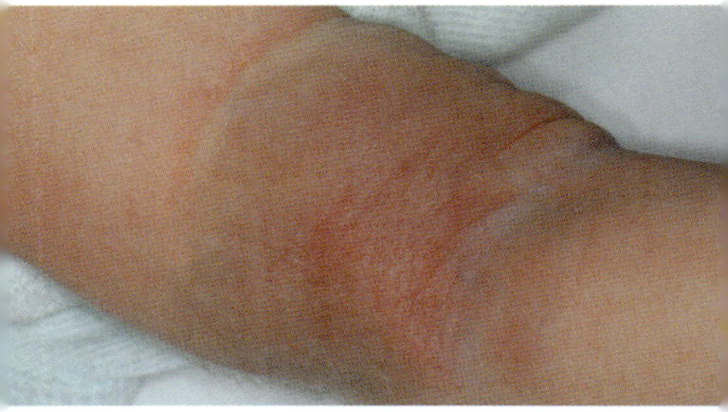

Solitary tufted angioma on the leg.

DDx ref 55 • 42 • 60

CLINICAL FEATURES

Tufted angiomas are described histologically by discrete, dermal, cannonball-like tufts of endothelial cells.

The classic type is that of a slowly expanding, dusky, reddish-blue vascular plaque. More than 50% occur on the head, neck, upper arms, and upper back. Satellite lesions may be seen. The majority of lesions arise within the first two decades of life. Regression in this type of tufted angioma is not expected.

The other type is a solitary vascular nodule presenting on an extremity at birth. This type of tufted angioma does not exhibit the slow expansion seen in the other clinical type and satellite lesions are not seen. Regression of this type of tufted angioma has been reported, although it may have been confused with a RICH (rapidly involuting congenital hemangioma).

Nodular type tufted angiomas may be confused clinically with nodular venous malformations, RICH and NICH (non-involuting congenital hemangioma).

Kasabach–Merritt syndrome may be seen in association with tufted angiomas and it has been argued that tufted angiomas may be in the spectrum of hemangioendotheliomas.

TREATMENT

Vascular-specific pulsed dye lasers have been used with variable success for the plaque-like type.

Nodular types may be removed by surgical excision.

If Kasabach–Merritt syndrome occurs this should be treated appropriately. Optimal first-line treatment is controversial and based on case reports. Oral steroids, vincristine, surgical excision (if the lesion is small), radiotherapy, and propranolol have been used. Recently, mTOR inhibitors have been gaining favor over older therapies.

42 DDx ref

RED PAPULES AND NODULES

Hemangioendothelioma

41 • 55 • 39

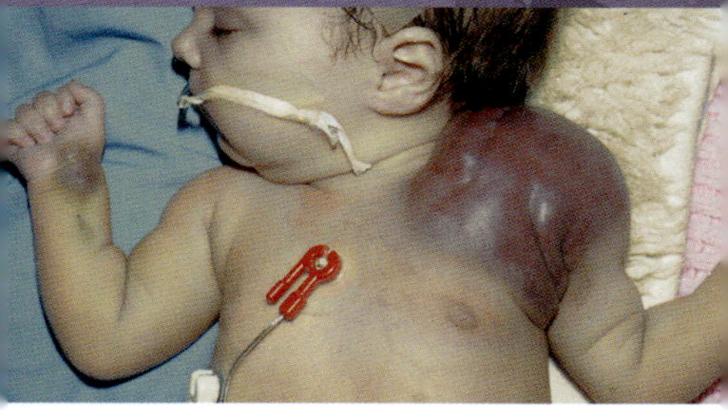

Sudden change of a hemangioendothelioma to deep purple in Kasabach–Merritt syndrome.

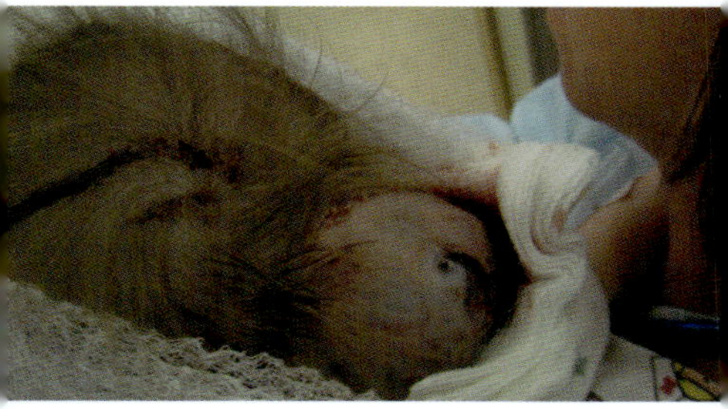

Kaposiform hemangioendothelioma of a baby.

43 DDx ref

RED PAPULES AND NODULES

Congenital self-healing reticulohistiocytosis

136 • 89 • 39

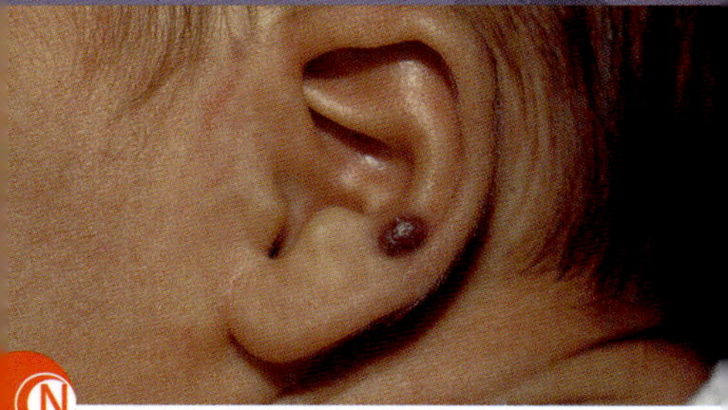

Congenital self-healing reticulohistiocytosis. Reddish-brown papule on the ear of a neonate.

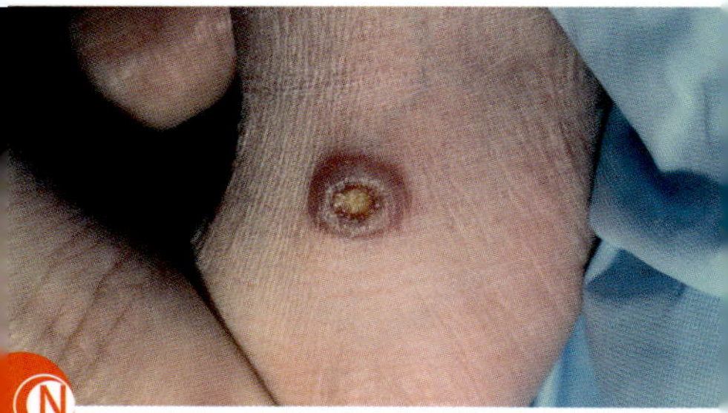

Congenital self-healing reticulohistiocytosis. Nodule present at birth with crateriform central erosion.

42 DDx ref

RED PAPULES AND NODULES

Hemangioendothelioma

41 • 55 • 39

CLINICAL FEATURES

Kaposiform hemangioendotheliomas (KHE) are rare vascular tumors that may be present at birth and are usually seen before 2 years of age. Lesions are usually solitary.

Mature lesions have a nodular infiltrative growth pattern and a characteristic purple hue. They have also been described as occurring in the peritoneum.

KHE are very aggressive locally and, although not malignant, may be fatal.

Fatalities are usually associated with the Kasabach–Merritt syndrome. Spontaneous regression is not expected.

TREATMENT

Optimal treatment for small lesions is surgical excision, but unfortunately very few lesions present at a small enough size to be amenable to this therapy. Some KHE respond well to methylprednisolone 1–2 mg/kg per day.

Vincristine is a second-line therapy for steroid treatment failures.

Kasabach–Merritt syndrome should be treated aggressively.

43 DDx ref

RED PAPULES AND NODULES

Congenital self-healing reticulohistiocytosis

136 • 89 • 39

CLINICAL FEATURES

Congenital self-healing reticulohistiocytosis (CSHR) is a variant of Langerhans cell histiocytosis (LCH). CSHR presents at birth as red to reddish-brown papules up to 2 cm. Usually, multiple lesions are present.

Lesions may be present anywhere on the body. Central ulceration of lesions is common. Lesions resolve rapidly with the majority healing before 6 months of age. By definition, no other organ system is involved.

TREATMENT

CSHR resolves spontaneously and therefore no treatment is necessary. However, histologically, the lesions of CSHR cannot be differentiated from any of the other types of LCH. The neonate should be followed closely and if new lesions continue to appear or any signs of systemic illness develop, a thorough evaluation for disseminated LCH should be performed.

RED PAPULES AND NODULES

Malignant tumors

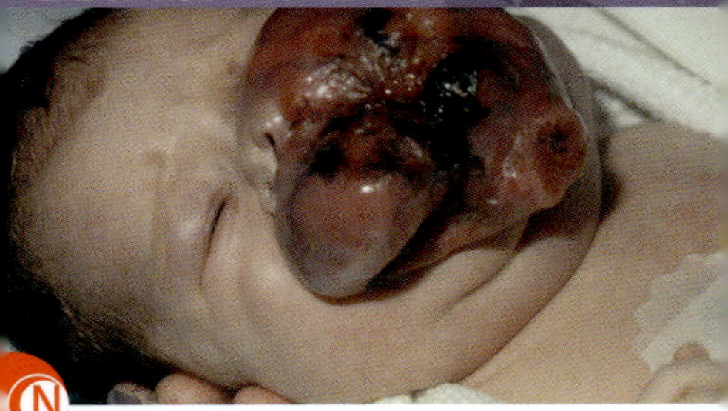

N

Red, firm lobulated masses on the face of a newborn with embryonal rhabdomyosarcoma.

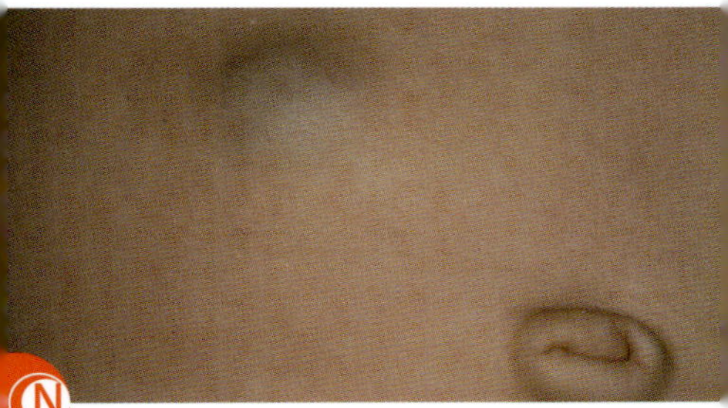

N

Pale firm nodule on the abdomen of a newborn with neuroblastoma.

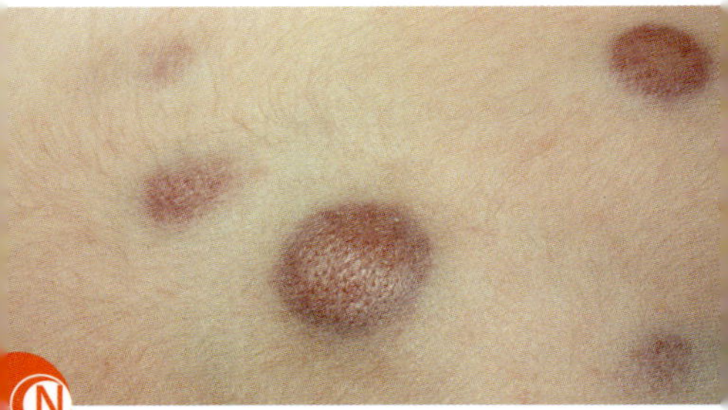

N

Red-purple firm nodules on the trunk of a newborn with leukemia cutis.

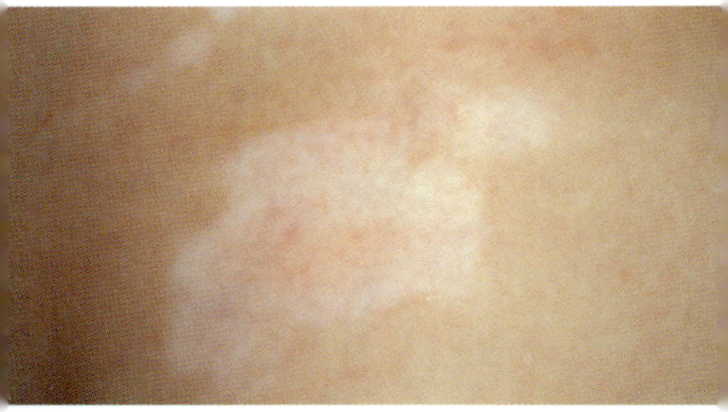

Red nodules, hypopigmentation, and eczematous plaques on an 8-year-old boy with cutaneous T-cell lymphoma (mycosis fungoides).

CLINICAL FEATURES

Malignant tumors in newborns and children are quite uncommon. Rapid progressive growth of red or purple nodules is a valuable clue. Also, suspicion of malignancy should be high if nodules are firm and fixed to deeper tissue. In suspected childhood malignancies, biopsy of the nodule is indicated. The most frequent soft tissue malignant tumor is rhabdomyosarcoma. They are seen in the head and neck and genital areas as lobulated red nodules and tumors. They are seen between the ages of 0–5 years and again in teen years. There is no hereditary pattern. There are two types determined by histologic analysis, embryonal rhabdomyosarcomas and alveolar rhabdomyosarcomas. Rhabdomyosarcomas spread by local extension, by lymphatics or hematogenously to lungs, liver, bone marrow, bone, and brain.

Neuroblastomas appear in newborns as red-purple nodules on the trunk that blanch when stroked. Abdominal ultrasound or CAT scan for internal involvement may be necessary. In older children, they appear as a lateral abdominal mass. Serum ferritin, lactic dehydrogenase, and neuron-specific enolase levels are helpful in prognosis. Gene analysis of tumors provides important clues to clinical outcome and may guide therapy selection.

Newborns with acute myelogenous leukemia will have red-purple nodules on the skin. Skin lesions are common in acute myelogenous leukemia but seen in only 1% of the more common acute lymphatic leukemia. A peripheral blood smear examination and a bone marrow evaluation are key in the evaluation.

Cutaneous T-cell lymphoma (mycosis fungoides) initially presents in childhood as hypopigmented patches that develop over months to red nodules and red, eczematous-appearing plaques. It is frequently misdiagnosed as atopic dermatitis. In any persistent dermatitis unresponsive to therapy, a skin biopsy to evaluate for possible T-cell lymphoma is indicated.

TREATMENT

Referral to a children's oncology center is required for selection of the most appropriate cancer therapy. Some tumors such as neuroblastoma and leukemia cutis may have spontaneous regression, but such predictions depend upon thorough tissue analysis.

45 FLAT VASCULAR LESIONS, BLANCHING
Mottling

DDx ref 46 • 47 • 72

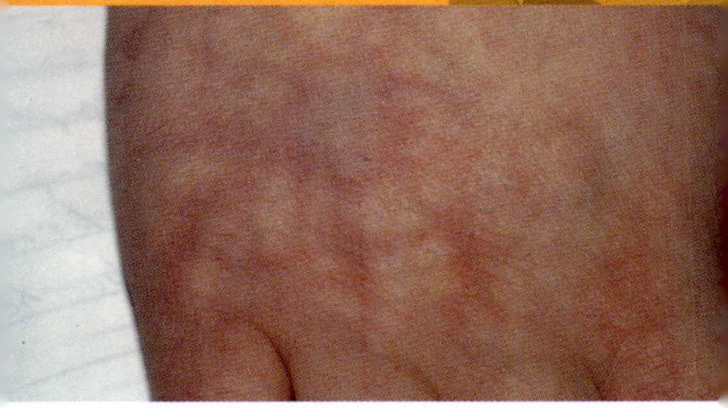

Permanent mottled appearance of cutis marmorata telangiectasia congenita.

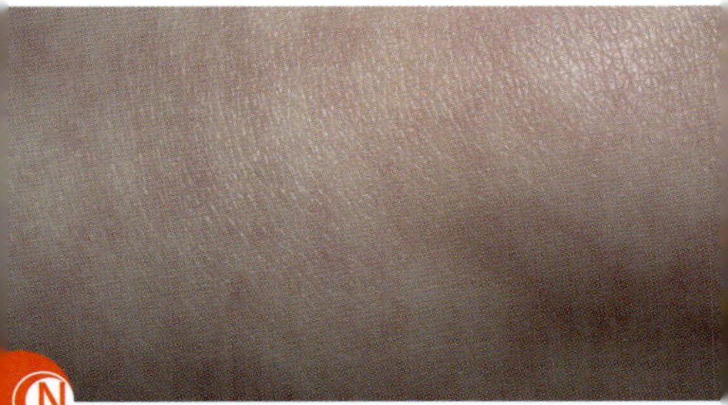

(N) Transient mottling of newborn, which disappeared on warming of the skin.

46 FLAT VASCULAR LESIONS, BLANCHING
Cutis marmorata telangiectasia congenita

DDx ref 45 • 47 • 72

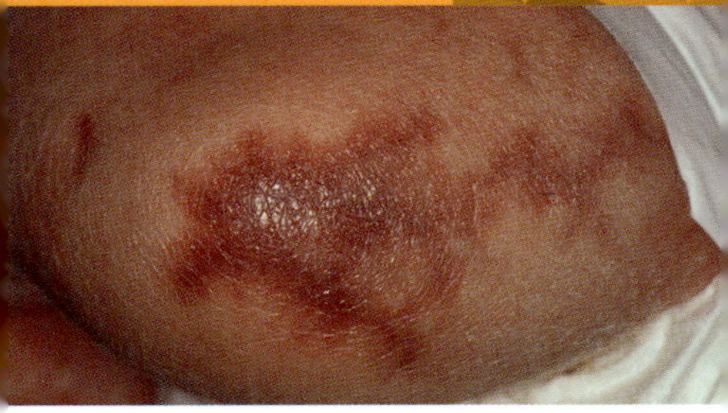

Venous pattern of cutis marmorata telangiectasia congenita (congenital phlebectasia).

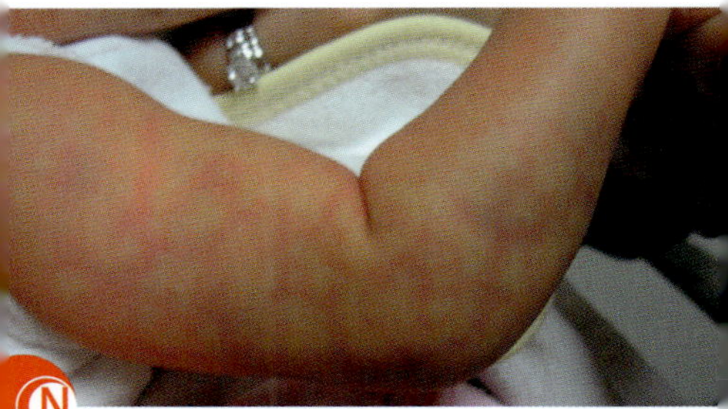

(N) Cutis marmorata telangiectasia congenita on the right arm of a neonate.

45 DDx ref

FLAT VASCULAR LESIONS, BLANCHING

Mottling

46 • 47 • 72

CLINICAL FEATURES

Mottling is an evanescent, lacy, reticulated red and/or blue cutaneous vascular pattern covering most of the body surface in a newborn when exposed to low environmental temperatures. Mottling represents an accentuated physiologic vasomotor response that disappears with increasing age, although it is sometimes discernible even in older children.

Cutis marmorata telangiectasia congenita may appear similar, but is persistent and usually localized to a portion of the body (see DDx ref 46 Cutis Marmorata Telangiectasia Congenita).

Livedo reticularis has a similar pattern, but is acquired, usually seen on the lower extremities and may be associated with systemic illness (see DDx ref 47 Livedo Reticularis and Periarteritis Nodosa).

TREATMENT

No treatment is necessary.

46 DDx ref

FLAT VASCULAR LESIONS, BLANCHING

Cutis marmorata telangiectasia congenita

45 • 47 • 72

CLINICAL FEATURES

In cutis marmorata telangiectasia congenita (CMTC) two clinical presentations may be seen. One is a mottled, reticulated pattern of blue and dusky-red erythema. In the other form, there is atrophy of the skin and larger, depressed, blue venous malformations (congenital phlebectasia). Both types may be seen in the same patient. The lesions may be restricted to a single limb and a portion of the trunk, or may be more widespread. Ulceration may occur within the depressed area. A gradual increase in size is expected as the child grows, but the lesions become less noticeable within the first few years of life. They may be seen in association or confused with reticulate port-wine stains. Rarely, defective growth of the underlying bone and other congenital anomalies may be present.

Adams–Oliver syndrome and CMCT-macrocephaly syndrome are rarely associated.

TREATMENT

No treatment is necessary.

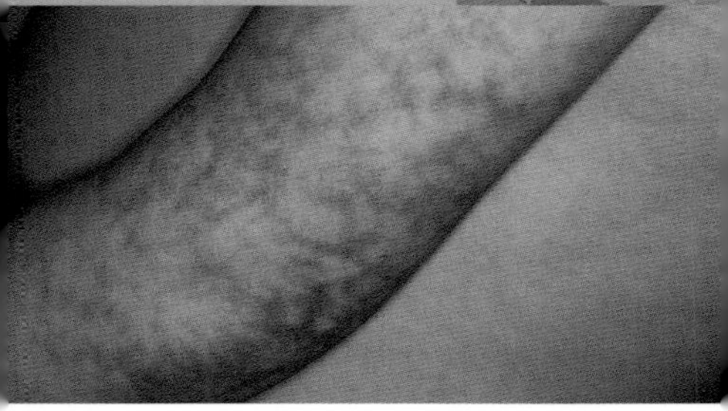

Livedo reticularis pattern on the arm of a teenage boy.

Livedo reticularis pattern plus linear red nodules in a child with periarteritis nodosa.

Linear dusky-red nodules on the leg of a child with periarteritis nodosa.

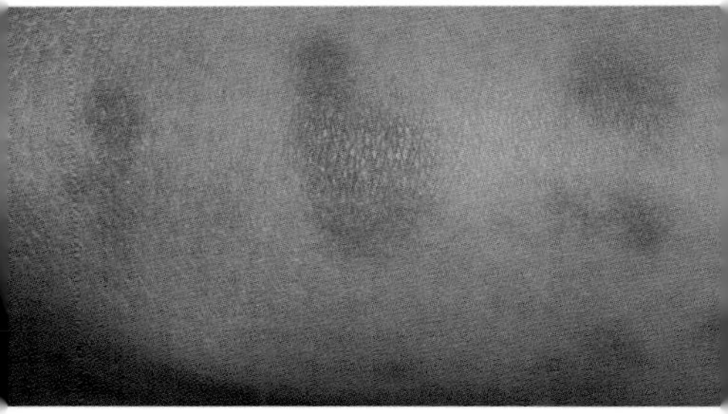

Linear and oval dusky-red nodules on the leg of a child with periarteritis nodosa.

CLINICAL FEATURES

Children with chronic cutaneous polyarteritis nodosa develop livedo reticularis (a lacy, purple-red pattern of skin) and tender, linear, dusky-red nodules in a symmetrical distribution. The livedo pattern does not improve with warming of the skin. Skin lesions persist for weeks with new crops appearing. Focal areas of skin infarction and ulceration may accompany the nodules. Fever, myalgias, arthralgias, and gastrointestinal symptoms are observed in 70%. Some develop hypertension, renal disease, pulmonary involvement, and localized neuropathy (mononeuritis multiplex). A positive ANCA test and elevated erythrocyte sedimentation rate are almost always present. Mixed cryoglobulinemia may be found.

Newborns of mothers with periarteritis nodosa may suffer a transient disease with skin lesions lasting up to 3 months. The segmental vasculitis is best diagnosed by skin biopsy of a linear nodule. The segmental vasculitis of periarteritis has been associated with certain infections such as parvovirus B19, hepatitis B & C, and streptococcus.

In some children, livedo patterns are associated with other connective tissue diseases such as **lupus erythematosus** (see DDx ref 72 Lupus Erythematosis) and, rarely, the periarteritis form can be asymmetrical and quite localized.

TREATMENT

Low-dose oral prednisone at 0.5 mg/kg per day will often result in clearing of lesions. Steroid-sparing immunosuppressive drugs may additionally be required in some children. This includes once-weekly methotrexate, TNF-α blockade, pulsed intravenous cyclophosphamide, or azathioprine.

Urticaria and dermographism

36 • 17 • 72

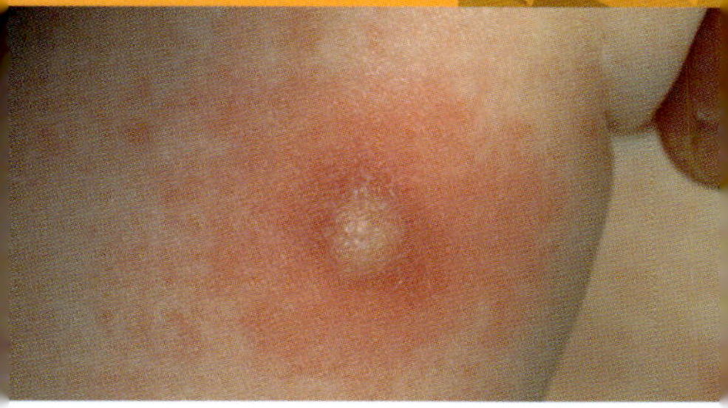

Central wheal with red border in acute urticaria.

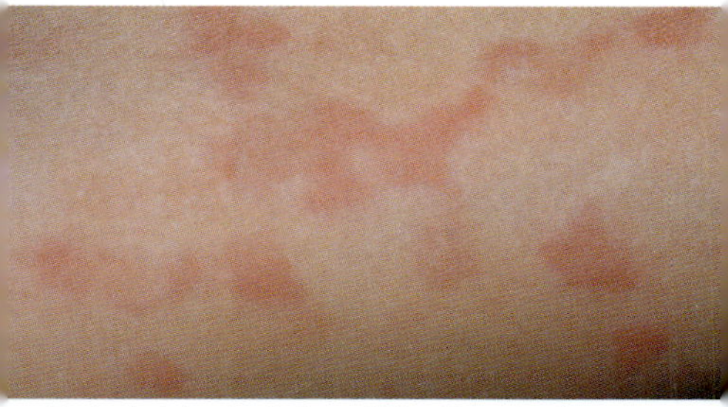

Typical pink wheals in a child with urticaria.

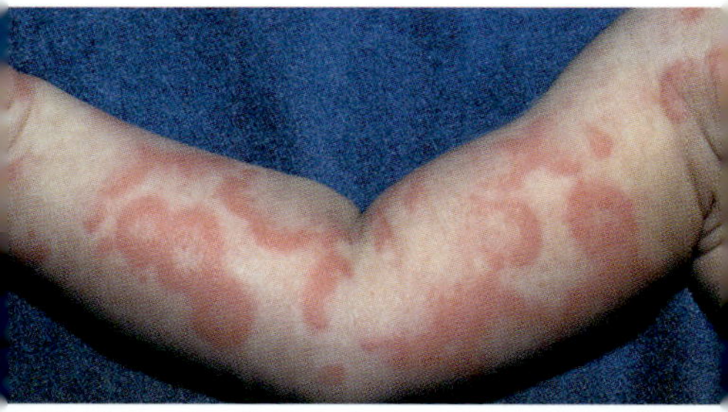

Multiple polycyclic red wheals of different sizes in a child with urticaria.

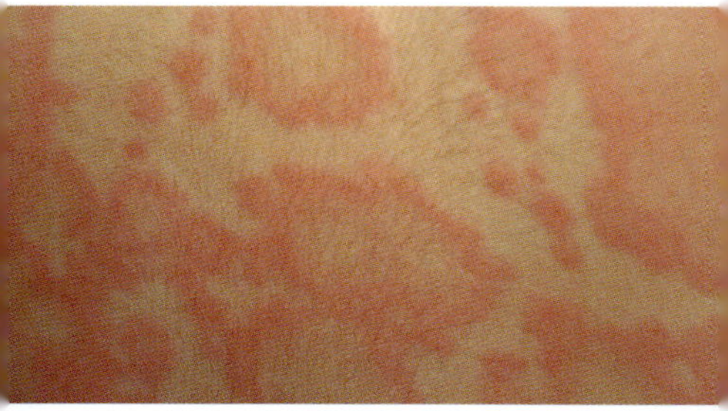

Multiple shapes of urticarial lesions in a child.

Urticaria and dermographism

DDx ref 36 • 17 • 72

CLINICAL FEATURES

Acute urticaria is the sudden onset of pruritic, erythematous raised wheals scattered over the body. The wheals are usually 2–15 mm in diameter, flat-topped with tense edema. The edema can be demonstrated by stretching the skin lightly to demonstrate whitish centers. The erythematous borders with pale centers can be quite large and mistaken for target lesions of erythema multiforme. Some experts use the term 'urticaria multiforme' to describe the type of lesion. Occasionally, giant urticarial lesions up to 30 cm in diameter with polycyclic borders will appear. More typical are pink wheals scattered on the skin. As the urticaria resolves, flat, dusky areas that resemble purpura may be left. Swelling of deep tissue with indistinct borders is called 'angioedema'. Some 85% of patients with angioedema will have swelling of the face, hands, and feet, although the trunk and genitalia can be involved. Up to half of children with acute urticaria may have angioedema at some time during the urticaria, with swelling of the hands and feet most commonly seen. Individual wheals commonly last from 20 minutes to 3 hours. Most episodes of urticaria last 2–3 days. The vast majority of cases of acute urticaria in childhood are caused by infections, medications, and foods.

Chronic urticaria is urticaria that lasts longer than 6 weeks. Chronic urticaria often lasts 3–5 years. Most cases of chronic urticaria in childhood are idiopathic. However, approximately 30–50% will have autoimmune urticaria (AIU). AIU is characterized by the presence of antibodies directed against the high-affinity IgE receptor or the IgE molecule itself.

Physical urticarias consist of dermographism, heat- and exercise-induced urticaria (cholinergic), delayed pressure urticaria, and cold urticaria. Dermographism is characterized by wheal and erythema after minor stroking of the skin. The wheal reaches maximal size in 6–7 minutes and resolves within 15 minutes. A minority of children with dermographism will have severe pruritus. In most children, dermographism will last less than 2 years. Almost all newborns have dermographism that lasts until 6–8 months.

Heat- and exercise-induced urticaria is characterized by 10–20-mm blotchy red macules surrounding 1–3-mm central wheals. Heating of the skin or exercise sufficient to raise the body temperature 0.5°C will induce attacks. Delayed pressure urticaria appears after prolonged pressure from a heavy weight. Painful deep swellings begin 4–6 hours after pressure and last up to 24 hours. Cold urticaria may be associated with cryoglobulins or be idiopathic. Wheals form upon rewarming of skin exposed to cold.

Hereditary angioedema (HAE) is an autosomal dominant condition with repeated attacks of swelling of the extremities, face, and throat, accompanied by abdominal pain. Children with HAE do not get urticaria. Abdominal pain becomes a major complaint in most patients. Mortality is from airway edema. A persistently low C4 level is a rapid screening test. A lack of C1 esterase inhibitor is causative.

FLAT VASCULAR LESIONS, BLANCHING

Urticaria and dermographism

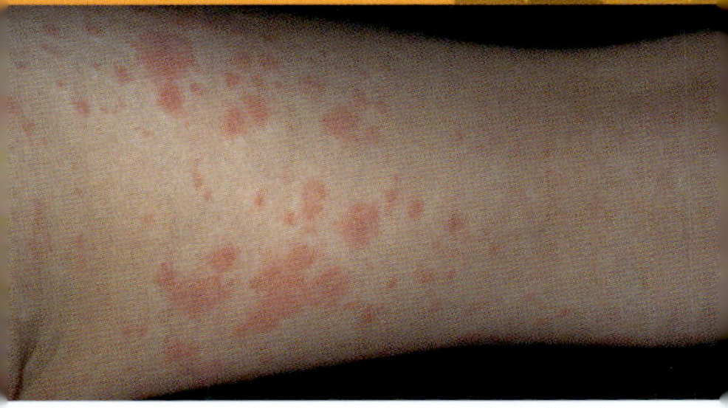

Pink wheals on the leg of a child with urticaria.

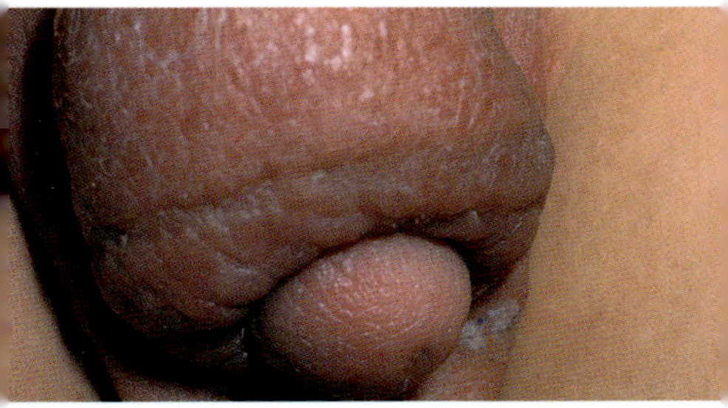

Angioedema of the scrotum and foreskin in an infant.

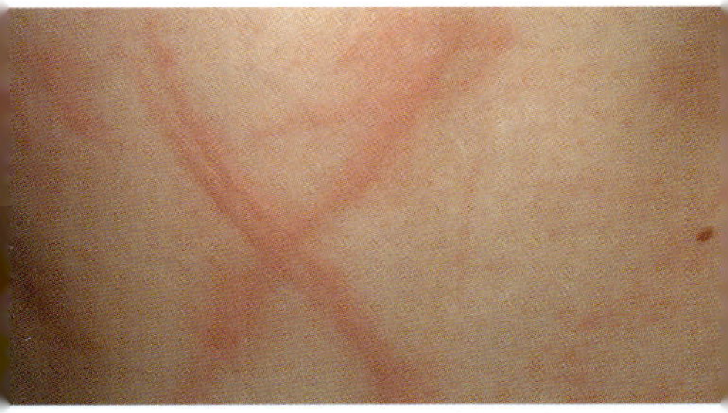

Dermographism. Light stroking of the skin evokes intense wheal and flare reaction.

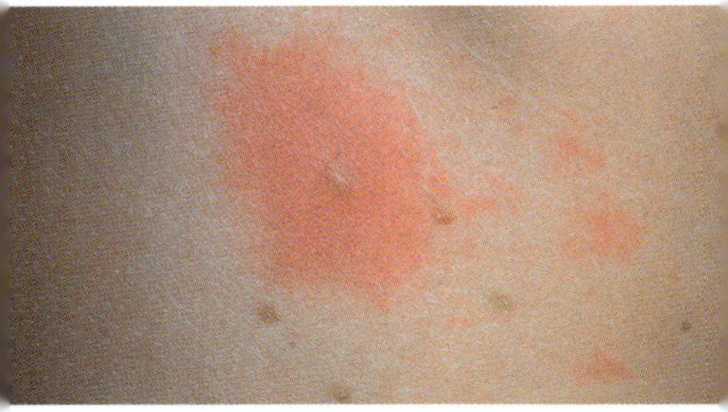

Heat and exercise (cholinergic) urticaria. Central wheal within large blotchy erythema.

Autoinflammatory urticaria syndromes include familial cold urticarias, Muckle–Wells syndrome and neonatal-onset multisystem inflammatory disease (NOMID). Mutations in the cold-induced autoinflammatory syndrome gene (CIAS1) that encode the protein cryopyrin are the cause. These syndromes overlap in severity and are characterized by fever, urticaria, arthralgias, and neutrophil-mediated disease.

Urticarial vasculitis is characterized by fixed wheals distributed symmetrically over the extremities. Lesions remain fixed in the same areas for days. Mild arthralgias and malaise may accompany the rash. Urticarial vasculitis may be associated with systemic lupus erythematosus or juvenile idiopathic arthritis.

TREATMENT

Acute urticaria is treated by removal and avoidance of the offending agent if identified. Oral H1 antihistamines are effective therapy. Cetirizine 2.5–10 mg every morning combined with hydroxyzine 1 mg/kg before bed is the optimal treatment. Oral glucocorticoids should not be used.

Chronic urticaria is treated in the same manner as acute urticaria. The offending agent is usually difficult to identify. There is controversy regarding the effectiveness of adding H2 antihistamines or leukotriene inhibitors to H1 therapy. Sulfasalazine starting at 500 mg/day and increasing to a maximum of 1 gram twice a day may be effective for those children not responding to H1 antihistamines. Children with autoimmune urticaria do not respond as well to antihistamine treatment. Omalizumab, a monoclonal antibody that inhibits IgE binding to the high-affinity IgE receptor on mast cells is approved for the treatment of chronic urticaria for patients at least age 12 years that have failed antihistamine therapy.

Physical urticaria treatment depends on the type. Dermographism is treated similarly to chronic urticaria. Delayed pressure urticaria does not respond to antihistamines, but may respond to prednisone 1–2 mg/day for 5 days, but treatment is usually not necessary in most affected children. H1 antihistamines may be used for cold urticaria, although cold avoidance is the preferred therapy.

Hereditary angioedema is best treated with C1 esterase inhibitor. Other treatments include ecallantide (DX-88, a plasma kallikrein inhibitor) and icatibant (a bradykinin B2 receptor antagonist) to decrease the severity of acute attacks. Androgens are now used only for those patients who cannot get any of the above treatments.

Autoinflammatory urticaria are best treated with the IL-1 antagonist anakinra.

Urticarial vasculitis has been treated with antihistamines, indomethacin, dapsone, colchicines and low-dose prednisone, with variable success.

FLAT VASCULAR LESIONS, BLANCHING

Port-wine stains

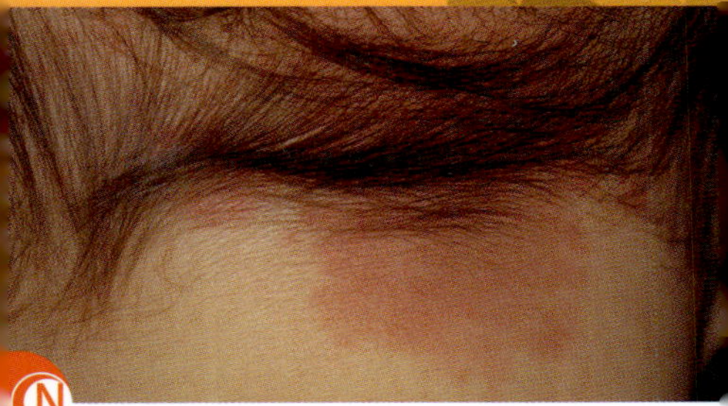

Nevus simplex on the nape of the neck.

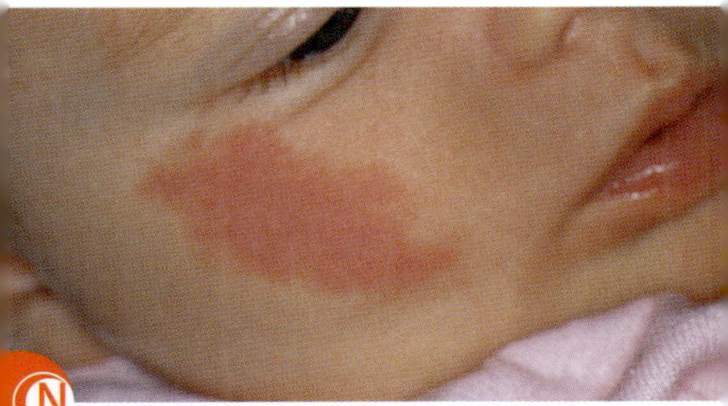

Port-wine stain (capillary malformation) on the cheek of a newborn.

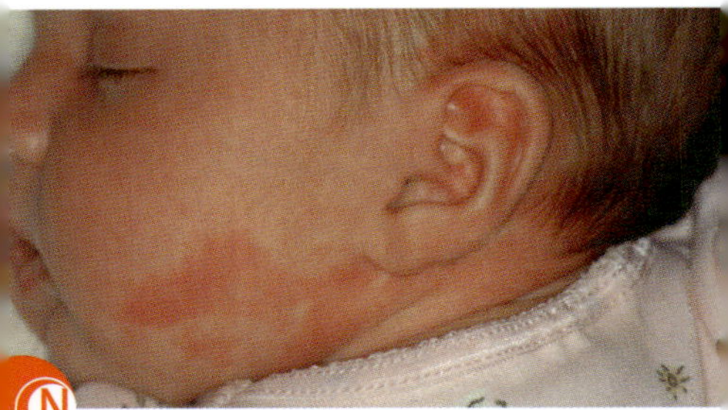

Port-wine stain (capillary malformation) over the mandibular skin and ear in a newborn.

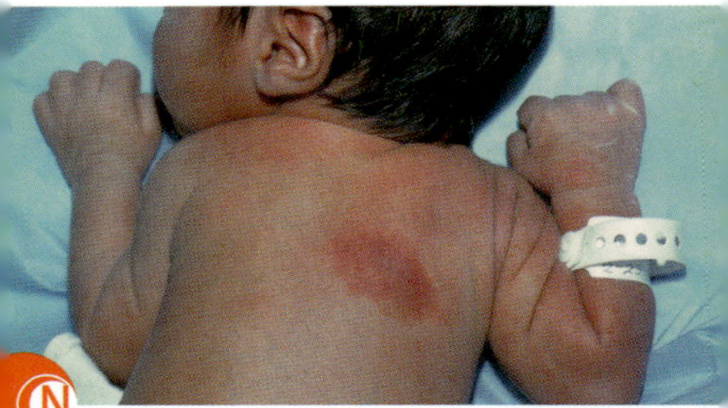

Port-wine stain (capillary malformation) over the back of a newborn.

CLINICAL FEATURES

Capillary malformations are the most common type of vascular malformation. Eyelid, central forehead, occipital, nuchal, and lower back lesions are common in light-skinned newborns. They differ from true port-wine stains and have been called 'nevus simplex'.

Newborns that have lesions in all or most of these areas are said to have the nevus simplex complex. The eyelid and small central forehead lesions will fade during the first year of life, but lesions in the other areas will remain. The nevus simplex type of vascular malformation is not associated with any other syndromes or abnormalities.

Excluding nevus simplex, port-wine stains occur in 3–5/1000 births. The name port-wine stain derives from the dark red color that is common in mature capillary malformations. However, most port-wine stains present at birth as light pink macules. The dark red color (port wine) slowly develops as the child ages. Along with the darkening in color, maturing port-wine stains develop progressive nodularity with blebbing and may lead to overgrowth of the underlying soft tissue and bone. The rate of progression of any individual port-wine stain cannot be predicted, but two thirds of patients with facial port-wine stains will develop these changes by the fifth decade. In patients with facial port-wine stains, **Sturge–Weber syndrome (SWS)** should be considered. SWS is the association of a facial port-wine stain with central nervous system (seizures, mental retardation, hemiplegia) and ophthalmologic (glaucoma) abnormalities. The overall risk of a facial port-wine stain having the associated abnormalities of the SWS is 8%, but the risk increases with increasing size of the facial port-wine stain. To be at risk for the SWS, the first branch of the trigeminal nerve must be involved, although there is debate about the exact distribution of this nerve. Patients with a port-wine stain, venous malformation, or mixed capillary venous malformation covering an extremity are at risk for the development of overgrowth of that extremity (**Klippel–Trenaunay syndrome, KT**). As the child gets older, he or she can develop cold intolerance, severe varicosities, venous stasis, ulceration, and recurrent infection leading to a state of chronic lymphedema. In any individual it is unknown how much of the extremity must be affected to lead to these changes or how rapidly they will occur. Occasionally, port-wine stains are extensive and cover large areas of the skin. Telangiectatic malformations are capillary malformations in which individual telangiectasia, rather than confluent vasculature are the presenting feature. They should be considered variants of port-wine stains. The risk of development of SWS or KT in association with a telangiectatic malformation is unknown, but unlikely.

TREATMENT

The vascular-specific pulsed dye laser (PDL) is the treatment of choice for port-wine stains. Treatment should be started as early in life as possible. It can be safely started as early as 2 weeks of life. The limitation of PDL therapy is the minimal depth of penetration of the laser light into the skin. The depth of the dermis doubles in the first year of life so it is best to perform as many treatments as possible during this time. PDL that emit two different wavelengths (585 nm and 595 nm) are available.

FLAT VASCULAR LESIONS, BLANCHING

Port-wine stains

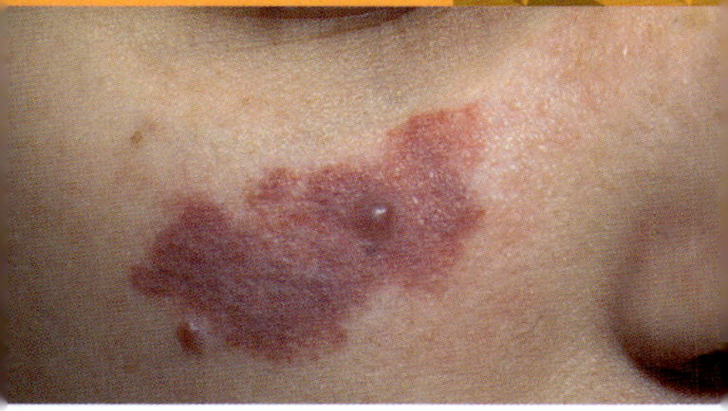

Dark red port-wine stain with central blebbing in a 14-year-old girl.

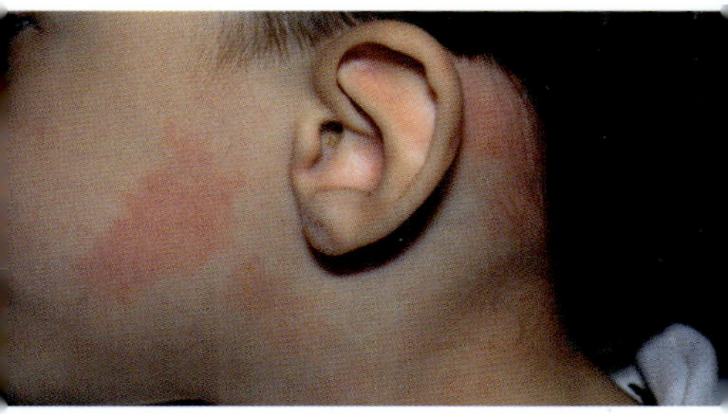

Typical light pink port-wine stain in a 3-year-old boy.

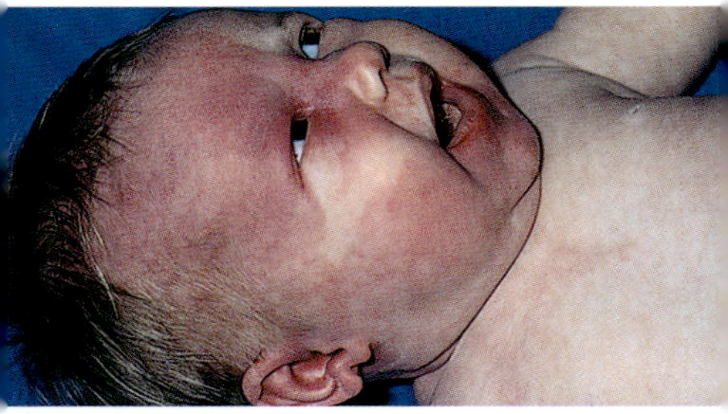

Port-wine stain on an infant with the Sturge–Weber syndrome.

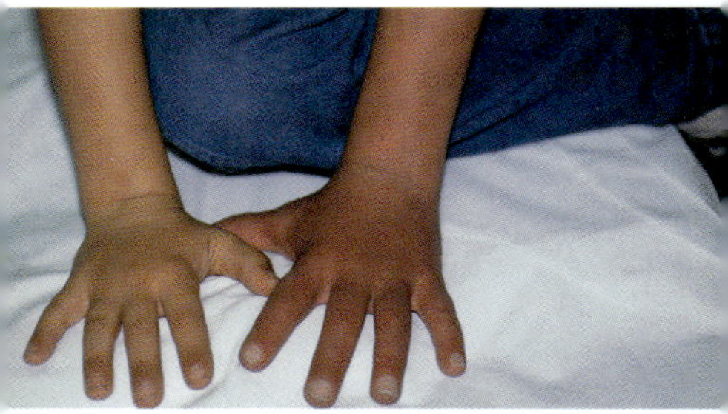

Hypertrophy of the left arm and hand in a 6-year-old boy with Klippel–Trenaunay syndrome.

Various pulse durations (0.5 msec, 1.5 msec, and longer) can also be used. Comparative studies of different wavelengths and pulse durations are few, in only a small number of patients. We recommend that the optimal settings are 585 nm wavelength with either a 0.5-msec or 1.5-msec pulse duration. **Response of port-wine stains** to laser treatment depends on the age of the patient being treated and the size and location of the lesion. The younger the child and the smaller the lesion, the more increased the likelihood of complete removal. Large lesions are improved by treatment and the risk of later blebbing and nodularity decrease, but total removal is unlikely. Response to treatment is slow and even small lesions in very young infants will frequently take 2–4 years for complete removal. PDL treatments are very safe and side-effects are minimal. Treatment has been greatly enhanced by the introduction of topical anesthetics and skin cooling during treatment, which significantly reduces the pain associated with the procedure. Study has begun on the use of anti-angiogenesis factors along with laser treatment to decrease rebound new vascular growth following laser treatment. At this time, this is not being used in general practice and the optimal agent and timing of delivery have yet to be elucidated. Unlike port-wine stains, **telangiectatic malformations** have a much smaller vessel load to destroy to return the skin to normal. Most telangiectatic lesions will be completely removed in three to six treatments.

All children with a port-wine stain in the distribution of the first branch of the trigeminal nerve and those with a port-wine stain in the distribution of the second branch of the trigeminal nerve with lower eyelid involvement should be referred for ophthalmologic evaluation for **glaucoma**. Glaucoma may be congenital or develop at any time in life. There is debate about the need for referral to a neurologist in the normally developing child.

Treatment of KT is difficult. Compression therapy is the mainstay of treatment. Referral to a multidisciplinary vascular malformation clinic is optimal.

Neonatal lupus erythematosus

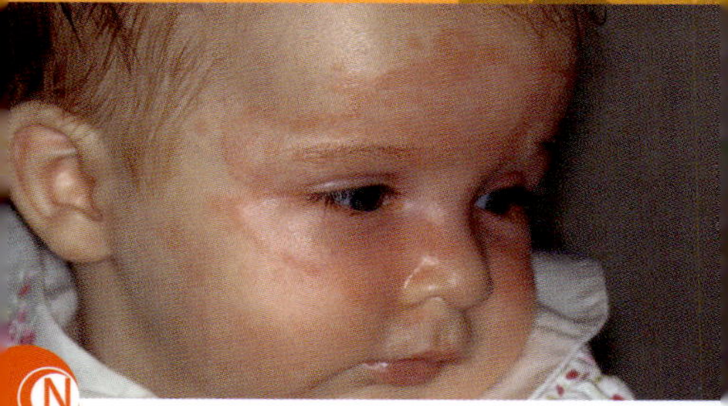

N 'Owl-eye' pattern of redness in neonatal lupus.

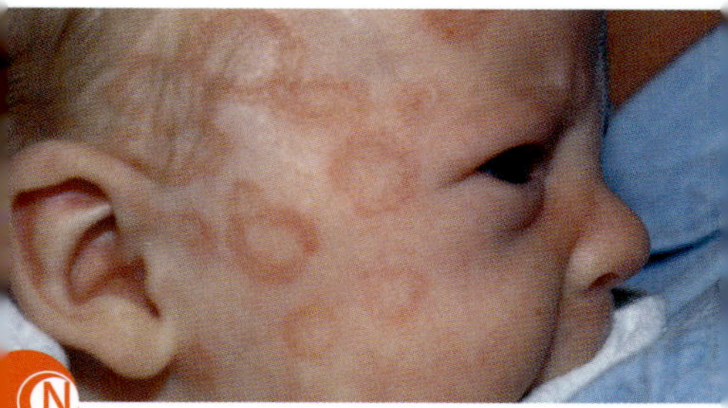

N Multiple annular red macules with clear centers in a baby with neonatal lupus.

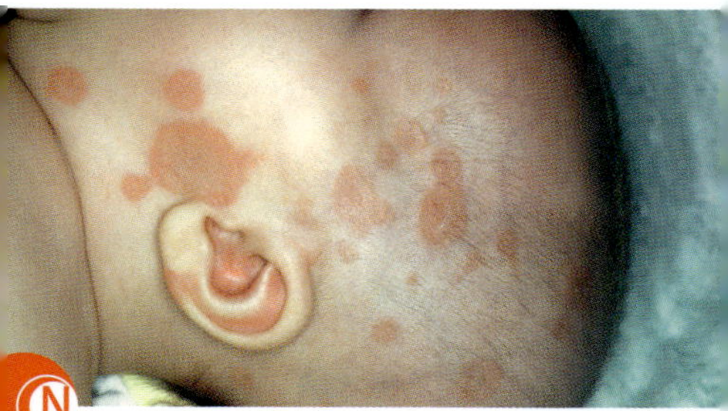

N Multiple red macules on the face of a baby with neonatal lupus.

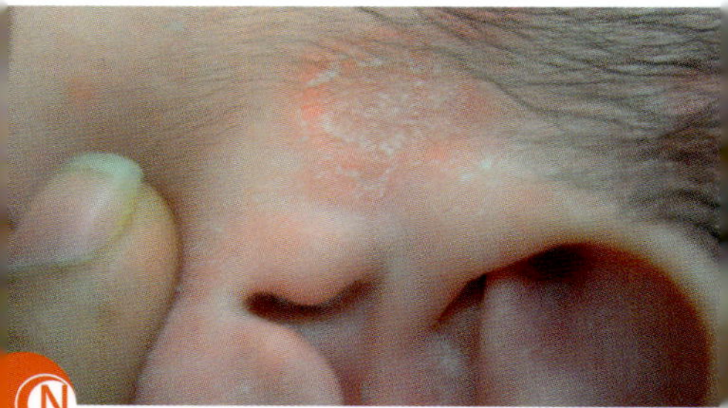

N Preauricular round red patch with fine white scale in a baby with neonatal lupus.

CLINICAL FEATURES

Round red macules or congenital heart block or both characterize neonatal lupus. Periorbital redness giving an 'owl-eye' pattern is a particularly characteristic skin finding and lesions on the head, upper trunk, and arms are most frequent. Round lesions may or may not clear in the center and may mimic ringworm. Some skin lesions will have fine white scale. Rarely, crusted lesions are seen. Mothers delivering an affected baby will often be asymptomatic or will have mild and easily overlooked symptoms of Sjögren's sicca syndrome. In babies with skin lesions, transient thrombocytopenia and abnormal liver studies are more common than heart block. An ANA may be negative and diagnosis is best made by analysis of mother's sera for anti-Ro and anti-La autoantibodies. Congenital heart block may be diagnosed by ultrasound as early as 18 weeks. Skin lesions will fade by 7 months of age, but congenital heart block will persist.

TREATMENT

Skin lesions will resolve spontaneously, but treatment with low potency topical steroids will rapidly hasten resolution. Residual telangiectasia at involved skin sites has been reported. A mother with a previous child with congenital heart block who is considering another pregnancy should be referred to a maternal/neonatal health program.

Kawasaki disease

DDx ref 31 • 54 • 48

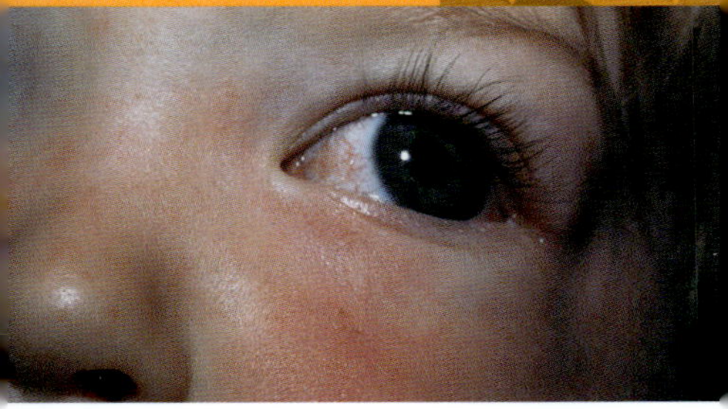

Conjunctival injection in early Kawasaki disease.

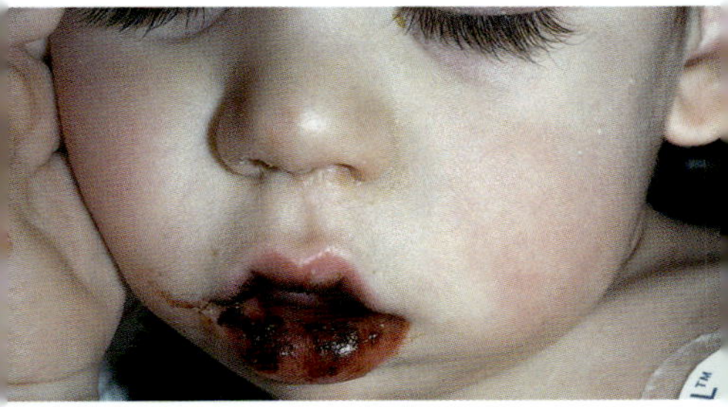

Red, swollen, dry crusted lips in a child with Kawasaki disease.

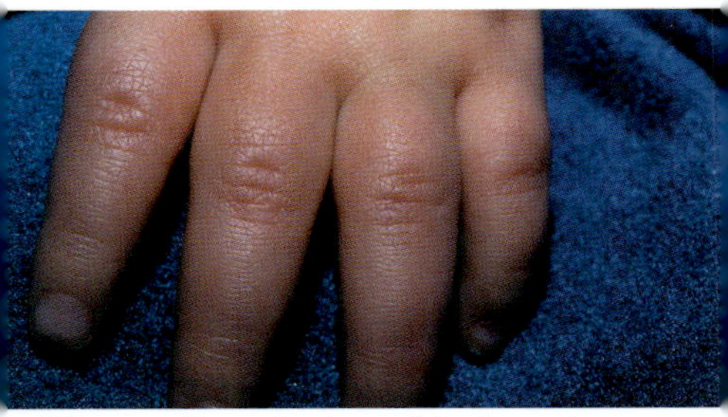

Diffuse swelling and redness of the fingers in Kawasaki disease.

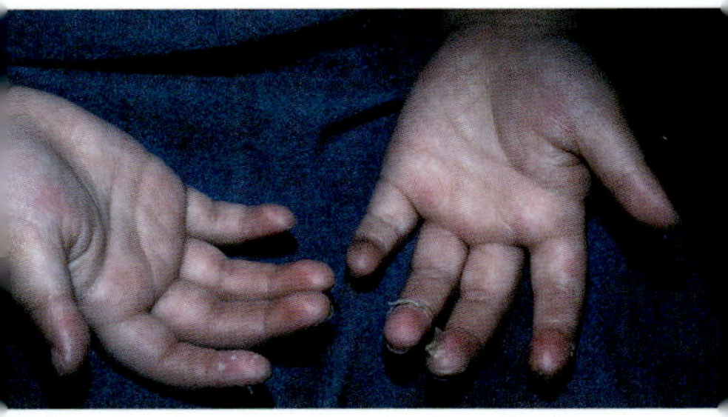

Typical peeling of the fingertips from distal to proximal in a toddler with Kawasaki disease.

Kawasaki disease

DDx ref 31 • 54 • 48

CLINICAL FEATURES

An abrupt onset of high fever with conjunctival redness is seen in Kawasaki disease. The fever persists for at least 5 days.

One of three oral changes can occur (1) dry, red, swollen, and fissured lips; (2) redness of the entire oropharynx; or (3) strawberry tongue. Skin changes of the extremities include swelling of the hands and feet; red palms and soles; generalized red skin with some polymorphic lesions; peeling of the fingertips from distal to proximal; and erythema of the groin followed by peeling. The fingertip peeling can be recurrent after the febrile phase. Lymph node enlargement greater than 1.5 cm may be noted, especially in cervical lymph nodes. It is particularly seen in **toddlers and young children** and may cluster in winter and spring outbreaks.

The serious complication of Kawasaki disease is the development of coronary artery aneurysms secondary to segmental vasculitis and are found in 25% of affected children. The mortality rate is 0.2%. Kawasaki disease is recurrent in less than 1% of children. Acute adenovirus infections, measles, leptospirosis, scarlet fever, drug eruptions, and toxic shock syndrome may mimic.

Laboratory changes are nonspecific with elevated sedimentation rate, C-reactive protein, lactic acid dehydrogenase, plus mild anemia and thrombocytosis can be seen.

TREATMENT

Intravenous immune globulin (IVIG) and low-dose aspirin if given within 10 days of onset of fever, reduce the incidence of coronary artery aneurysms to less than 5%. All children with presumed Kawasaki disease should be referred to a regional Pediatric center for IVIG therapy and pediatric cardiology evaluation.

52

FLAT VASCULAR LESIONS, BLANCHING

Scarlet fever

DDx ref 6 • 79 • 65

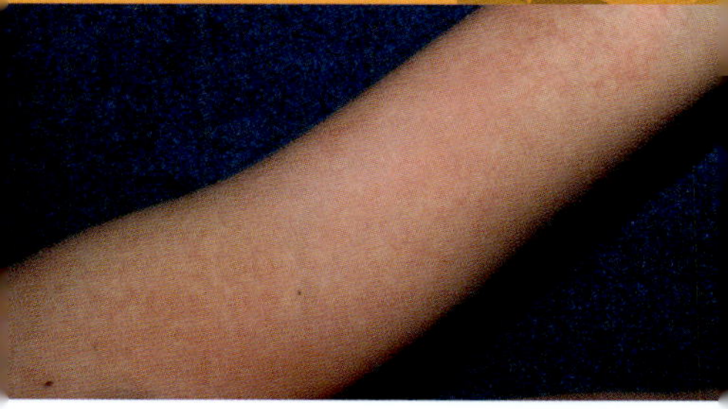

Red, rough maculopapular rash in a child with scarlet fever.

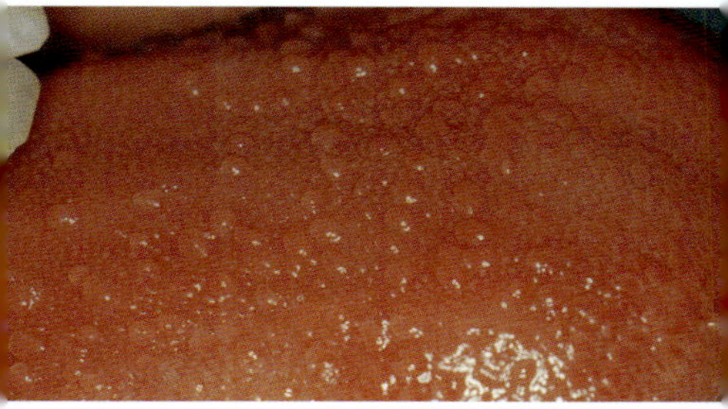

Bright red (strawberry) tongue with prominent papillae in streptococcal scarlet fever.

53

FLAT VASCULAR LESIONS, BLANCHING

Fixed drug eruptions

DDx ref 80 • 53 • 124

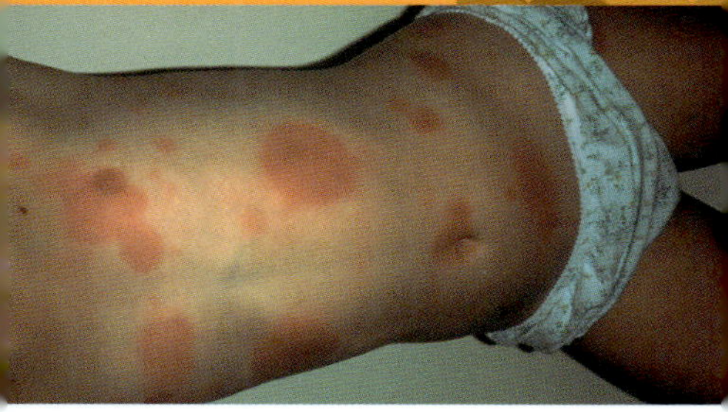

Fixed drug eruption to trimethoprim-sulfamethoxazole.

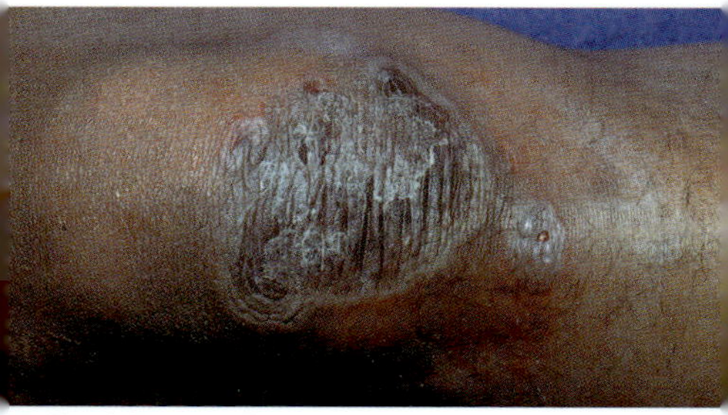

Fixed drug eruption to tetracycline. Hyperpigmentation developed as solitary lesion evolved.

52 Scarlet fever

DDx ref 6 • 79 • 65

CLINICAL FEATURES

Scarlet fever occurs in children between 2 and 10 years of age. Streptococci bacteria from pharyngitis or a skin wound are responsible. At 24–48 hours after the onset of clinical infection, a generalized red skin change of macules, rough papules, and some petechiae appears. **Linear petechiae** in the axillary and antecubital skin folds are seen as Pastia's sign. The rough feel to the red skin is the result of goose bumps (arrector pili muscle contraction). Circumoral pallor is common. Palms and soles are uninvolved. **A dry, red tongue** with prominent papillae comprises a 'strawberry tongue'. Generalized lymphadenopathy may be observed. As the eruption fades, fine desquamation appears. A severe septicemic form with hypotension is rarely seen. Scarlet fever is caused by various streptococcal exotoxins.

TREATMENT

Penicillin V 125–250 mg twice daily for 10 days is recommended. If staphylococci are suspected, then dicloxacillin 15–50 mg/kg per day for 10 days may be used. The association of scarlet fever with rheumatic fever can be prevented by prompt antibiotic administration. Fever control is essential and, for the desquamative stage, bland ointments applied to the skin will relieve pain and restore skin surface integrity. Tonsillectomy may be considered in the rare patient whose symptomatic episodes do not diminish in frequency over time and for whom no alternative explanation for recurrent GAS pharyngitis is evident. However, tonsillectomy has been demonstrated to be beneficial only for a relatively small group of these patients, and any benefit can be expected to be relatively short-lived.

53 Fixed drug eruptions

DDx ref 80 • 53 • 124

CLINICAL FEATURES

Fixed drug eruptions may present as single or multiple red macules that evolve over a few days into hyperpigmented macules. Occasionally, lesions are edematous or, rarely, bullous in appearance. The hyperpigmented areas may persist for several months.

The most common drug causes are trimethoprim-sulfamethoxazole combinations, acetaminophen, barbiturates, and sulfonamides. Rechallenge with the offending drug results in lesions at the original skin site(s) and, occasionally, new areas of involvement as well.

TREATMENT

The usual first therapeutic step is avoidance of the suspected drug. Potent topical steroids applied twice daily help shorten the course of fixed drug eruptions.

54

Morbilliform and urticarial drug eruptions

DDx ref 31 • 48 • 66

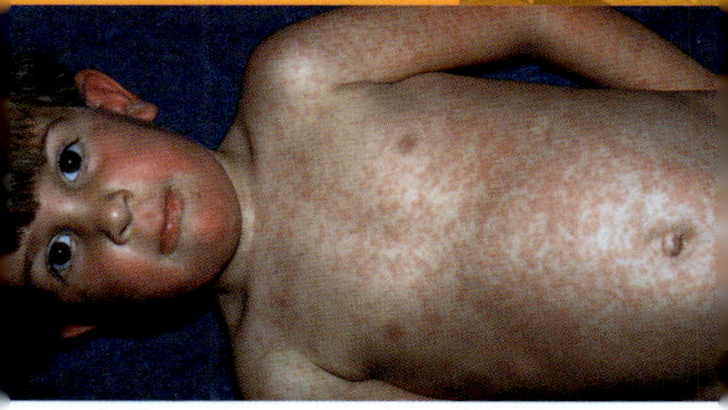

Morbilliform drug eruption due to trimethoprim-sulfamethoxazole (front view).

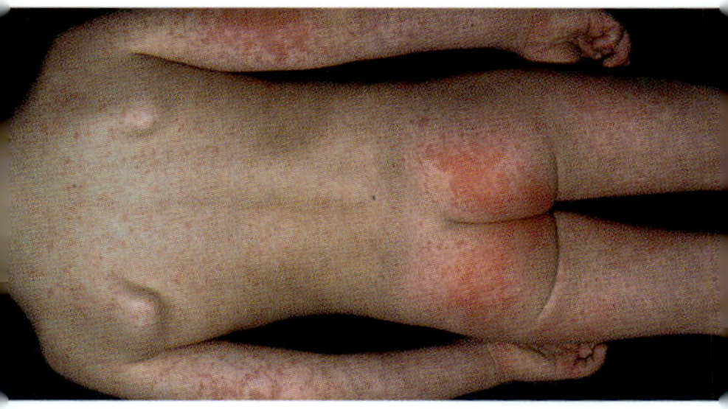

Morbilliform drug eruption due to trimethoprim-sulfamethoxazole (back view).

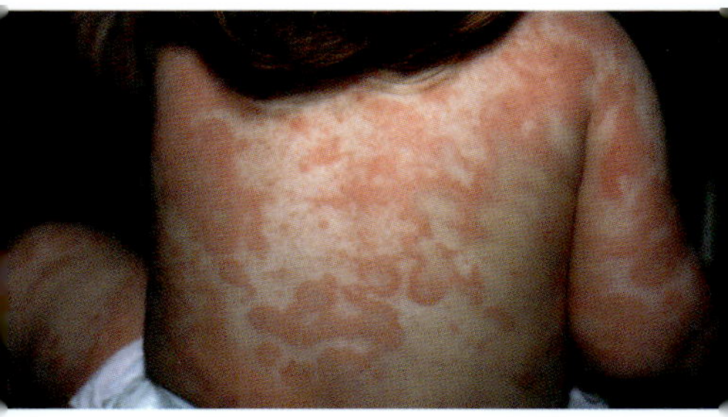

Urticarial drug eruption with partially clearing areas due to ceclor.

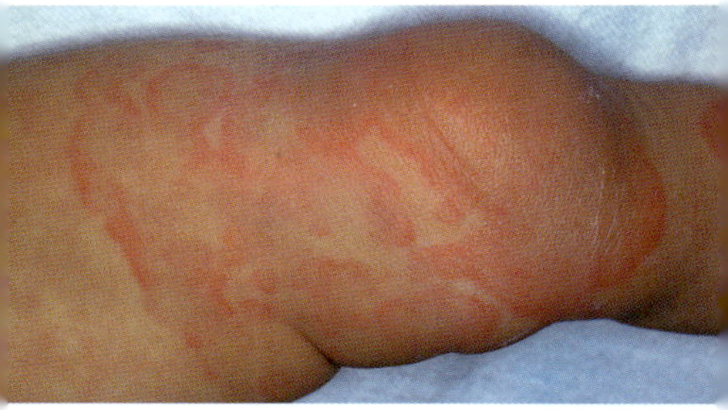

Urticarial drug eruption due to phenobarbital or trimethoprim.

54

Morbilliform and urticarial drug eruptions

DDx ref 31 • 48 • 66

CLINICAL FEATURES

Widespread itchy red macules following ingestion of a drug constitute a morbilliform drug reaction. The rash becomes confluent in areas with clearing of adjacent areas of skin. The eruption lasts 7–14 days and may be associated with malaise and arthralgias. The most likely responsible drugs are **non-steroidal anti-inflammatory drugs**, penicillins, cephalosporins, and sulfonamide antibiotics (including trimethoprim-sulfamethoxazole combinations), anticonvulsants and oral fluconazole, or ketoconazole antifungal drugs. Morbilliform drug eruptions often mimic viral exanthems.

Urticarial drug eruptions are characterized by hives that move from skin site to skin site within hours, with new areas of involvement appearing almost continuously. Giant hives with clear centers may be seen.

Angioedema is rarely seen but can be accompanied by fever and arthralgias. Cephalosporins are most responsible for the angioedema-type reaction. The same drugs responsible for morbilliform reactions also are implicated in urticarial drug reactions, with ibuprofen and ceclor the most common. The urticarial response usually lasts 7–14 days but occasionally lasts 4–6 weeks.

TREATMENT

Removal of the suspected offending drug is necessary.

In a child on multiple medications eliminating the most often associated may result in stopping more than one medication, and sorting out the responsible medication can be difficult. Oral antihistamines may help suppress the urticarial eruptions and those with angioedema may require 1 : 1000 aqueous epinephrine administered subcutaneously 0.2–0.5 mL, followed by oral antihistamines, and, if severe, the addition of oral steroids until the edema subsides.

55 DDx ref

RAISED BLANCHING VASCULAR LESIONS

Hemangiomas

41 • 42 • 60

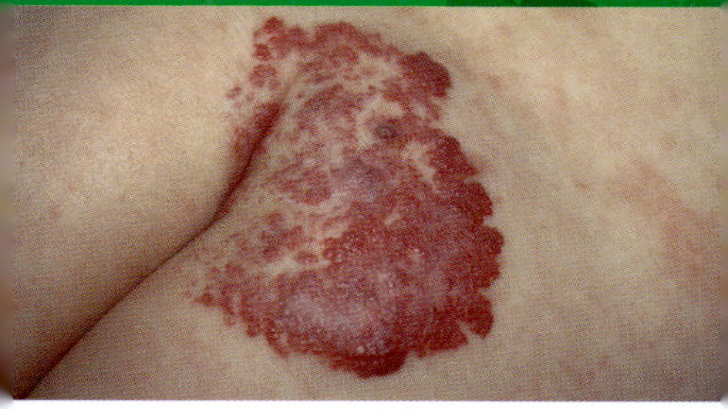

Mixed superficial and deep HOI.

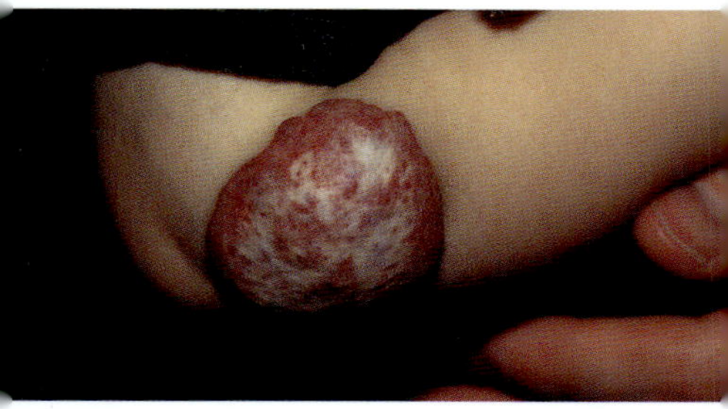

Paling as the initial sign of regression in a mixed superficial and deep HOI.

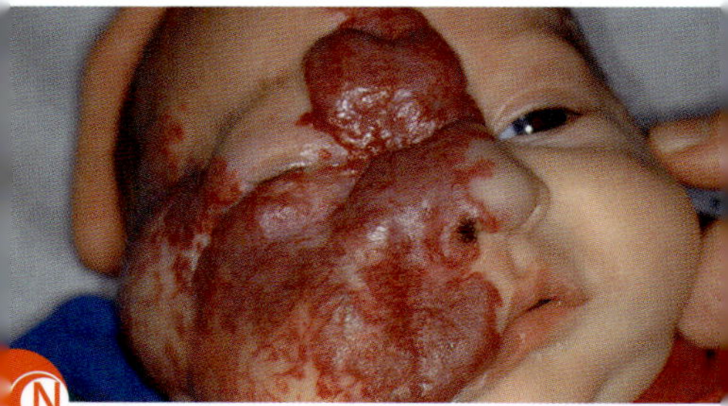

Widespread (segmental) facial HOI in the PHACE syndrome.

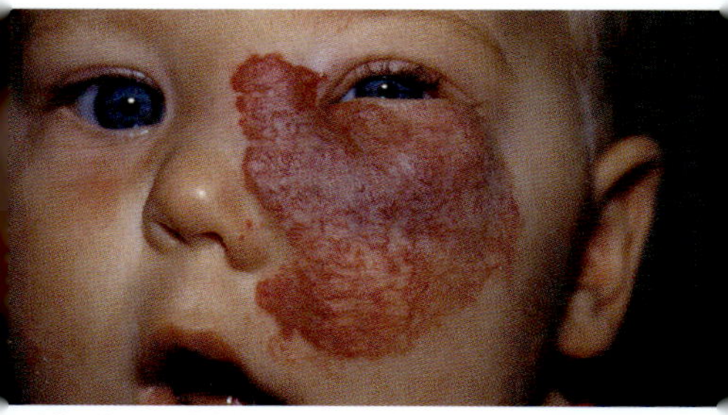

Mixed superficial and deep HOI in a 4-month-old infant leading to partial visual obstruction.

CLINICAL FEATURES

Hemangiomas of infancy (HOI) are proliferative hamartomas of vascular endothelium that may be present at birth (20%), or more commonly, become apparent in the first 2 months of life. HOI are common with estimates of up to 10% of term infants eventually being affected. They are more common in females and in preterm infants.

There are three major types of HOI presentation. The most common is a pale white to gray-blue macule. The other types are the telangiectatic and the papular. Rarely, HOI present as areas of ulceration surrounded by a thin red vascular rim. At presentation, it is impossible to predict what form the HOI will eventually take or its final size. HOI should be classified as superficial, deep, or mixed. The terms 'strawberry' and 'cavernous' should not be used to describe HOI. **Superficial HOI** are bright red, papular, and sharply demarcated from normal skin.

Deep HOI are compressible and the overlying skin may appear normal in color or may have a bluish hue. Deep HOI are more diffuse and less well-defined than superficial HOI. Most HOI are mixed, having both superficial and deep components. HOI undergo a phase of rapid expansion, followed by a stationary phase and then finally by spontaneous involution. The rapid growth phase lasts for 2–4 months.

The stationary growth phase usually lasts until about 1 year of age and is heralded by a change of the superficial component from red to maroon. The involution or regressive phase begins during the second year of life.

The regressive phase begins with paling of the HOI, followed by flattening. This phase slowly continues and by 5 years of age, 50% of HOI will have reached maximal regression. By 9 years of age, 90% of HOI will have reached maximal regression. Overall, the amount of regression of an HOI is minimal after 5 years of age. Rate of regression of an individual HOI cannot be correlated with size or location, although lip lesions persist most often. Maximal regression of HOI does not define return of the skin to normal. Residual post-HOI regression includes hypopigmentation, telangiectasia, fibrofatty deposits, and scarring if the HOI has previously ulcerated.

Local complications of HOI include ulceration, secondary infection, and, rarely, hemorrhage. Ulcerations are most common in the diaper area, although they may occur in an HOI in any location, and usually occur in mixed superficial and deep HOI during the rapid growth phase.

RAISED BLANCHING VASCULAR LESIONS

Hemangiomas

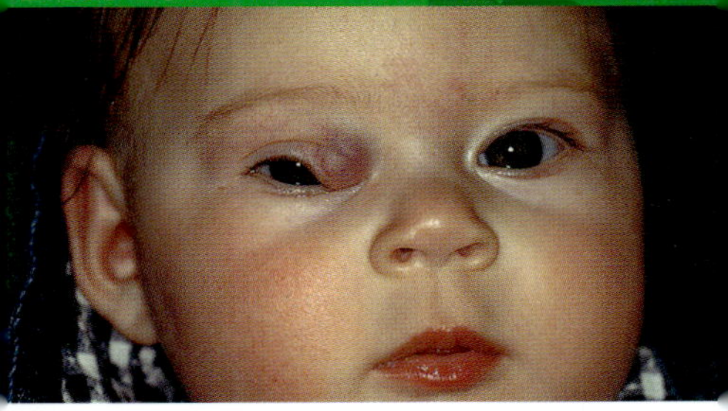

Deep HOI obstructing vision.

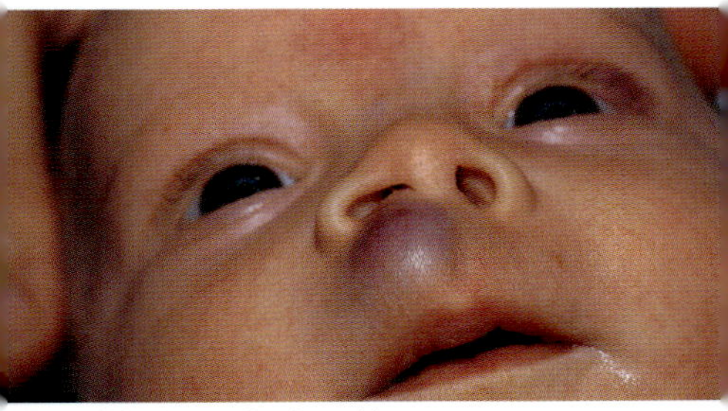

Deep HOI obstructing breathing.

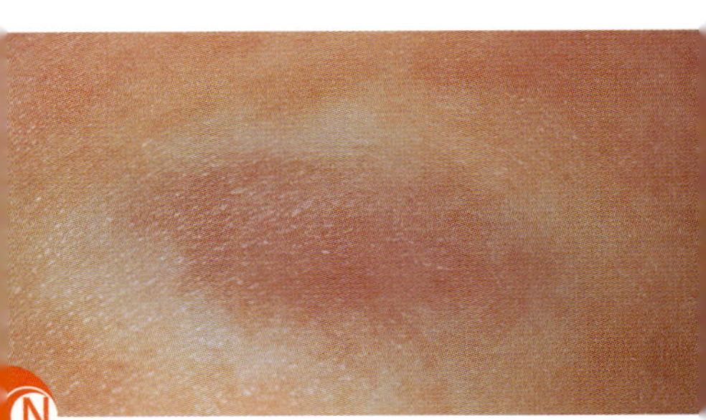

N Dull red plaque with surrounding halo in a non-involuting congenital hemangioma (NICH).

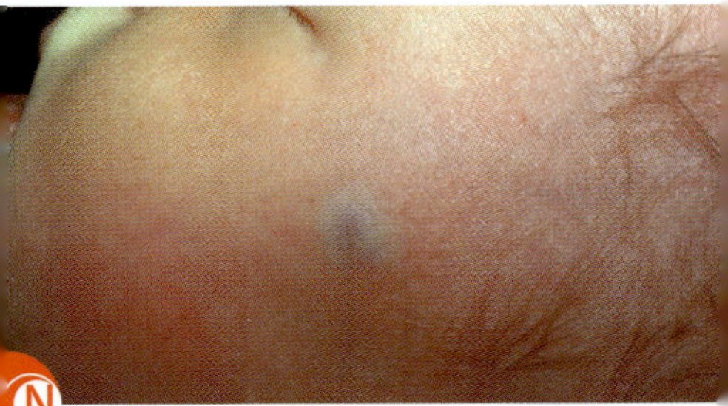

N Gray-blue precursor of an HOI. Later the lesion will become raised.

Infection is usually with *Staphylococcus aureus*, but *Pseudomonas aeruginosa* and *Klebsiella pneumoniae* may also be seen.

The location of an HOI may interfere with a vital function (vision, breathing, eating, urination, defecation). Infants with periorbital HOI should always be referred for ophthalmologic evaluation. HOI in a 'beard' distribution may be associated with upper airway or subglottic involvement. Large lumbosacral HOI spanning the midline may be associated with underlying anomalies of the spine and/or spinal cord. Large facial (segmental) HOI may be associated with central nervous system malformation (most commonly Dandy–Walker posterior fossa malformations and cerebellar hypoplasia), abnormal central nervous system arteries, cardiac and large vessel defects, and ophthalmologic abnormalities (PHACE syndrome (posterior fossa malformations, HOI, arterial anomalies, coarctation of the aorta and other cardiac defects, and eye abnormality)). Large perianal HOI can be associated with congenital anomalies, including anorectal, urinary tract, spine, and external genitalia malformations.

There are two other types of vascular lesions that are classified as hemangiomas. These are rapidly involuting congenital hemangioma (RICH) and non-involuting congenital hemangioma (NICH). Their clinical appearance and natural history are markedly different from an HOI.

RICH are present at birth and appear as violaceous nodules with ectatic veins, as a grayish nodule with overlying telangiectasias surrounded by a pale rim of vasoconstriction, or as flat violaceous infiltrative lesions. They do not undergo a rapid growth phase and involute rapidly with complete involution, usually by 1 year of age.

NICH are also present at birth and present as round plaques with central or peripheral pallor and overlying telangiectasias. They do not undergo a rapid growth phase, but they do not involute. They are better considered as vascular malformations.

TREATMENT

In the usual child with an HOI who has no serious complications, treatment consists of expectant observation. Therapy is rarely indicated and may cause further harm. Parents require repeated reassurance and support.

RAISED BLANCHING VASCULAR LESIONS

Hemangiomas

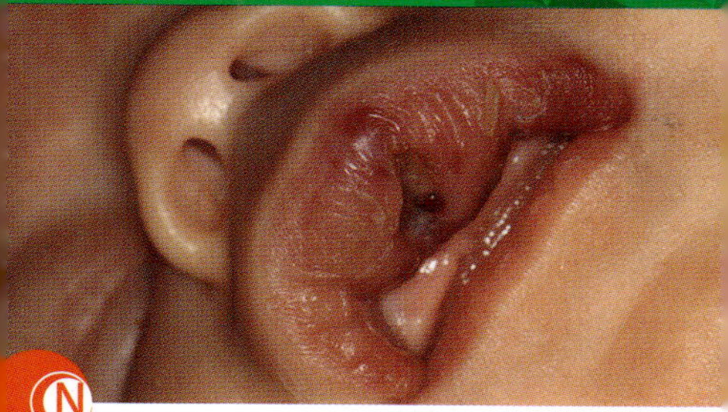

HOI of the upper lip with ulceration interfering with eating.

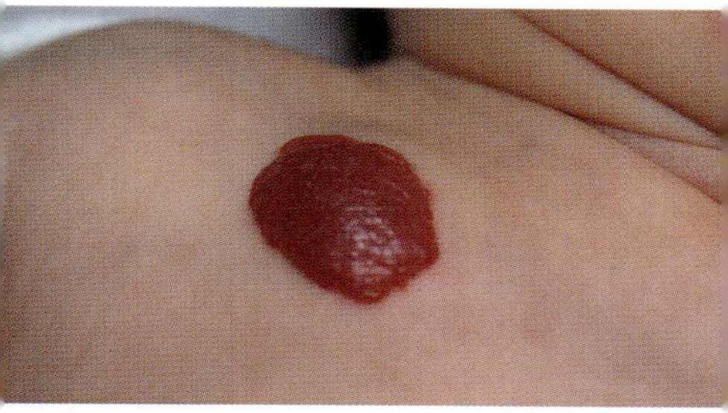

Superficial HOI.

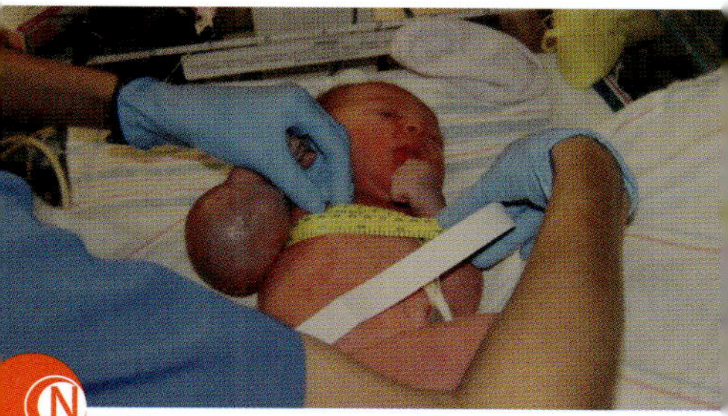

RICH presenting at birth.

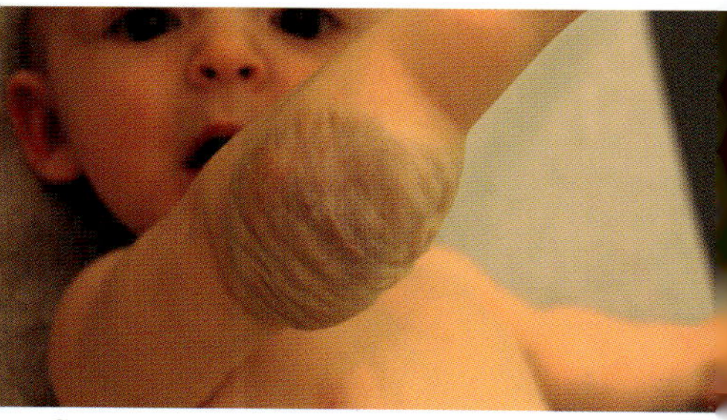

Same child at 6 months of age.

Small ulcerations (<5 cm) are often amenable to pulsed dye laser therapy (PDL). Secondary infection should be treated with the appropriate antibiotic.

For larger ulcerations frequent wound cleansing and dressing is necessary, although optimal methods remain unknown.

Superficial HOI in the early growth phase may also respond well to PDL, as will telangiectasias persisting post-regression. Small scars and areas of fibrofatty deposits can be treated or minimized by judicious surgical repair if desired.

Magnetic resonance imaging should be performed on large lumbosacral HOI and if any abnormalities are noted, the patient should be referred to neurosurgery.

Infants with PHACE syndrome or large perineal lesions should be referred to the appropriate specialist.

For other HOI which require treatment (usually periorbital HOI but any HOI interfering with a vital function) propranolol 2–3 mg/kg per day divided in two or three doses. Hypoglycemia and hypotension may complicate propranolol therapy. If no response to propanolol, second-line therapy with prednisolone 1–3 mg/kg per day has been effective and Vincristine has also been used.

RICH & NICH Although RICH involute rapidly, there is almost always residual skin and fibrofatty deposits remaining post-involution. These can be removed by surgical excision. The only option for treatment of NICH is surgical excision.

56
DDx ref

RAISED BLANCHING VASCULAR LESIONS

Diffuse neonatal hemangiomatosis

55 • 59 • 43

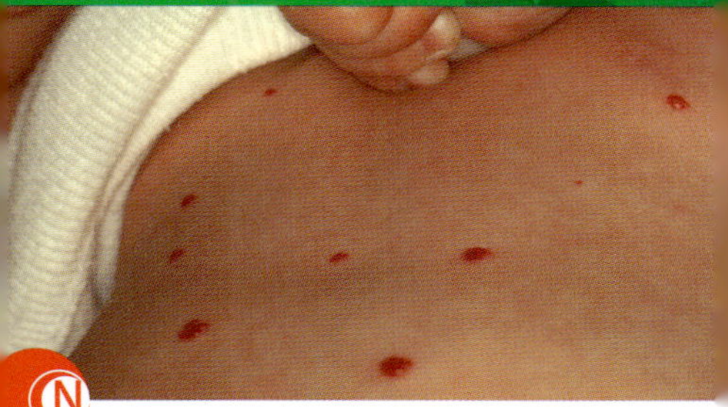

Benign neonatal hemangiomatosis. Multiple small red papules on the trunk of a neonate.

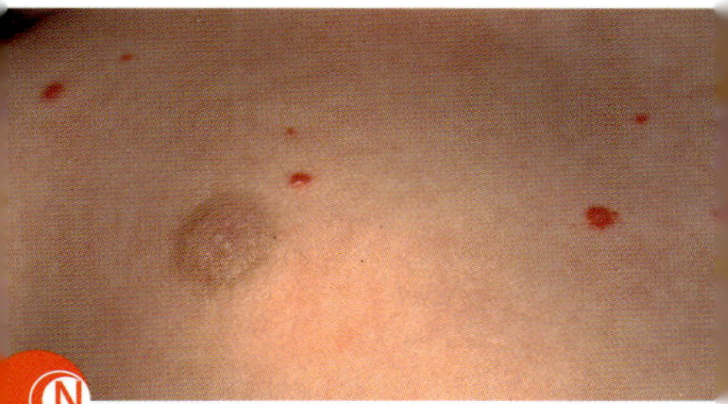

Blanching red papules of diffuse neonatal hemangiomatosis.

57
DDx ref

RAISED BLANCHING VASCULAR LESIONS

Pyogenic granuloma

55 • 59 • 129

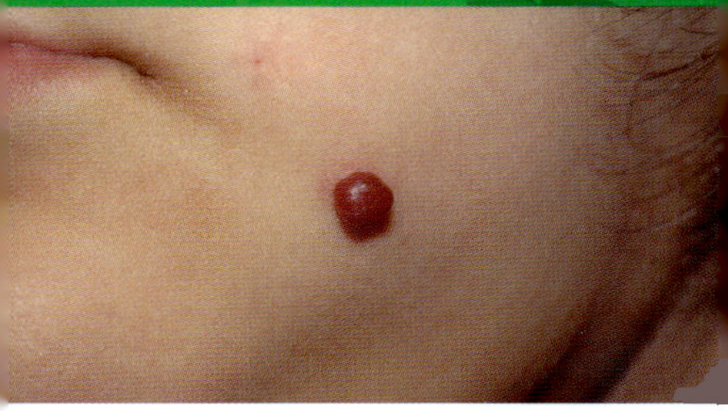

Pyogenic granuloma. Smooth, glistening, red papule on the face.

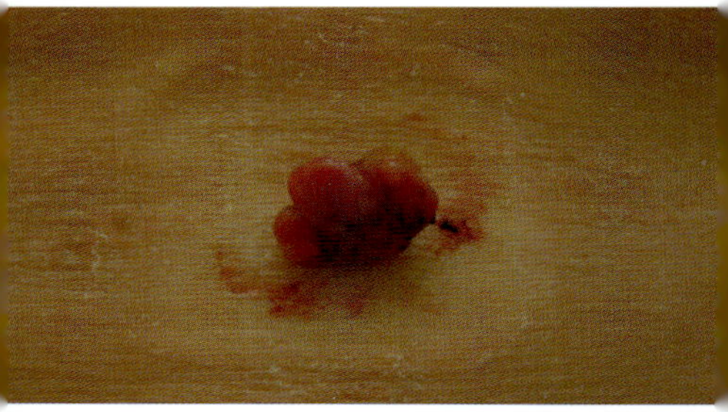

Multilobular red papule of pyogenic granuloma.

56

RAISED BLANCHING VASCULAR LESIONS

Diffuse neonatal hemangiomatosis

DDx ref 55 • 59 • 43

CLINICAL FEATURES

Diffuse neonatal hemangiomatosis is the association of multiple cutaneous hemangiomas of the skin with similar lesions in internal organs. The skin usually has many small red superficial hemangiomas. The internal hemangiomas may involve any of the viscera: the liver, gastrointestinal tract, central nervous system, and lungs are the most common sites involved. Infants with diffuse neonatal hemangiomatosis are usually ill at birth. The disorder is often fatal secondary to high-output cardiac failure, visceral hemorrhage, obstruction of the respiratory tract, or compression of the central nervous system. Most infants with multiple hemangiomas have benign neonatal hemangiomatosis with widespread cutaneous hemangioma without internal organ involvement. In our experience, any asymptomatic infant over 2 months old brought to the dermatology clinic with multiple hemangiomas will not develop systemic disease that requires treatment.

Treatment Most infants have benign neonatal hemangiomatosis, and the hemangiomas will regress as any other hemangioma of infancy and do not require therapy. Prednisolone has been the initial treatment of choice for symptomatic diffuse cutaneous hemangiomatosis, but we believe that propranolol 2–3 mg/kg per day divided in two or three doses will now be used as the primary therapy (see topic 55).

57

RAISED BLANCHING VASCULAR LESIONS

Pyogenic granuloma

DDx ref 55 • 59 • 129

CLINICAL FEATURES

Pyogenic granuloma is misnamed, given that the lesions are neither pyogenic nor granulomatous. Microscopically, they resemble a capillary hemangioma and should best be called 'acquired lobular capillary hemangiomas' to differentiate from a hemangioma of infancy. They are common in children and appear as 3–10-mm solitary, dull red firm papules predominantly on the face, arms, and hands. The surface may be smooth or glistening, but is often ulcerated and crusted. The lesions bleed easily when traumatized. Daily bleeding from even small lesions can result in anemia. They may arise at sites of injury, but a history of trauma is usually not elicited.

TREATMENT

Removal with an open curette followed by cauterization of the base is the most successful therapy. Facial lesions less than 5 mm in size in young children may be treated with PDL (pulsed dye laser), but multiple treatments are often necessary and the treatment is not always successful. When PDL therapy is successful scarring is often prevented. Pyogenic granulomas should not be surgically excised and sutured, because this frequently leads to the formation of multiple lesions on and around the surgical scar.

RAISED BLANCHING VASCULAR LESIONS

Lymphatic malformations

41 • 55 • 100

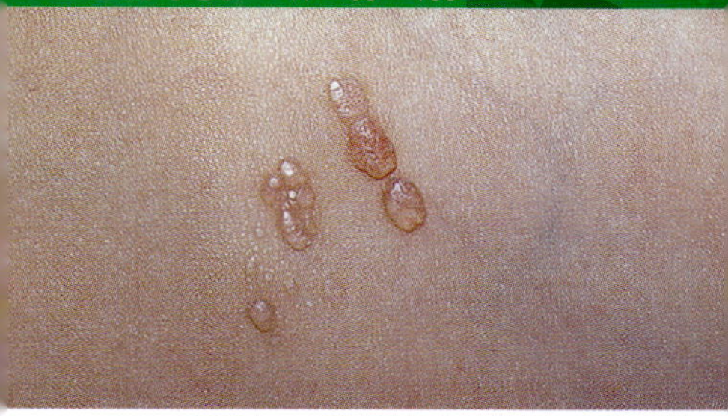

Superficial lymphatic malformation. Grouping of gelatinous flesh-colored papules on the abdomen.

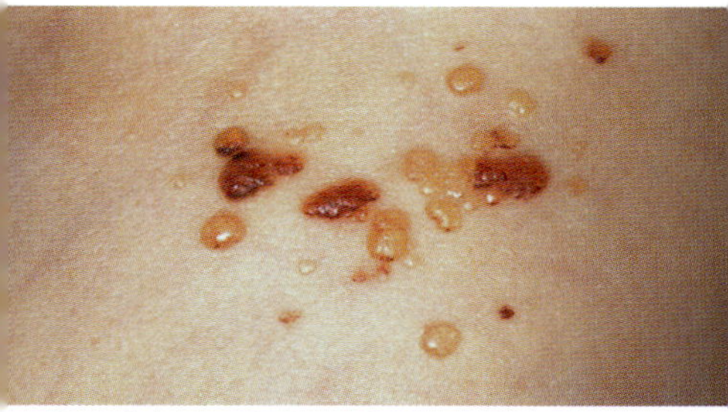

Superficial lymphatic malformation. Darkening from bleeding into the lesions.

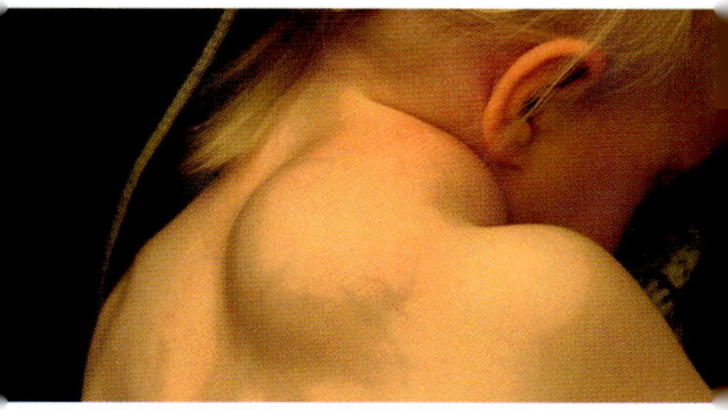

Deep macrocystic lymphatic malformation seen as a compressible nodule on a girl's shoulder.

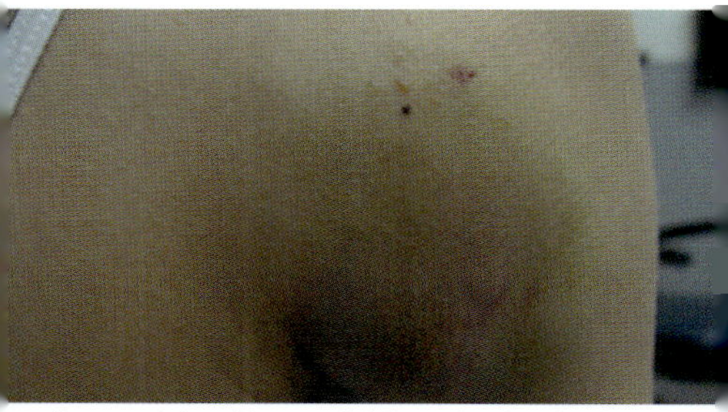

Deep nodule with superficial venules in mixed lymphatic malformation.

Lymphatic malformations

DDx ref 41 • 55 • 100

CLINICAL FEATURES

Lymphatic malformations are developmental errors in lymphatic vessel development. They should not be referred to as lymphangiomas because they are not tumors. There are two clinical types of lymphatic malformations: superficial and deep.

Superficial lymphatic malformations consist of multiple clusters of small vesicles covering limited areas of skin.

Deep lymphatic malformations present as flesh colored dermal or subcutaneous, squishy nodules. They vary in size from a few centimeters to large ill-defined grotesque rubbery flesh-colored subcutaneous nodules that may underlie more superficial lymphatic malformations. They are usually solitary and involve the face, trunk, and upper extremities. They may either consist of one or a few large cysts (macrocystic–cystic hygroma) or many small cysts (microcystic).

TREATMENT

Referral to a vascular malformations center may be beneficial.

Superficial lymphatic malformations should not be treated because following surgical excision they always recur along the scar and the end result is worse than the initial lesion.

Microcystic deep lymphatic malformations may be surgically excised if they are affecting vital structures. They otherwise should be left untreated due to recurrence deep and along the scar line as with superficial lesions.

Macrocystic deep lymphatic malformations are best treated by sclerotherapy with doxycycline or some other irritating agent.

Vascular spiders

DDx ref 40 • 57 • 55

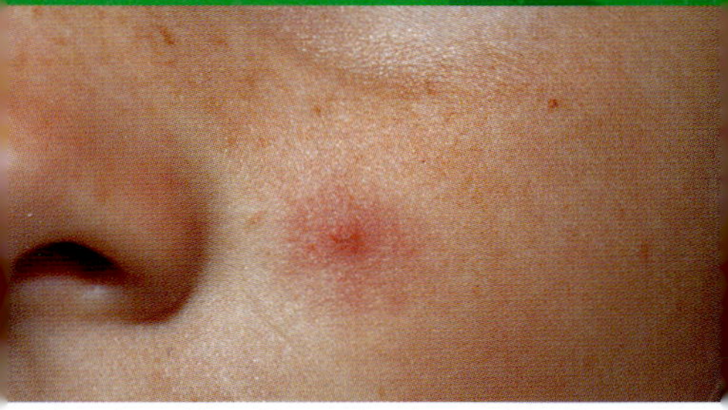

Vascular spider with prominent central feeding vessel on the cheek.

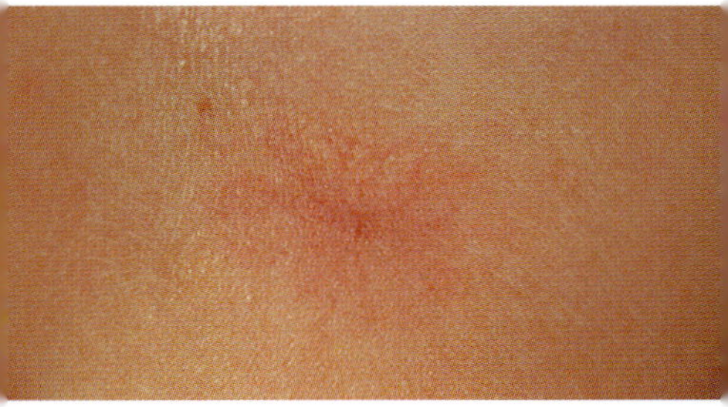

Large vascular spider.

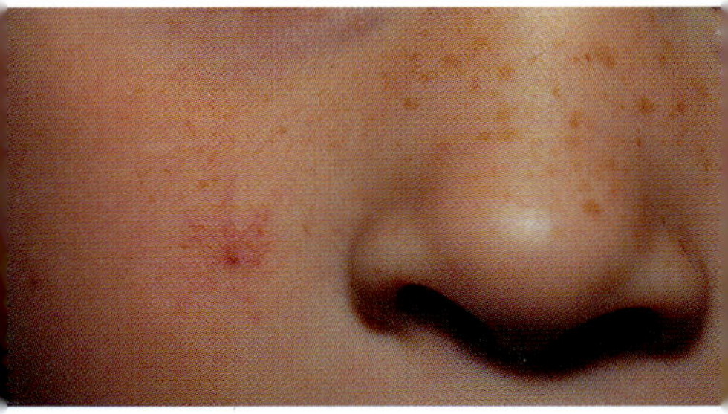

Vascular spider on the face of a child.

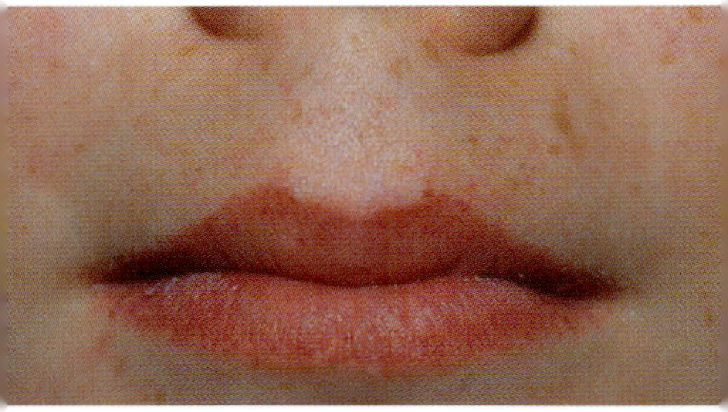

Vascular telangiectasias on the lips of a child with HHT (Osler–Weber–Rendu).

Vascular spiders

DDx ref 40 • 57 • 55

CLINICAL FEATURES

Vascular spiders (spider angioma – spider telangiectasia – nevus araneus) consist of a central arteriole with many dilated radiating telangiectasias and a surrounding flush area, varying from a few millimeters to several centimeters in diameter. Sometimes the central arteriole may be raised and prominent and may be pulsatile on diascopy. Pressure on the central vessel causes blanching. Vascular spiders occur in up to 45% of light-skinned children. They are seen most commonly on sun-exposed areas, usually the cheeks, nose, dorsa of the forearms, and hands. Lesions resolve spontaneously at puberty. Children with hereditary hemorrhagic telangiectasias have multiple lesions of the skin and mucosa. A history of severe epistaxis and gastrointestinal bleeding may be obtained. Telangiectasias in connective tissue disorders are also seen on the face and arms, but are more numerous and mat-like.

TREATMENT

Treatment is not necessary. If treatment is desired for cosmetic purposes, a single treatment with the PDL is 70–80% effective.

60 DDx ref

RAISED BLANCHING VASCULAR LESIONS

Venous malformations

41 • 46 • 55

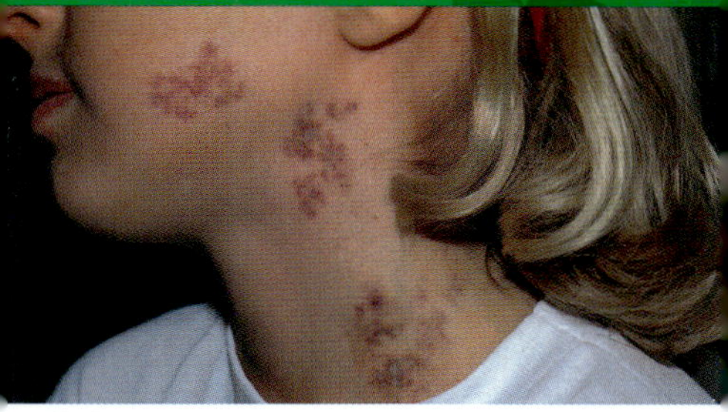

Distinct blue venous pattern of a venous malformation in an 11-year-old girl.

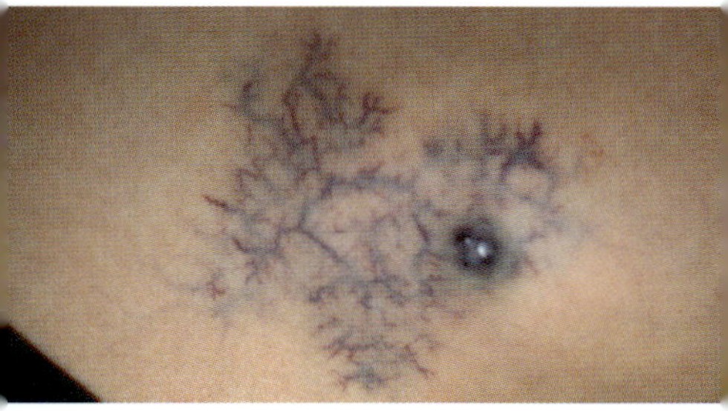

Venous malformation with a large nodule in a 9-year-old boy.

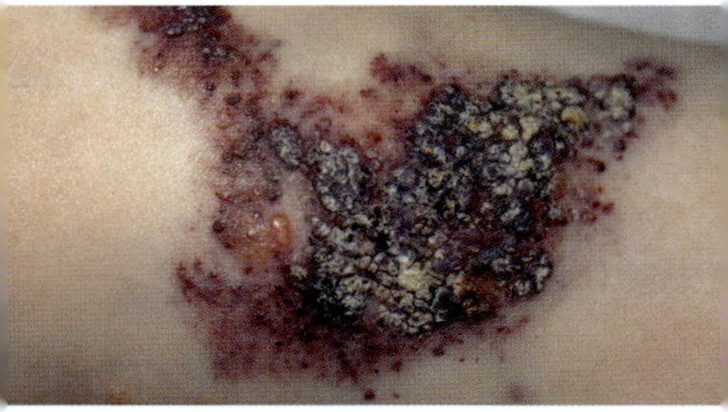

Venous–lymphatic malformation with superficial angiokeratomas.

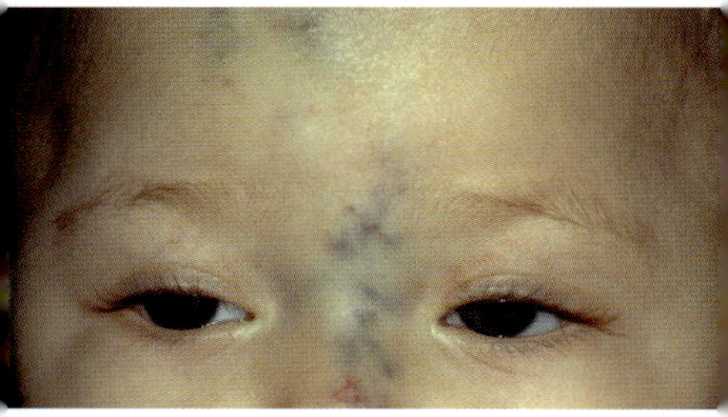

Prominent dilated veins in a child with venous malformation.

Venous malformations

DDx ref 41 • 46 • 55

CLINICAL FEATURES

Venous malformations are developmental errors in vein formation. Venus malformations vary from discrete nodules containing a mass of venules to diffuse large vein abnormalities resembling varicose veins. The distinct venous pattern in larger vessel lesions is obvious. Lesional pain is common. Nodular venous malformations are frequently confused with hemangiomas. Rapidly involuting congenital hemangiomas (RICH) and non-involuting congenital hemangiomas (NICH) may both be confused. Nodular venous malformations may be differentiated from hemangiomas by their presence at birth, lack of a rapid growth phase, and no tendency toward regression. They are differentiated from NICH histologically, and RICH by the rapid involution of the latter.

TREATMENT

Superficial nodular venule malformations may be surgically excised. The treatment of larger venous malformations is at best difficult and often impossible. Sclerotherapy with ethanol, ethylcellulose-ethanol, or polidocanol may be of use for symptomatic lesions or prior to surgery. Sclerotherapy is associated with numerous side-effects and should be used judiciously.

61

Vasculitis (Henoch–Schönlein purpura)

DDx ref 31 • 72 • 54

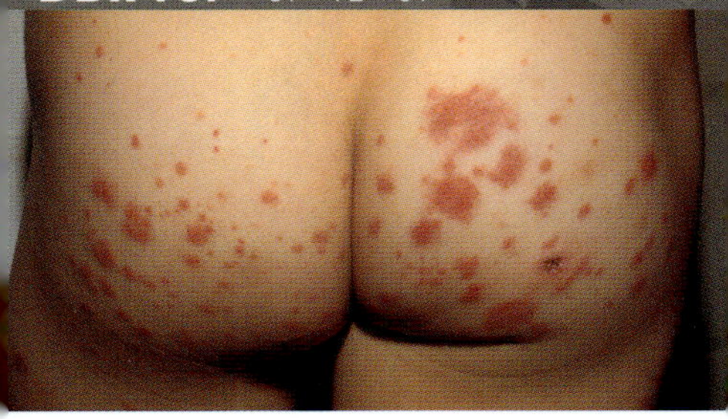

Purpuric macules and papules on buttocks of a child with necrotizing venulitis.

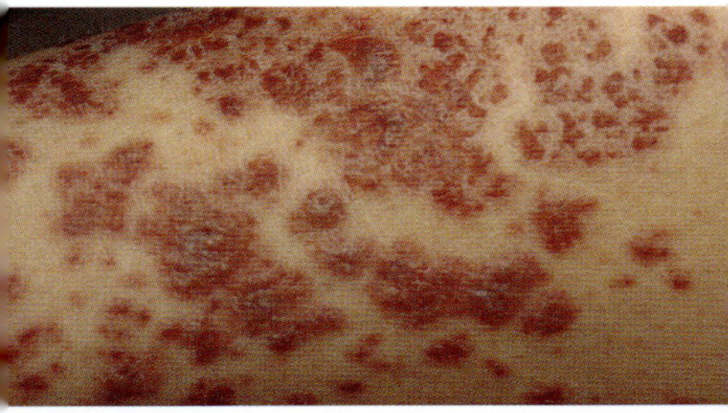

Multiple purpuric papules on the leg of a child with necrotizing venulitis.

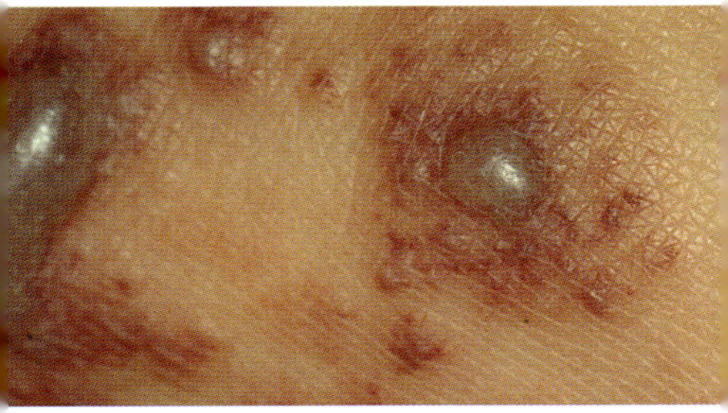

Severe necrotizing venulitis with purpuric papules and bullae on a child's leg.

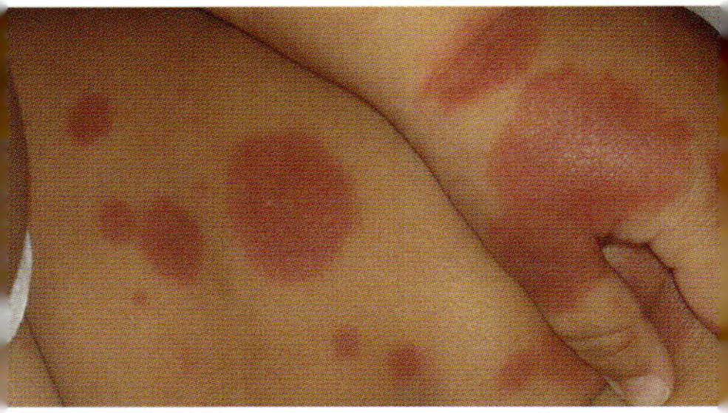

Large purpuric plaques on an infant's hand and leg in acute hemorrhagic edema of infancy.

CLINICAL FEATURES

The presence of dozens of symmetric non-blanching purpuric papules characterizes the most common form of childhood vasculitis, necrotizing venulitis (Henoch–Schönlein purpura, IgA vasculitis). Following a prodrome of upper respiratory symptoms, early lesions appear that resemble urticarial wheals, then red papules with a petechial center develop. Skin lesions evolve within 24–48 hours to completely purpuric papules. **Lesions** are seen mostly on the lower legs or buttocks. Severe involvement results in cutaneous infarcts, seen as purpuric bullae and gangrene. The severe lesions heal with scarring. Although the predominant signs are cutaneous, necrotizing venulitis should be considered a systemic vasculitis as renal, gastrointestinal, joint, and cerebral venules can be involved. Joint pains and abdominal pains often accompany the skin lesions.

Arthralgias or overt arthritis of knees and ankles is seen in 60–80% of children. **Cramping abdominal pain**, vomiting, hematemesis, and melena signify gastrointestinal involvement.

The kidney is involved in up to 50% of children as asymptomatic microscopic hematuria. Of children with renal involvement, 10% may progress to renal failure over the next 3–6 months, including those whose initial urine tests were normal, and 5% will develop chronic renal disease.

Seizures, paresis, coma are rarely found and signify cerebral vessel involvement.

A skin biopsy will reveal fibrinoid necrosis of venule walls with intact and fragmented neutrophils present. With immunofluorescence staining, IgA deposits are seen surrounding superficial skin blood vessels.

A variant in infancy presents with ≥10 cm purpuric plaques with prominent edema mostly on the genitalia and buttocks (acute hemorrhagic edema of infancy), with some involvement of the extremities. Despite the different clinical appearance of acute hemorrhagic edema of infancy, skin biopsy results are the same as the classic form of necrotizing venulitis. A variety of precipitating factors have been associated, including strep throat, parvovirus B19, hepatitis B and C, and immunization to pneumococci, hepatitis B, measles, and influenza.

Other uncommon conditions that may have papular purpura include chronic meningococcemia, gonococcemia, Gram-negative bacterial septicemia, subacute bacterial endocarditis, lupus erythematosus, juvenile rheumatoid arthritis, and periarteritis nodosa. Antineutrophilic cytoplasmic antibodies will help distinguish periarteritis from necrotizing venulitis; blood cultures will help distinguish bacterial infections.

NON-BLANCHING VASCULAR LESIONS (PETECHIAE AND PURPURA)

61

Vasculitis (Henoch–Schönlein purpura)

DDx ref 31 • 72 • 54

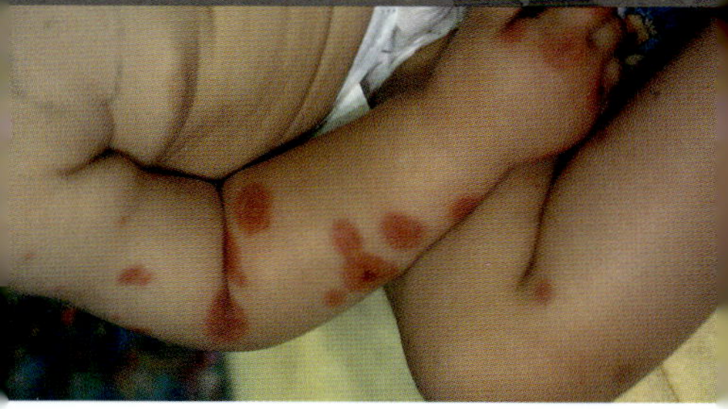

Arm of an infant with acute hemorrhagic edema of infancy.

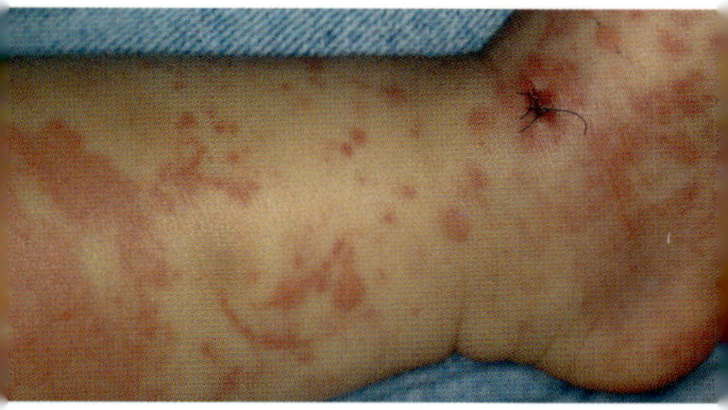

Non-blanching red-purple areas in acute hemorrhagic edema of infancy.

NON-BLANCHING VASCULAR LESIONS (PETECHIAE AND PURPURA)

62

Pernio

DDx ref 47 • 44 • 61

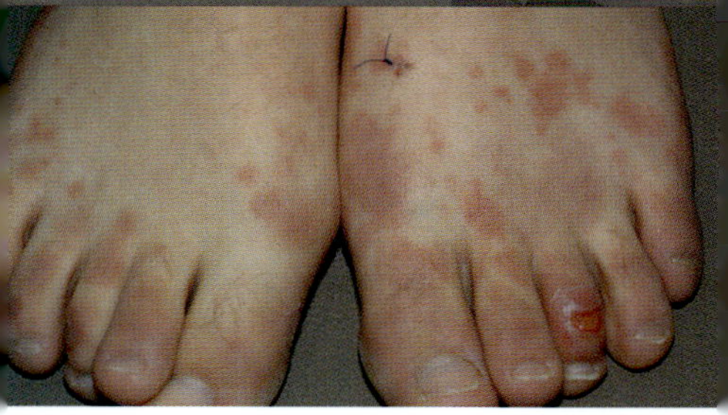

Purple, oval, nontender nodules on the toes in a child with pernio.

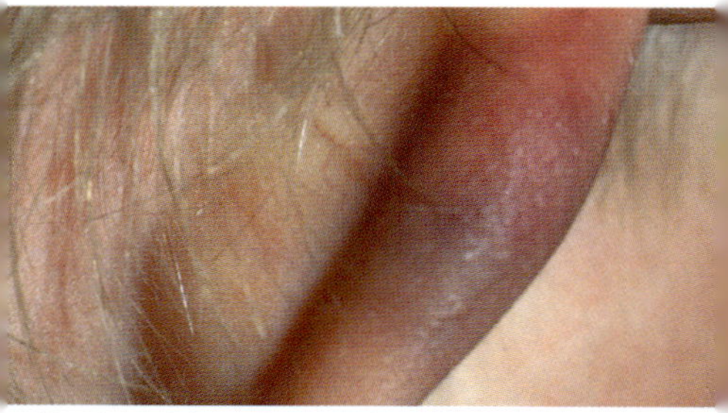

Purple nodule on the ear of toddler with pernio.

NON-BLANCHING VASCULAR LESIONS (PETECHIAE AND PURPURA)

61

Vasculitis (Henoch–Schönlein purpura)

DDx ref 31 • 72 • 54

TREATMENT

With only skin involvement, no treatment is necessary. Skin lesions are unlikely to respond to corticosteroids. With gastrointestinal or renal involvement, prednisone 2 mg/kg per day may be helpful although the skin lesions will not improve. Skin changes last 4–6 weeks and resolve in most children. Non-steroidal anti-inflammatory drugs may be used for the joint symptoms. With severe cutaneous infarcts or prolonged disease, intravenous methylprednisolone plus plasmapheresis has been effective, as has cyclophosphamide. Microscopic analysis of urine every 2 weeks for 3 months may detect microscopic hematuria not found on initial evaluation.

NON-BLANCHING VASCULAR LESIONS (PETECHIAE AND PURPURA)

62

Pernio

DDx ref 47 • 44 • 61

CLINICAL FEATURES

Asymptomatic red-purple to purple nodules that develop several days to weeks after cold exposure characterize pernio. The nodules are on the fingers, toes, or ears and are accompanied by a livedo pattern on adjacent skin. Uncommonly, the nodules ulcerate and become painful (kibes). The amount of cold exposure may seem trivial and associated wetness is required to develop pernio. Adolescent girls with anorexia nervosa are susceptible to pernio. Cryoglobulins or other cryoproteins may be present. Pernio is frequently recurrent. ANA is occasionally positive.

TREATMENT

Avoidance of wet and cold may prevent new lesions but there is no effective treatment for established pernio.

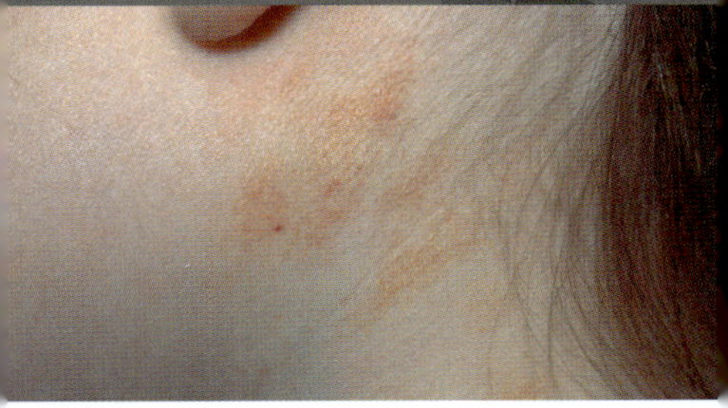

Diffuse generalized progressive pigmented purpura (PPP). Golden-brown and cayenne-pepper macules on the neck of a child with progressive pigmented purpura.

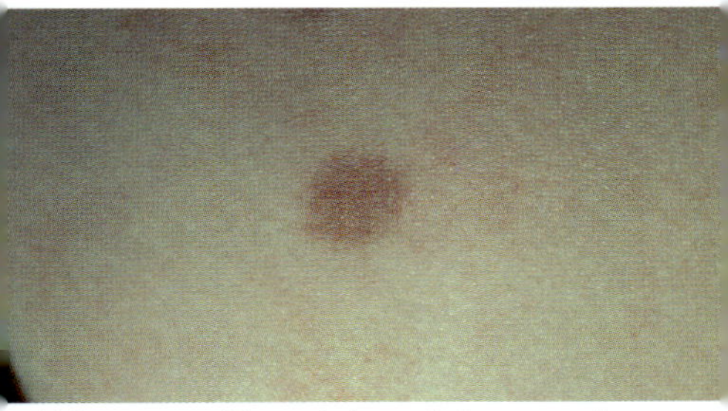

Lichen aureus. Pigmented macule in progressive pigmented purpura.

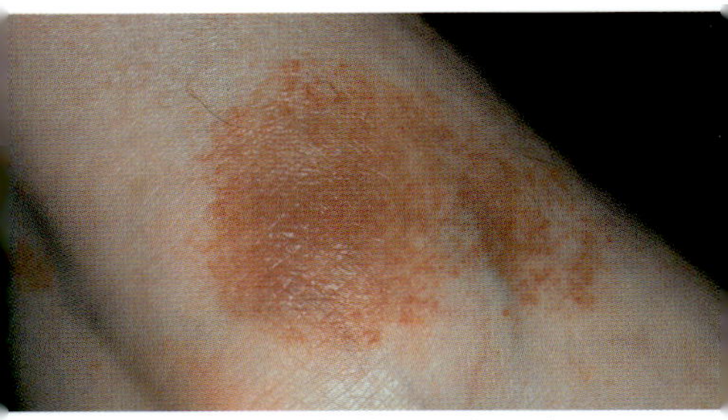

Lichenoid PPP. Lichenified brown plaque in a child with progressive pigmented purpura.

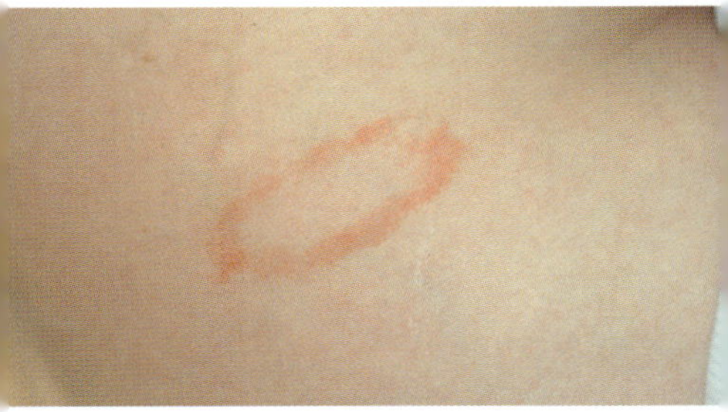

Annular PPP. Annular pigmented macules in progressive pigmented purpura.

CLINICAL FEATURES

The pigmented purpuras are characterized by the appearance of non-palpable petechiae over the extremities, trunk, or neck. Individual lesions consist of fresh and old petechiae with a mix of red, brown, and yellow spots. There are five clinical types: diffuse generalized, lichenoid, annular, eczematoid, and lichen aureus. Different types of lesions may be seen in the same child. The lower extremities are most commonly involved, with more lesions in dependent areas. Lesions may progress to involve the entire trunk and upper extremities. Pruritus is usually mild or absent and there are no associated systemic symptoms. Spontaneous remission in a few years is the norm, but there are no long-term studies evaluating risk of recurrence. Platelet and clotting abnormalities are not associated.

TREATMENT

Treatment is not necessary.

64 Purpuric gloves-and-socks syndrome

DDx ref 62 • 61 • 72

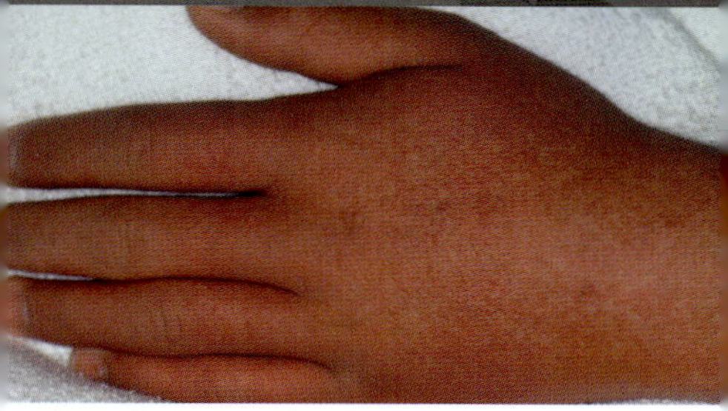

Purpuric gloves-and-socks syndrome in parvovirus B-19 infection. (Photo courtesy J. Burch MD.)

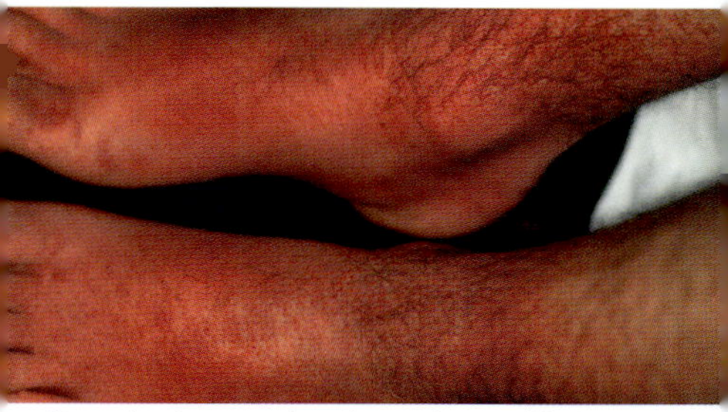

Purpuric gloves-and-socks syndrome. (Photo courtesy J. Burch MD.)

65 DRESS syndrome

DDx ref 18 • 20 • 31

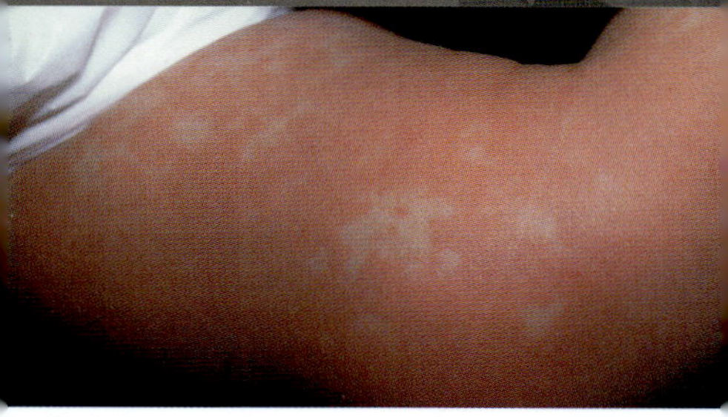

Red skin with islands of sparing in early DRESS syndrome.

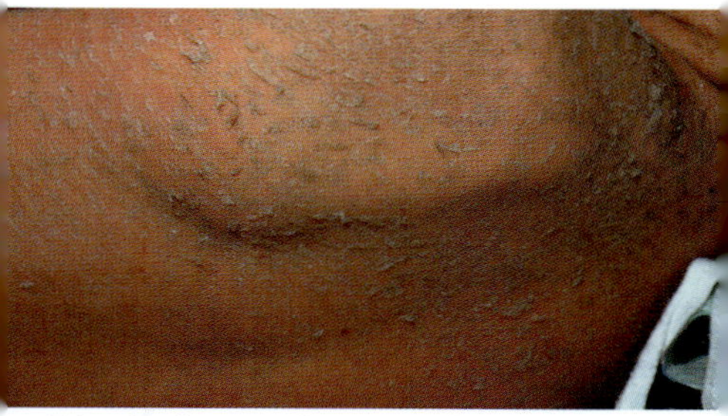

Extensive desquamation eventually develops in DRESS syndrome.

64 Purpuric gloves-and-socks syndrome

DDx ref 62 • 61 • 72

CLINICAL FEATURES

Purpuric gloves-and-socks syndrome is a rare manifestation of parvovirus B19 infection. It is heralded by the acute onset of fever, pruritus, painful edema, and purpura of the distal extremities in a 'gloves-and-socks' distribution. It may be accompanied by oral and facial lesions.

TREATMENT

Treatment is unnecessary because the illness resolves spontaneously within a few weeks.

65 DRESS syndrome

DDx ref 18 • 20 • 31

CLINICAL FEATURES

DRESS syndrome (drug rash with eosinophilia and systemic symptoms) historically has gone by many names. It was initially called the 'anticonvulsant pseudolymphoma' or 'hypersensitivity' syndrome. It has also been called the 'exfoliative dermatitis/fever/hepatitis/lymphadenopathy' syndrome. DRESS syndrome is characterized by progressively widespread erythema with subsequent extensive desquamation, accompanied by fever, pronounced eosinophilia, atypical lymphocytes in the blood and skin, elevated liver enzymes, generalized lymphadenopathy, renal and pulmonary involvement. Not all organ systems are affected in every individual. Progressive malnutrition and weight loss may occur. It can be life-threatening. Onset occurs 1–3 weeks after starting the offending agent. Anticonvulsants (hydantoins, carbamazepine, lamotrigine) and antibiotics (sulfonamides, dapsone, vancomycin) are the most common causes, but DRESS syndrome can also be caused by other drugs.

TREATMENT

The offending agent must be stopped immediately. Prednisone 1–2 mg/kg is the treatment of choice for the systemic symptoms. Hospitalization for supportive care is usually necessary.

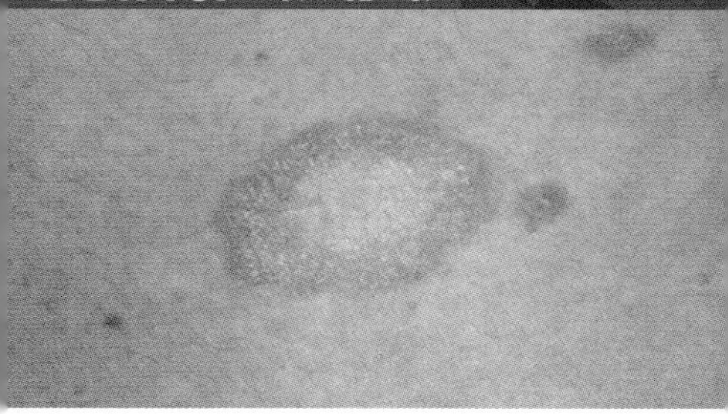

Herald patch of PR larger than adjacent generalized papules.

Oval pink papules of PR in a fir tree distribution.

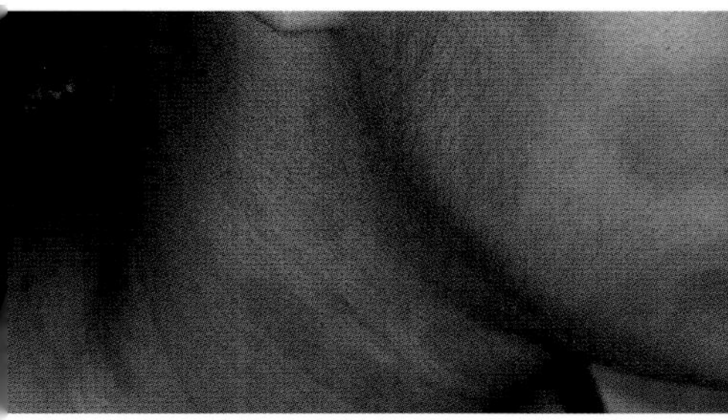

Inverse PR with neck and lower face lesions in a dark-skinned child.

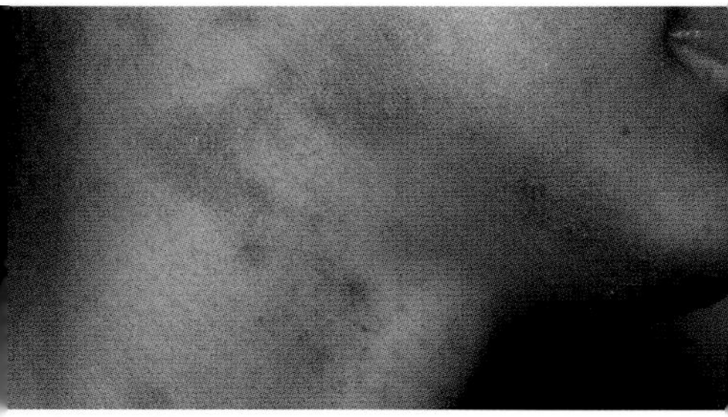

Inverse PR on the neck.

CLINICAL FEATURES

Pityriasis rosea (PR) is a unique eruption characterized by the sudden appearance of dozens of symmetrical, pink-red, round 1–3-mm papules on the trunk in a distribution of a fir tree. The papules enlarge and become oval over the next few days and develop a central scale with the long axes of oval lesions parallel to adjacent lesions. Some children complain of itching. Approximately 1 week (range: 1–30 days) before the generalized eruption, there is the appearance of a 'herald' patch. Although the generalized eruption is predominantly truncal, the herald patch can appear anywhere on the skin.

The 'herald' patch consists of a large 2–10-cm oval, pink, scaly border surrounding a center of normal skin. Easily confused with tinea corporis, the herald patch is often treated with antifungals and the subsequent eruption of typical PR lesions is misinterpreted as a reaction to the antifungal medication. Some 80% of children will have a herald patch and some will have more than one. PR usually occurs **in older children and teens** and may be preceded by a prodrome of pharyngitis, lymphadenopathy, headache, and malaise, leading to the presumption that PR may be caused by an infectious agent. Streptococcal infections, HHV-7 infections, and most recently, the influenza A H1N1 variant have been implicated as possibly responsible. Distribution **in children with dark skin** differs with involvement predominantly on the neck, lower face, and proximal extremities, with the trunk mostly spared. This pattern has been termed 'inverse PR'.

Children with a nontruncal distribution have the same course and outcome as those with truncal involvement. Secondary syphilis (see DDx ref 32 Syphilis) may mimic PR and sexually active older children and teens should be screened with a syphilis serology, especially if they demonstrate lymphadenopathy and fever. Mucosal lesions should increase the suspicion for syphilis although in PR, oral lesions are present in 16%.

As in all papulosquamous diseases, skin lesions persist, typically lasting for 2–12 weeks, increasing patient and parent concern. The skin lesions resolve without residua.

TREATMENT

Most children and teens require no treatment. For the child with itching, either natural sunlight exposure of affected areas or a single dose of UVB sunlamp to a minimal erythema dose will stop itching and hasten the disappearance of skin lesions. Clearing has also been reported with oral erythromycin 250 mg four times a day for 2 weeks. Oral antihistamines and topical steroids usually do not influence the skin lesions.

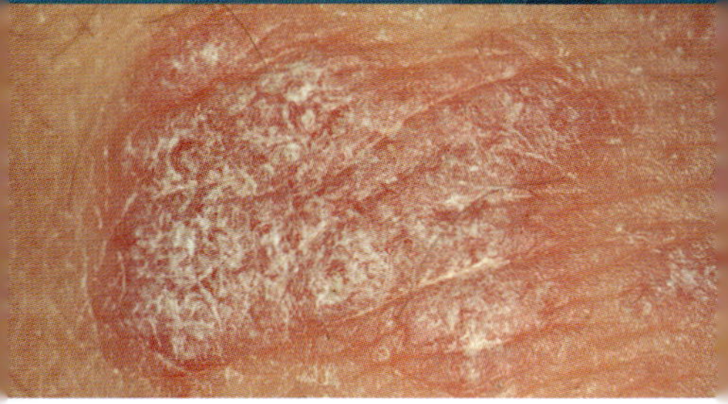

Red plaque with silvery scale in childhood psoriasis vulgaris.

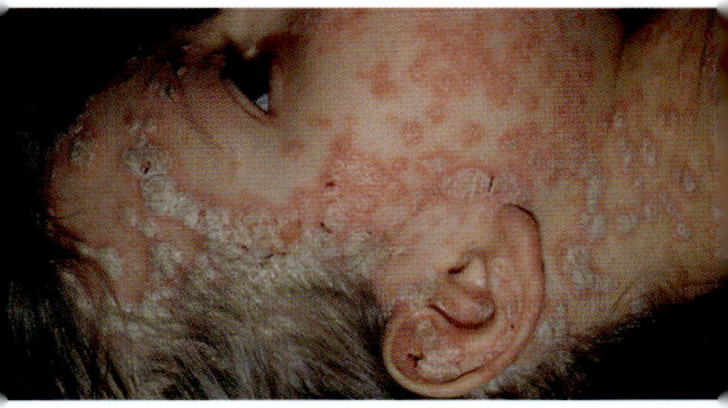

Thick silvery scale and red plaques, some nonscaly in a child with psoriasis vulgaris.

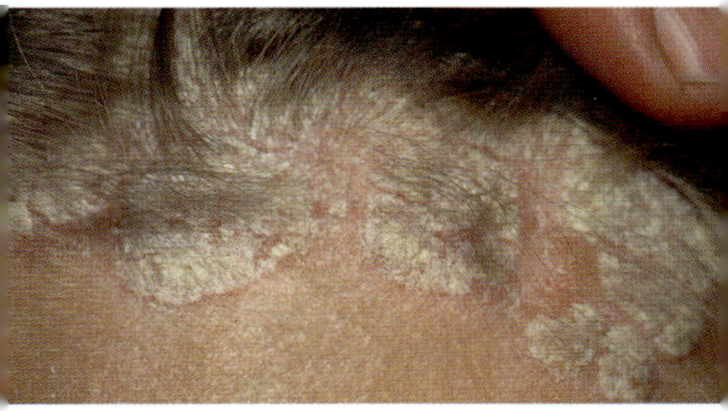

Diffuse thick scale throughout a child's scalp.

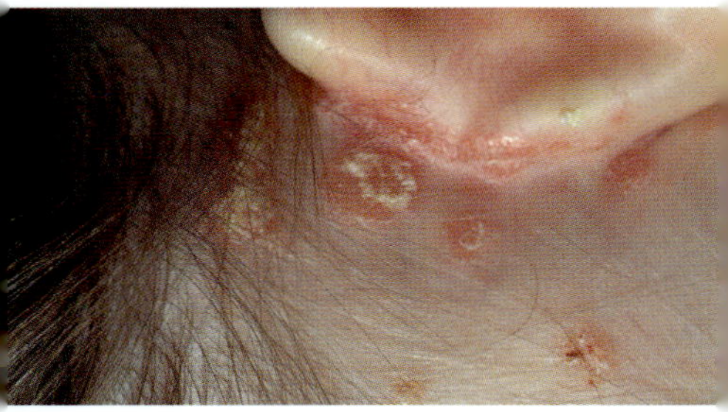

Scaly papules behind the ear in a child with psoriasis vulgaris.

CLINICAL FEATURES

Psoriasis is a hereditary heterogeneous disorder divided into type I psoriasis (beginning before age 40 years with a peak onset between 16 and 22 years) and type II psoriasis (beginning after age 40 years). Multiple susceptibility genes have been associated. Type I psoriasis has a stronger genetic basis with a greater proportion of psoriasis patients with a family history of psoriasis and stronger HLA-C*06 associations.

In childhood psoriasis is uncommon (0.4% of children). Psoriasis is a clinical diagnosis based on the presence of thick, silvery scales over red papules or plaques, a characteristic distribution, nail involvement, and the presence of the isomorphic (Koebner) phenomenon. Sites for predilection in psoriasis include the scalp, ears, eyebrows, elbows, knees, gluteal crease, umbilicus, genitalia, and nails. The most common clinical picture of psoriasis in childhood is involvement of ears, elbows, knees, and scalp with a few scaly plaques, and the anal crease by pink macules without scales.

Genital involvement occurs in 40% of children with the common form of psoriasis (psoriasis vulgaris). Nail changes are seen in only 15% of children with psoriasis vulgaris. Psoriasis may be rarely seen at birth and 10% of all psoriasis starts before puberty.

A subtype of psoriasis more common in children than adults, is guttate psoriasis. A history of guttate psoriasis is reported by 30% pf psoriasis patients and more likely in those with severe psoriasis. Guttate psoriasis begins with dozens of pink-red macules, scattered on the trunk, that mimic a viral exanthema. Individual lesions progress to red papules and develop a silvery-white scale. Follicular accentuation of lesions may be seen.

Children with guttate psoriasis should have a throat and rectal bacterial culture for streptococci as strep infection is the most common trigger of an episode of guttate psoriasis. A history of a sore throat in the previous 3 weeks is frequently obtained. Guttate psoriasis may spontaneously clear in 2–6 months but children who have had guttate psoriasis are likely to develop psoriasis vulgaris within 5 years.

The isomorphic phenomenon describes the development of psoriatic lesions restricted to sites of skin injury that occurred several days beforehand.

The psoriatic lesions are often linear at the site of a scratch, but can take on many shapes depending upon the skin trauma. They may result from lacerations, abrasions, sunburn, insect bites, or pressure sores. A curvilinear appearance may mimic epidermal nevi. Scratching off scales may leave fine bleeding points (Auspitz sign) and induce the isomorphic phenomenon, making the lesions worse. The isomorphic phenomenon offers insight into the pathogenesis of psoriasis, as skin injury is required prior to an abnormal genetic epidermal repair response.

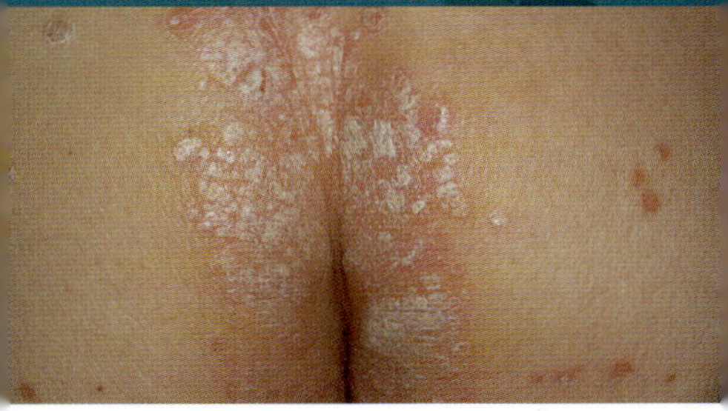

Scaly plaque on the anal crease in childhood psoriasis.

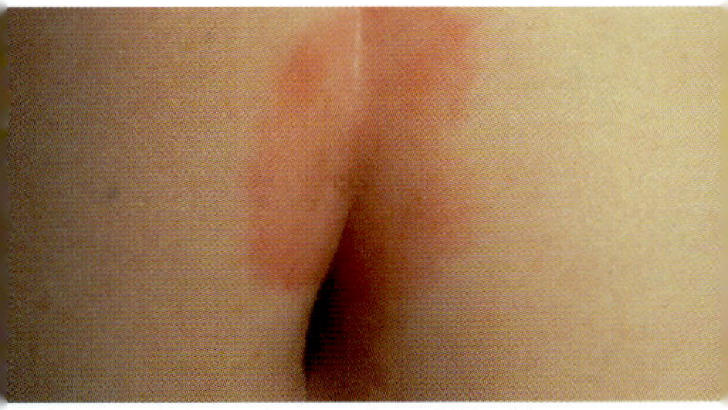

Pinking of the anal crease in a child with psoriasis.

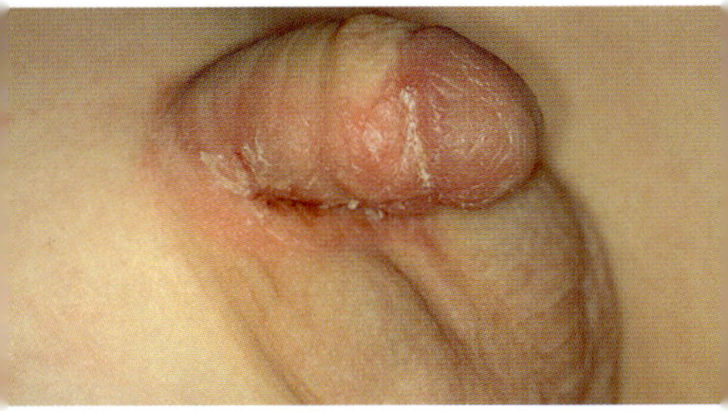

Scaly plaque of foreskin in an infant with psoriasis.

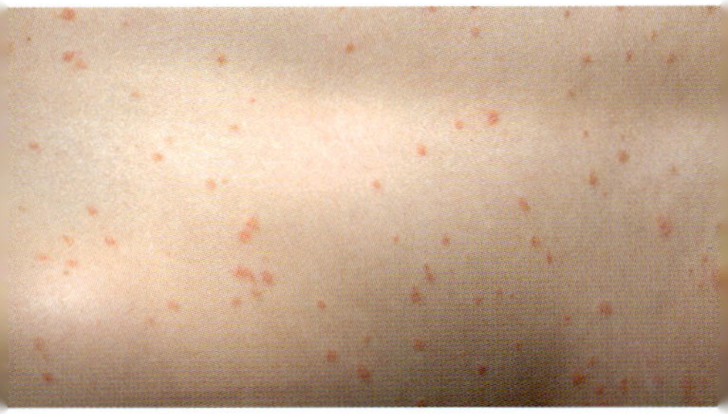

Dozens of red papules in a child with guttate psoriasis.

Scalp involvement is seen in 80% and is more severe in girls. It presents as thick white scales throughout the scalp without hair loss. Itching may be severe.

Nail signs of psoriasis include multiple tiny pits in the surface of the nail, yellowing of the distal nail due to separation of the distal nail plate from the nail bed (onycholysis), thickening of the distal nail, or crumbling and destruction of the entire nail. Nail pitting is most common. Nail involvement is seen in 39% and is more common in boys.

Involvement of palms and soles is most uncommon in childhood, but if present, may be severely uncomfortable for the child. Painful fissures may develop in the thick scaly plaques and small, sterile pustules may be seen.

A rare severe variant of psoriasis is generalized pustular psoriasis. This is seen as erythroderma accompanied by thousands of pinpoint pustules, which eventuate in sheets of desquamation. Pustular psoriasis can develop when psoriasis vulgaris is treated with systemic steroids and may be accompanied by lytic bone lesions. A rare pustular dermatosis found in children with mutations in the IL36RN gene can mimic pustular psoriasis.

TREATMENT

The choice of treatment depends upon the location and severity of disease; 75% of children with psoriasis respond to topical therapy.

For children with psoriasis vulgaris and few skin lesions, moderate-potency topical steroid ointments are helpful, although it may require 4–8 weeks to clear. OTC topical steroids are ineffective. Topical calcipotriene (vitamin D3 analog) is effective after 4–8 weeks of therapy and faster resolution may be obtained by alternating topical steroids with topical calcipotriene. A strategy of calcipotriene twice a day on weekdays and clobetasol once daily on weekends is a useful approach.

Anthralin a tricyclic hydrocarbon, is useful because it downregulates the TGF-α growth factor and its receptor. It is most effective when used in a short-contact fashion. The 1% ointment is applied once daily for 20 minutes, then washed off with a neutral pH soap such as Dove. If not washed off, skin irritation will develop. Anthralin also stains skin and clothing.

Tazarotene is a retinoid used topically for psoriasis. Because tazarotene is irritating, alternating it with topical steroids is useful. For nail involvement, massaging topical tazarotene gel into the nail cuticle is effective.

Scalp involvement requires additional treatment strategies. Soften the scales overnight by massaging in 3% salicylic acid in olive oil or mineral oil, or using a phenol and saline scalp solution. In the morning, a tar shampoo can be used and a mild brushing for scale removal. Either steroid or calcipotriene solutions can be massaged into the scalp following scale removal.

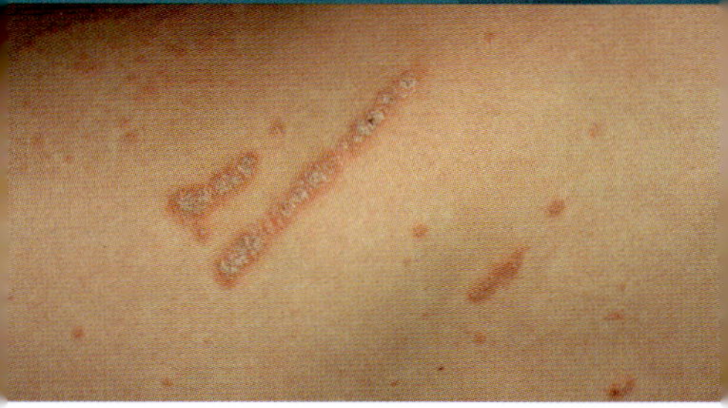

Linear scaly papules in a child with isomorphic phenomenon, 3 days after cat-scratch at the skin site.

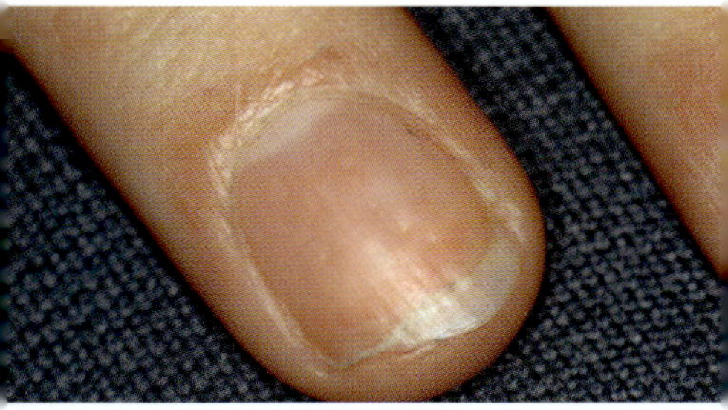

Nail pitting in a child with psoriasis.

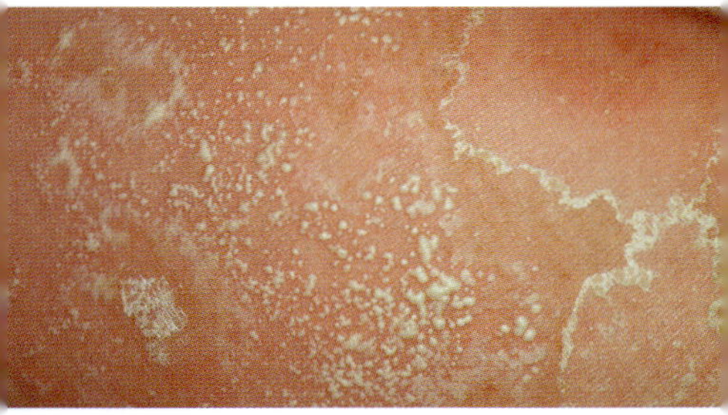

Erythroderma, pinpoint pustules and desquamation in pustular psoriasis.

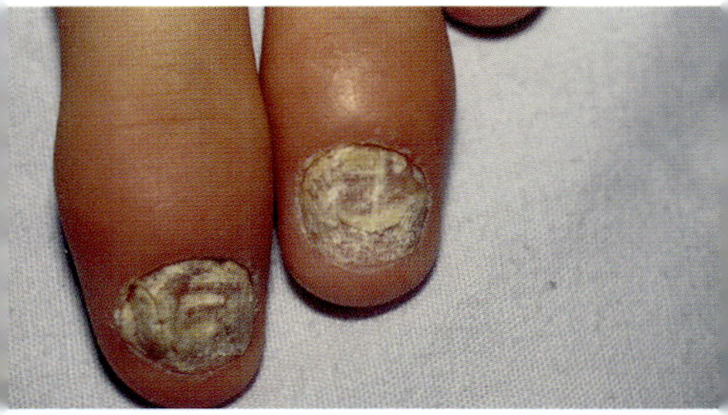

Diffuse redness and swelling of DIP joints and nail destruction in childhood psoriatic arthritis.

It is impractical to use topical agents for widespread disease.

UVL or a systemic agent can be considered. Natural sunlight may improve psoriasis through deliberate sunbathing. Alternatively, artificial sunlamps can be used. Narrow band UVB three times weekly or psoralen pills plus UVA (PUVA) can be used. Psoralen is difficult to administer to children and it can create severe sunburn in areas of skin where it is dribbled or regurgitated. If sunlamp therapy is not available, then systemic drugs such as oral retinoids, methotrexate, or anti-TNF-α biologics can be considered. All have significant side-effects and their use should be restricted to the child with severe forms of psoriasis, including psoriatic arthritis.

Staphylococcus aureus frequently colonizes psoriatic skin and a child hospitalized with psoriasis will shed billions of organisms into the hospital environment.

Children with guttate psoriasis and a positive streptococcus culture should be treated with penicillin although it may not influence the course of the guttate psoriasis.

Arthritis common in adults with psoriasis, is rarely seen is children. It is seen as oligoarticular disease involving the metacarpophalangeal, proximal interphalangeal joints, or the axial skeleton.

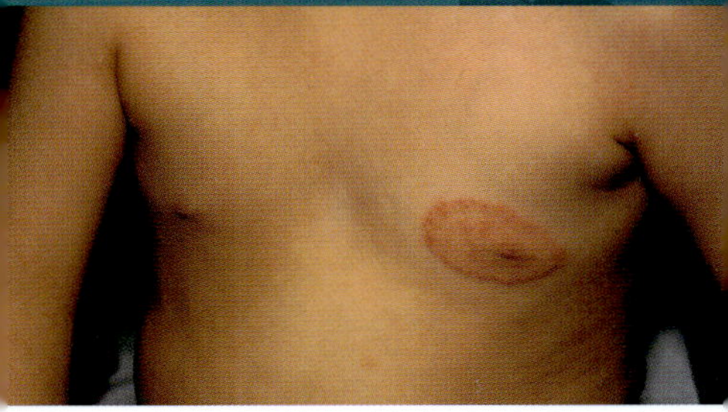

Red, scaly patch with partial clearing in the center in a boy with tinea corporis.

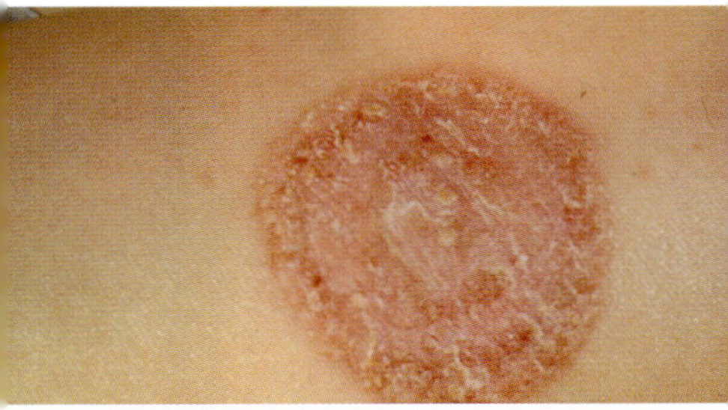

Red, scaly plaque on the leg of a teen from cattle ringworm, *T. verrucosum*.

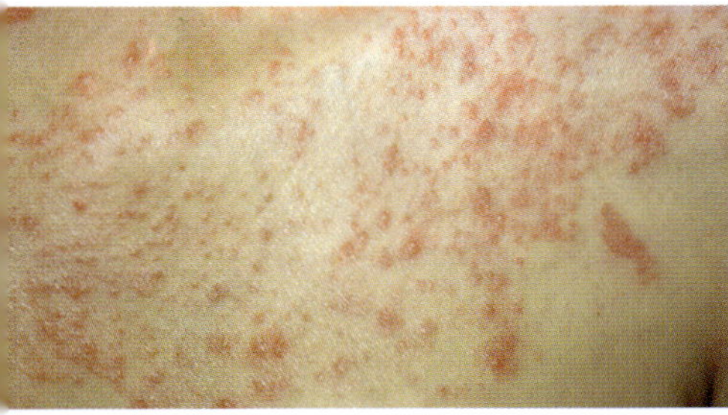

Red follicular papules without scale in tinea that was treated with super-potent topical steroids.

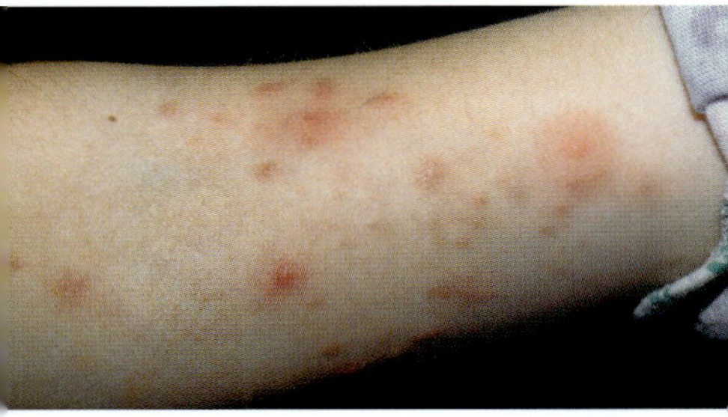

Red pustules and nodules on the leg of a child with leukemia (Majocchi's granulomas).

CLINICAL FEATURES

Classic tinea presents as asymmetrical annular scaly red plaques, at times clearing in the center (ringworm pattern). The appearance may change depending on location.

On the body (tinea corporis) lesions may not always clear in the center, instead being red throughout, sometimes with follicular pustules. This is particularly true of dog, cat, or cattle ringworm infection. The mistaken use of super-potent topical steroids on tinea corporis may permit dermatophyte invasion into the hair follicles, resulting in an area of follicular pustules without a distinct border (tinea incognito).

Children who have cancer or are immunosuppressed may develop scattered pustules and follicular red nodules (Majocchi's granulomas) without the red scaly borders of classic ringworm.

On the face (tinea faciei) red scaly areas may appear on one eyelid, one ear, or sometimes both cheeks. The rash on the cheeks mimics the butterfly rash of lupus erythematosus.

In the groin (tinea cruris) diffuse red, scaly areas are seen that may be confused with candidiasis.

On the feet (tinea pedis, athlete's foot) early infections of acute tinea pedis may demonstrate round areas of vesicles on the instep of the foot. After persistence for a few months, the infection evolves into a chronic pattern of diffuse scaling of the entire soles of the feet. Toe web redness and thickened nails are additional clues to the diagnosis of chronic tinea pedis. It is useful to remember that anything red and scaly could be tinea even without a ringworm pattern, and examination for tinea is always indicated in papulosquamous conditions. Scraping fine scale off the skin surface from the border of an involved area onto a microscope slide, then dissolving the scale in a 10% potassium hydroxide solution and covering with a coverslip, permits microscopic examination that will reveal branching hyphae. Demonstration of hyphae is best done by experienced microscopists. If this is not possible, then fungal culture screening of scales with dermatophyte test medium (DTM) culture is recommended. Inoculation of scales into the agar and incubation at room temperature will turn the agar red in 2 or 3 weeks, and exhibit a fuzzy growth on the surface. Direct dermatophyte invasion of the stratum corneum is responsible for tinea lesions.

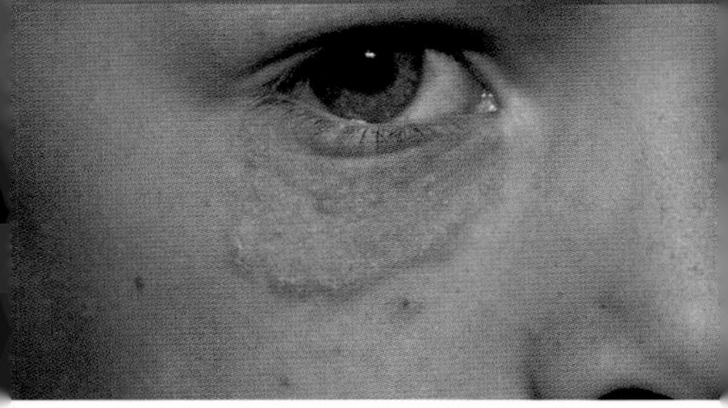

Annular red scaly area on one lower eyelid in a child with tinea faciei from a cat.

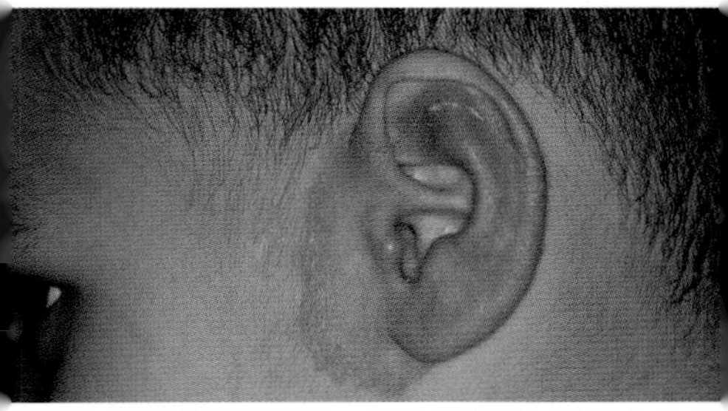

Annular red scaly area on one ear in tinea faciei.

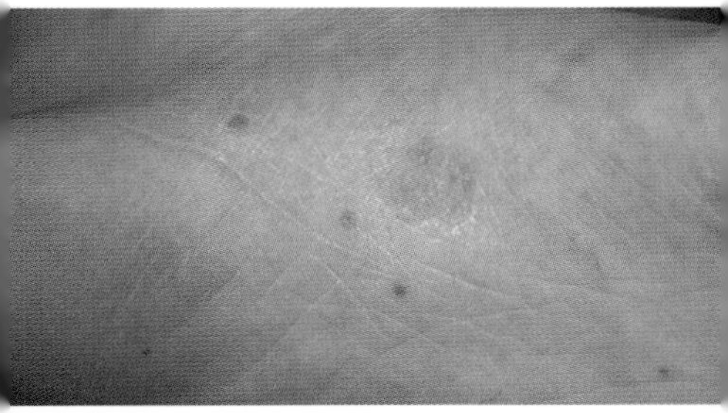

Annular red scaly patches on the instep of the foot (tinea pedis).

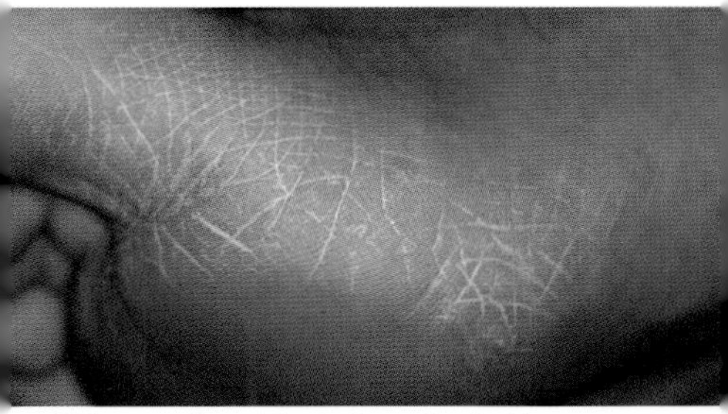

Diffuse scaling of the bottom of a foot in a teen with tinea pedis.

Responsible organisms include *Microsporum canis, Trichophyton mentagrophytes, T. rubrum, T. tonsurans, T. verrucosum, M. gypseum*, and *Epidermophyton floccosum*.

Animal source dermatophyte infection (*M. canis, T. verrucosum*) tends to be quite inflammatory.

TREATMENT

If hair or nails are not involved, then topical antifungals will suffice. Topical allylamine creams such as terbinafine, butenafine, and naftifine are fungicidal. The imidazole creams are fungistatic and include clotrimazole, econazole, ketoconazole, miconazole, and oxiconazole. These topical creams are applied twice daily, treating an area beyond obvious skin involvement. Therapy for 2–4 weeks is usually necessary. Rarely, oral antifungals are required such as terbinafine, griseofulvin, itraconazole, or fluconazole.

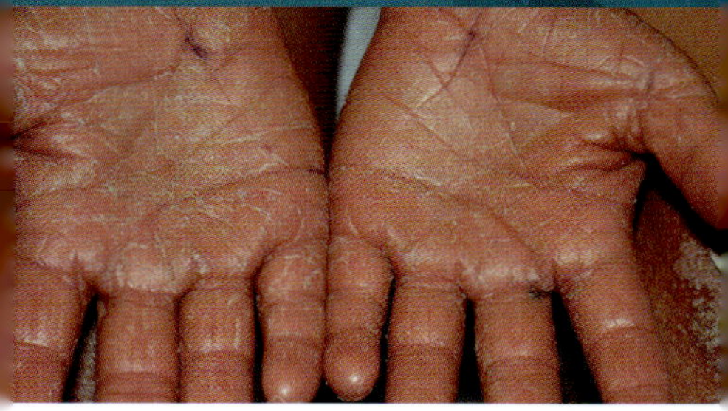

Salmon-colored scaly palms in a child with PRP.

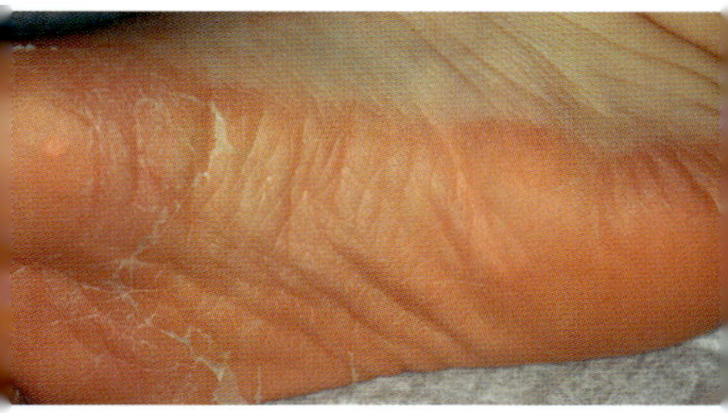

Salmon-colored thickening of the soles of the feet in a child with PRP.

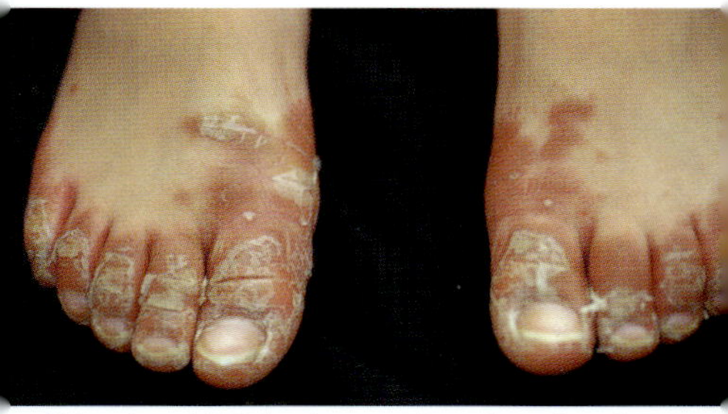

Extension of PRP involvement from the soles of the feet to the tops of the toes.

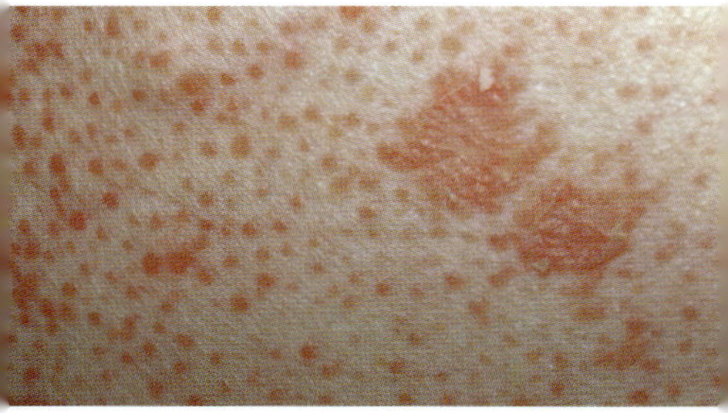

Salmon-colored follicular papules and plaques on an extremity of a child with PRP.

CLINICAL FEATURES

Juvenile PRP is an uncommon papulosquamous disorder with onset between 1 and 10 years of age. It has distinctive clinical features with scaly salmon-colored diffuse thickening of the palms and soles at onset of the eruption. Over the next few days, the skin change extends to involve the tops of the toes and the dorsa of the fingers. Some weeks later, 2–6-mm red follicular papules develop over the extremities and widespread involvement of the trunk. The disease may progress to **exfoliative erythroderma**. Islands of normal skin within the affected areas are commonly seen. Surprisingly, there is little or no itching with PRP. The skin is likely to spontaneously clear a few years after the onset. A dreaded, but rare, complication is the development of **ectropion**. A few children with juvenile PRP will have an autosomal dominant pattern of inheritance.

TREATMENT

PRP if well localized, may respond to topical calcipotriene (vitamin D_3) cream. Widespread disease may require oral retinoids such as isotretinoin 1 mg/kg per day for 4–5 months or acitretin. There are reports of good responses to methotrexate, and to anti-TNF-α biologics (etanercept and infliximab).

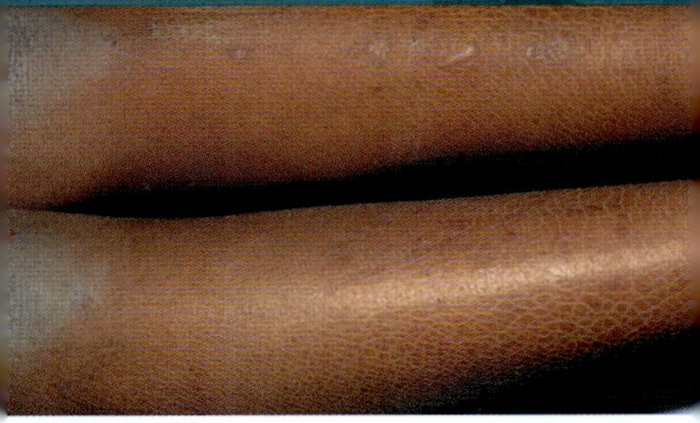

Scales over knees and anterior lower legs in ichthyosis vulgaris (IV).

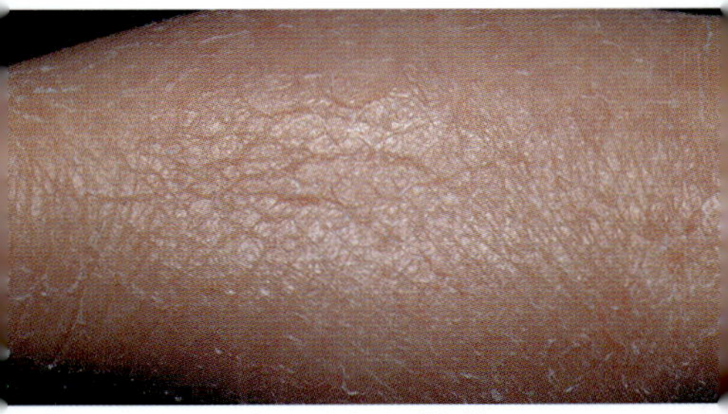

Fine, thin scales in an infant with IV.

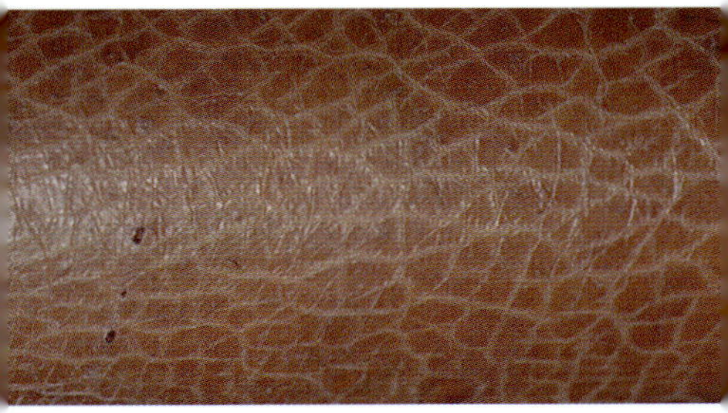

Scales in an older child with IV.

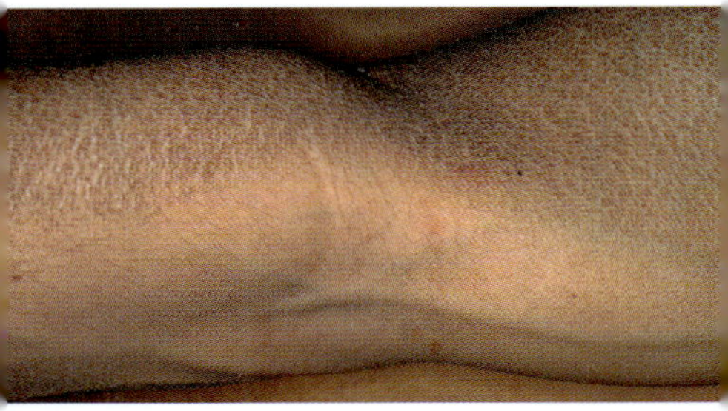

Darkened scales and sparing of the antecubital fossa in X-linked ichthyosis (XLI).

CLINICAL FEATURES

The hereditary ichthyoses are lifelong scaling conditions. The most common, **ichthyosis vulgaris (IV)**, is characterized by scaling and dry skin, with onset at about 6 months of age. The lower legs and buttocks have the most scales and prominent follicular papules consisting of horny plugs are seen over the extensor extremities (keratosis pilaris). Ichthyosis vulgaris and atopic dermatitis share a semidominant inheritance and alterations in the filaggrin gene, which is responsible for maintenance of the epidermal barrier. Half of children with IV will develop the eczematous skin of atopic dermatitis.

Recessive X-linked ichthyosis also has its onset in infancy with large scales over the extensor extremities, posterior neck, and upper trunk. The antecubital and popliteal fossae and palms and soles are unaffected. As the child ages, the scales become thicker and yellow-brown in color. It occurs in 1 of 6000 males. The gene for epidermal steroid sulfatase is abnormal. Placental steroid sulfatase deficiency in the mother results in low estrogen levels and a failure of initiation of labor. Asymptomatic corneal opacities will be seen in the affected boy and carrier mother. Cryptorchidism is common in 20%.

Lamellar ichthyosis is an autosomal recessive condition with red, scaly skin in the newborn.

Babies are often born with a collodion membrane – a taut, shiny, thickened stratum corneum that encases the baby.

The ears may be bound down and ectropion and eclabium are seen. Within hours, the membrane splits in many places and peels. After the separation leaving red skin, thick, plate-like scales develop over the next few days. Palms and soles are diffusely thickened leaving a yellowish appearance. The lamellar ichthyosis clinical pattern overlaps with that of congenital ichthyosiform erythroderma, and abnormal genes for epidermal transglutaminase 1 (most commonly) or ABCA 12, ALOX 12B, ALOX E3, CYP4f22, SLC 27A4, CER53, PNPLA1, and ichthyin are responsible. EHK (condition 16) also may begin as a collodion baby.

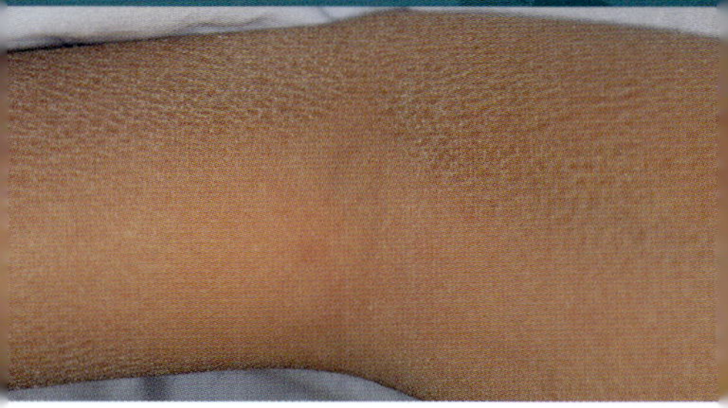

Large, brown plate-like scales in XLI.

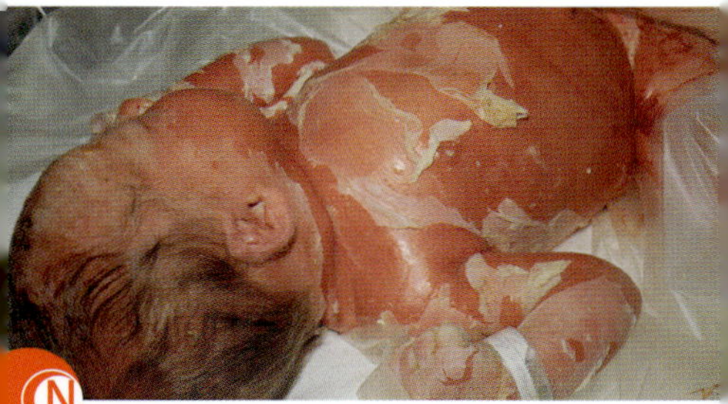

N Newborn with lamellar ichthyosis and peeling collodion membrane.

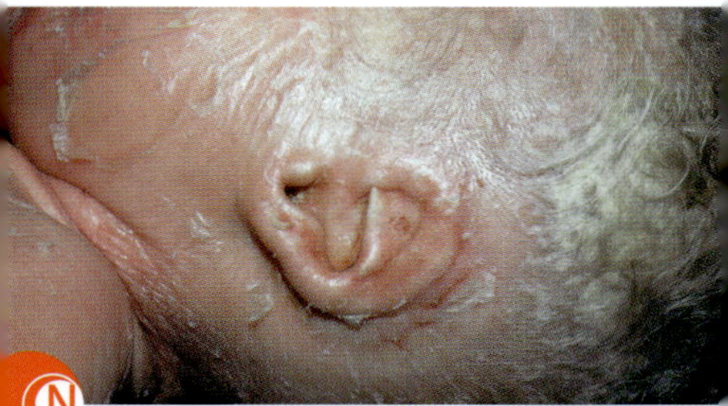

N Thick scales and bound-down ears in a baby with lamellar ichthyosis.

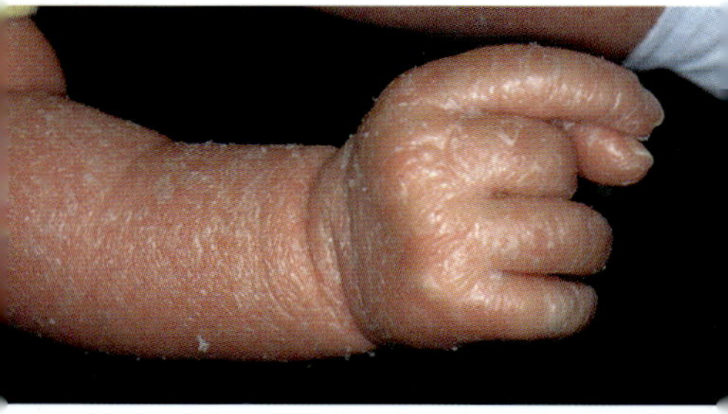

Red scaly skin of a child with Netherton's syndrome.

Netherton's syndrome is a severe autosomal recessive disorder with mutations in SPINK5 that encodes the serine protease inhibitor LEKT1. The epidermal barrier is severely compromised, leaving red, scaly skin and severe eczematous changes.

As newborns they may be collodion babies and demonstrate hypernatremic dehydration, skin infections, and eventually failure to thrive. The babies are often born with minimal eyebrows and no hair due to a diagnostic hair shaft defect of trichorrhexis invaginata that leads to hair breakage. Plucking broken eyebrow hairs in the newborn for microscopic examination will be an aid to the diagnosis. The severe eczema persists into adult life and the hair, as it grows, remains short, as it breaks off easily.

TREATMENT

There is no satisfactory treatment for the ichthyoses. Bland ointments help restore the epidermal barrier but must be applied twice daily. Infrequent and abbreviated bathing help keep the skin surface from excessive drying. Lactic acid 5% ointment, 12% ammonium lactate lotion, 10% urea creams, N-acetylcysteine, and propylene glycol have been beneficial.

These should not be used in **newborns or young infants** because of risk of systemic absorption and toxicity. In **lamellar ichthyosis**, oral retinoids may be useful but the risk:benefits ratio of their long-term use must be carefully considered.

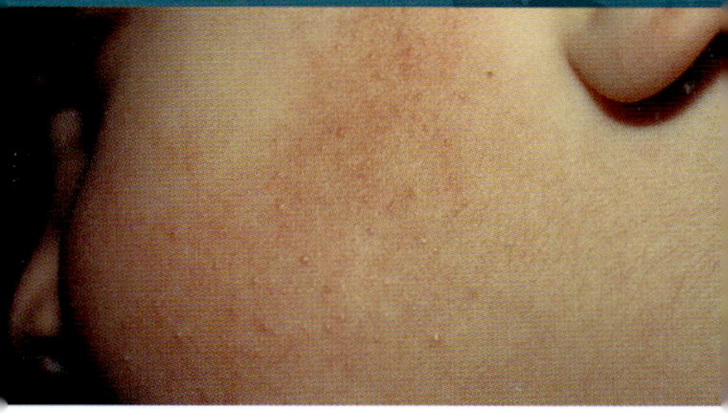

Follicular papules with surrounding redness on cheeks of a child with keratosis pilaris (KP).

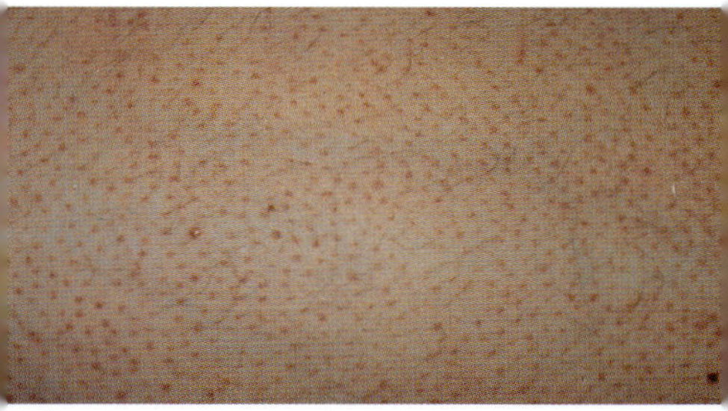

Rough follicular papules on the extensor arm of a teen with KP.

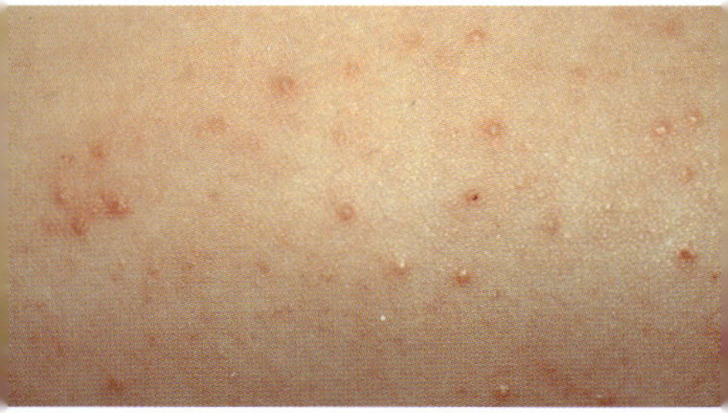

Scattered discrete follicular papules on the extensor arm of a child with KP.

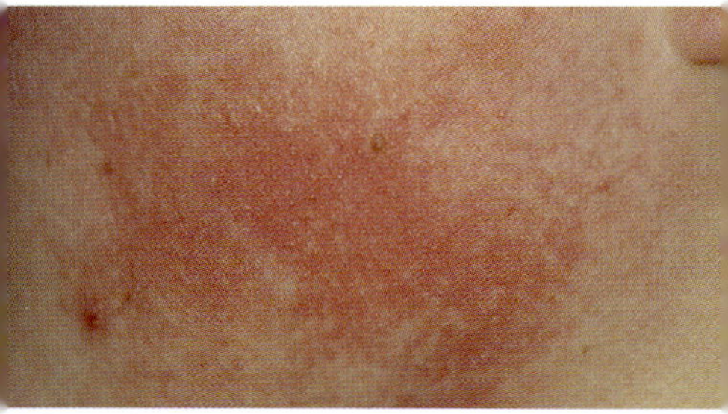

Rough follicular papules and surrounding red skin in a child with KP.

CLINICAL FEATURES

Keratosis pilaris is a common skin condition than can be found without other skin changes or accompanying **ichthyosis vulgaris** (see DDx ref 70 Ichthyosis) or **atopic dermatitis** (see DDx ref 79 Atopic Dermatitis). It is characterized by scaly follicular papules consisting of follicular keratin plugs seen on the extensor extremities, the cheeks, eyebrows, and buttocks.

The affected skin has a rough feel to the surface and follicles may be red and itchy.

On the cheeks the skin between keratotic follicles may be diffusely red. It is worsened by drying of the skin. Onset occurs in the first year of life and becomes more prominent throughout childhood.

TREATMENT

In mild disease the twice daily use of topical emollients applied to wet skin will result in improvement after several weeks. Lactic acid 12% cream or 10% urea cream, or combinations of lactic acid and urea creams can be helpful. Topical tretinoin creams may be too irritating. All creams must be continued to maintain improvement.

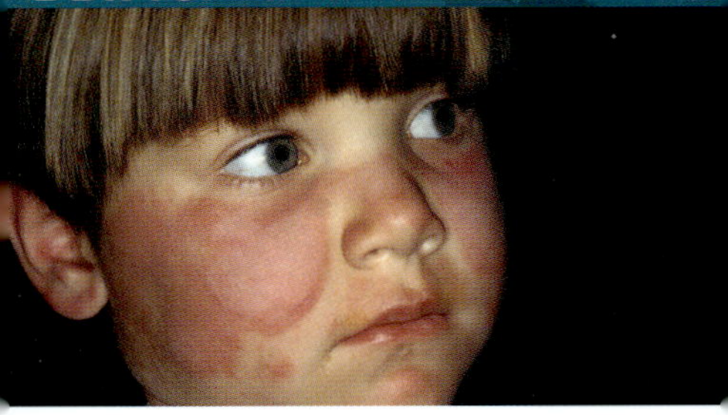

Butterfly rash of childhood acute systemic lupus erythematosus (SLE).

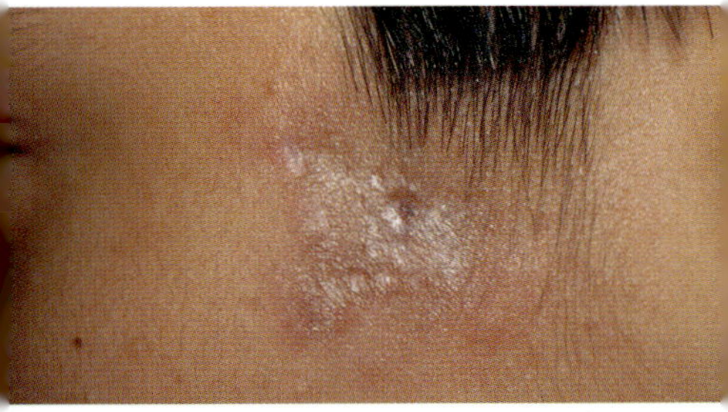

Slightly depressed scaly patch on the face of a girl with discoid LE.

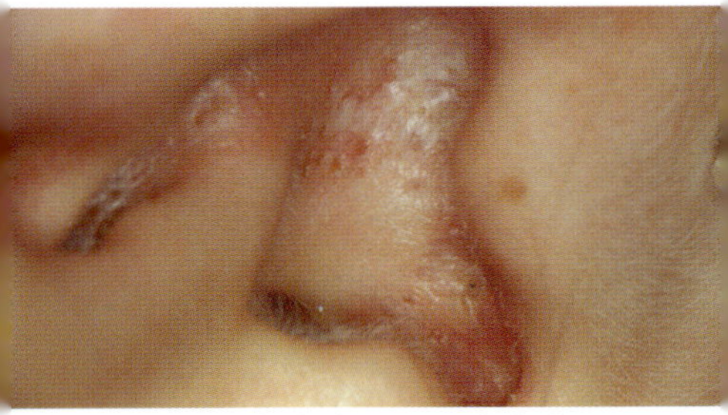

Scaling and atrophy in the ear canal of a teen with discoid LE.

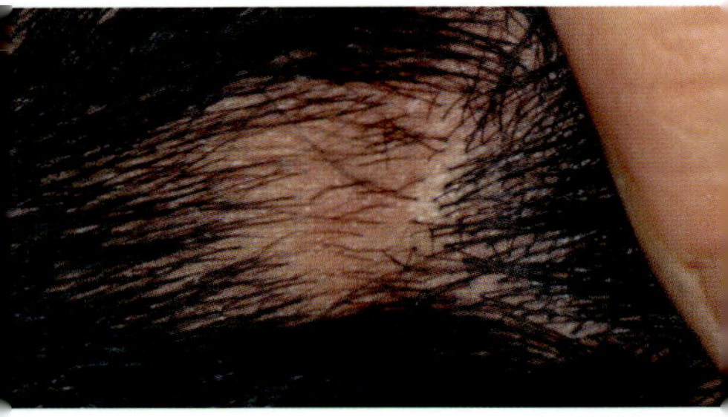

Scarring scalp hair loss in a child with discoid LE.

Lupus erythematosus (LE)

DDx ref 67 • 77 • 61

CLINICAL FEATURES

A cutaneous eruption (usually malar) is the presenting sign in 40–60% of children with lupus erythematosus (LE) and found in 80% of all affected children. Several distinct skin changes are seen. The classic malar butterfly rash of SLE is seen as red, slightly scaly plaques on both cheeks. A slightly depressed, red scaly patch indicates discoid LE. Discoid LE is found on the **face, scalp, and ears**. Scarring hair loss may also be found.

Subacute cutaneous LE (SCLE) demonstrates red scaly annular plaques on sun-exposed areas of skin.

Sun can also induce an acute phototoxic reaction with a blistering sunburn pattern. Large bullae may sometimes be seen.

Hand signs include red scaly plaques between knuckles on the dorsa of the hands or purpuric plaques on the finger pads.

Dermatomyositis by contrast, has red scaly patches over the knuckles. Skin biopsy of LE demonstrates liquefaction degeneration of basal cells of the epidermis and a patchy accumulation of lymphocytes around superficial blood vessels and hair follicles.

Rarely seen are livedo reticularis lacy patterns or the deep purple nodules of **lupus panniculitis**.

LE is a multisystem disease and **joint and kidney** involvement are common.

CNS, lung, and other systems may be involved.

72 DDx ref

PAPULOSQUAMOUS ERUPTIONS

Lupus erythematosus (LE)

67 • 77 • 61

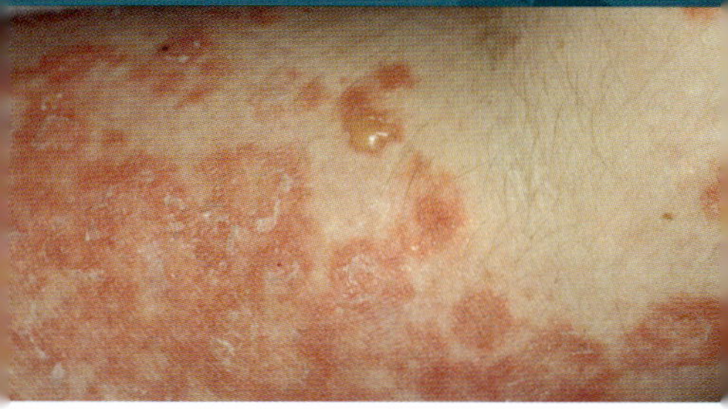

Annular papulosquamous eruption on sun-exposed skin in a child with SCLE.

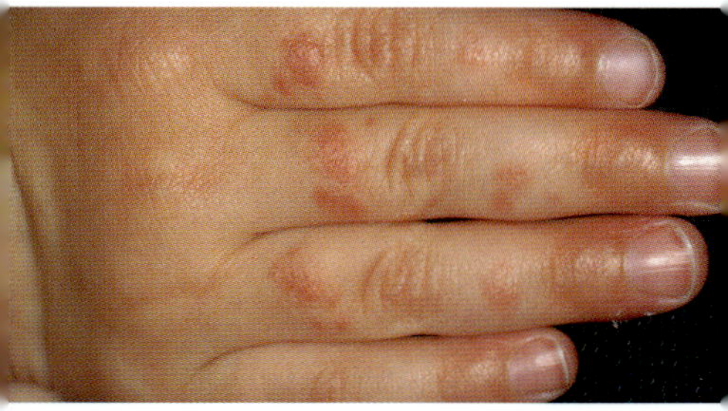

Scaly plaques between the knuckles on top of the hand of a child with SLE.

73 DDx ref

PAPULOSQUAMOUS ERUPTIONS

Darier's disease (keratosis follicularis)

69 • 67 • 23

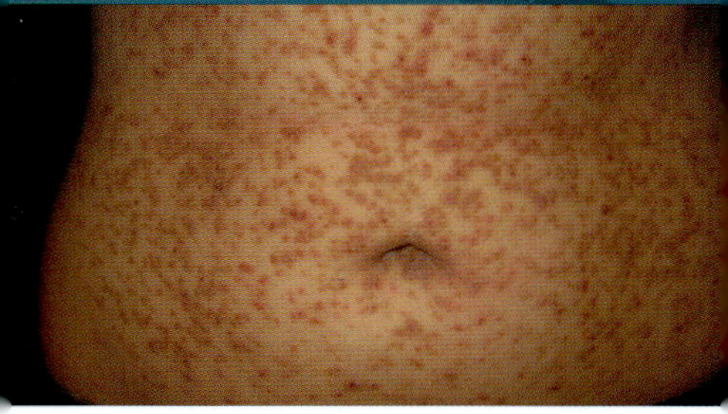

Darier's (keratosis follicularis). Discrete brown, 'greasy-feeling' keratotic papules.

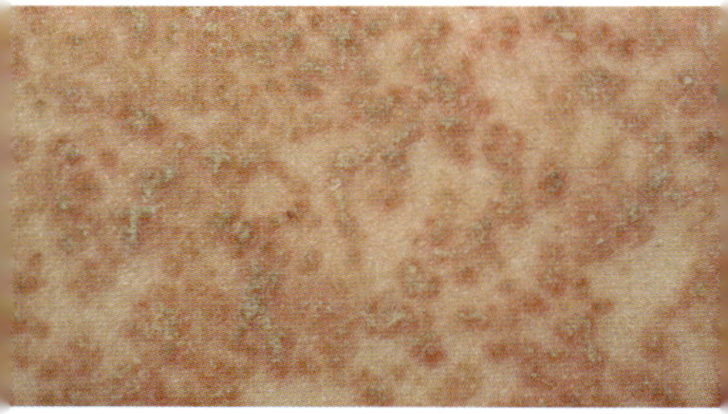

Darier's (keratosis follicularis). Confluent keratotic papules.

72

PAPULOSQUAMOUS ERUPTIONS

Lupus erythematosus (LE)

DDx ref 67 • 77 • 61

TREATMENT

For cutaneous disease mid to potent topical steroids applied twice daily is helpful. Sun protection with clothing, hat, and sunscreen use is a mainstay of therapy. For the very sun sensitive SCLE, sun avoidance between the hours of 10 a.m. to 4 p.m. may be necessary. Discoid skin lesions are difficult to treat. Hydroxychloroquine 5 mg/kg per day may be useful but requires careful ophthalmologic examination before and 1 month into therapy. The addition of quinacrine may also improve the response.

Children with multisystem disease require immunosuppressive therapy, which may also clear the skin. A variety of agents have been found to be effective with methotrexate, cyclophosphamide, glucocorticoids, mycophenolic acid, and anti-TNF biologics all being useful in some children with LE.

73

PAPULOSQUAMOUS ERUPTIONS

Darier's disease (keratosis follicularis)

DDx ref 69 • 67 • 23

CLINICAL FEATURES

Typical lesions of Darier's disease are skin-colored to red-brown keratotic 2–5-mm papules on the **face, neck, scalp, chest, back, and proximal extremities**. Lesions eventually coalesce to form large confluent crusted plaques. Flat-topped skin-colored papules are seen on the top of the **hands**, and punctuate tiny keratotic papules on the palms. Wedge-shaped nail dystrophy may occur. Severe pruritus, secondary infection with bacteria or herpes simplex virus, malodor, and heat and sun exposure aggravate the disease. Onset of disease is usually between **5 and 10 years of age** and worsens with adolescence. Autosomal dominant inheritance is associated with mutations in the ATP2A2 gene that encodes SERCA2 Ca^{2+} ATPase. Intellectual disability is frequently associated.

TREATMENT

Keeping the skin cool and using topical retinoids may be helpful in mild cases. Severe cases require oral retinoid therapy. Isotretinoin 0.25–1 mg/kg per day is very effective. Isotretinoin should be used only during periods of severe exacerbations to minimize the long-term side-effects. Oral antibiotics should be used for secondary bacterial infections. Intravenous or oral acyclovir is necessary to treat a widespread herpes simplex outbreak (Kaposi's varicelliform eruption).

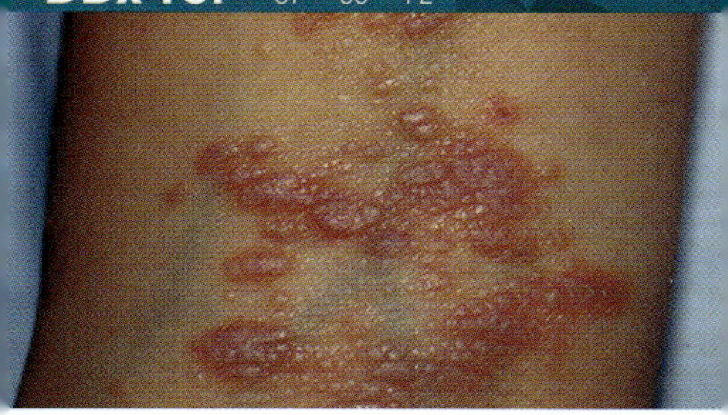

Itchy purple papules on wrist and forearm of a child with LP.

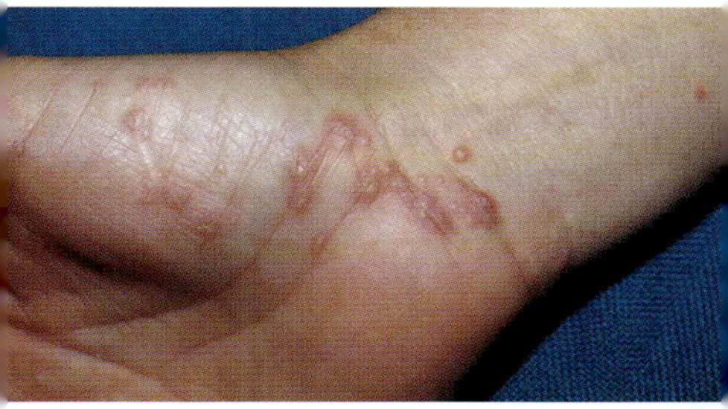

Itchy purple papules in a girl with LP.

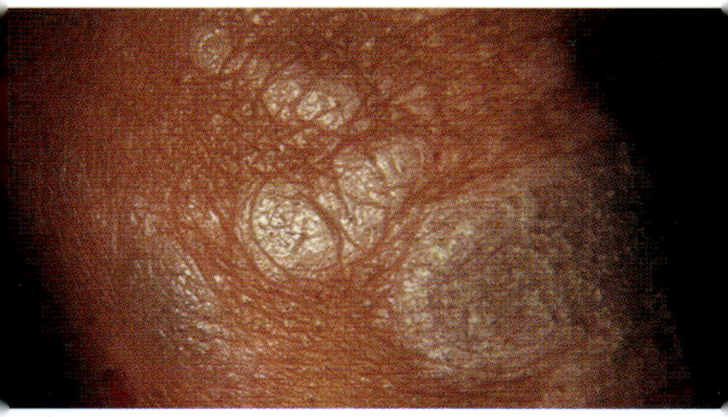

Purple papules and plaques with prominent scaling on the knee of a child with LP.

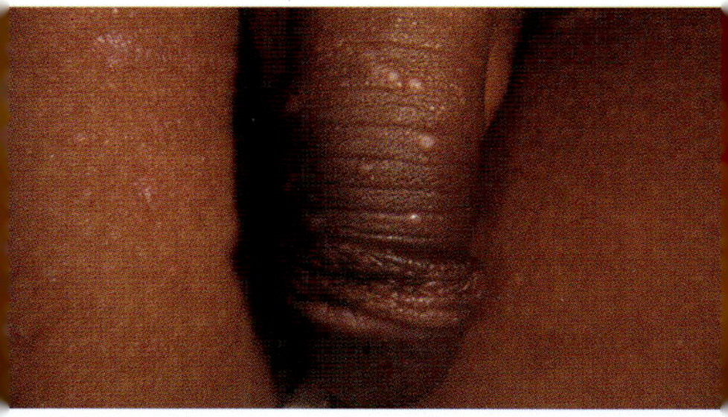

Flat-topped purple papules on the penis of a boy with LP.

CLINICAL FEATURES

The abrupt appearance of very itchy, flat-topped purple papules and plaques characterizes lichen planus. Papules frequently occur on the wrist and extensor surfaces of the extremities.

On the upper half of the body purple papules are not scaly but scale is prominent on the knees, lower legs, and feet. Involvement of the genitalia is common. The isomorphic (Koebner) phenomenon where LP lesions appear in sites of prior skin trauma is seen in LP as in psoriasis. Severe lesions may demonstrate bulla formation beneath the plaques. In contrast to many papulosquamous disorders, oral lesions are present in children with LP (15%). They appear as lacy white thickening of buccal mucosa and sometimes erosions of the sides of the tongue.

In the scalp scarring hair loss can uncommonly (8%) be found. Roughening of nail surfaces can sometimes be seen but severe nail changes are rare in childhood LP. The narrowed nail with medial fibrous bands or complete destruction and scarring are rare nail complications.

Roughening of the nails may precede, coincide with, or follow the development of skin lesions.

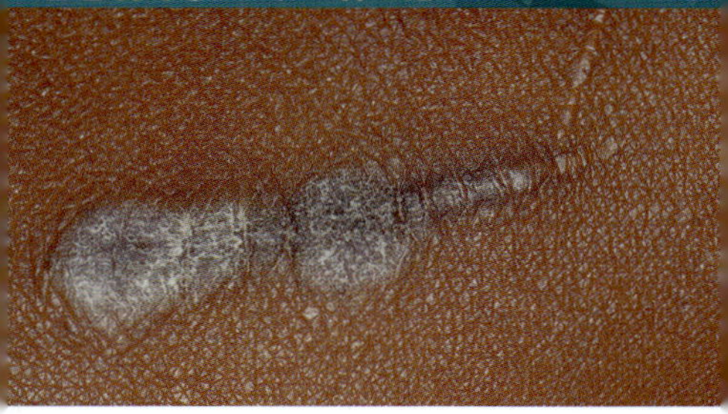

Isomorphic phenomenon in childhood LP. Linear LP in line of prior skin scratch.

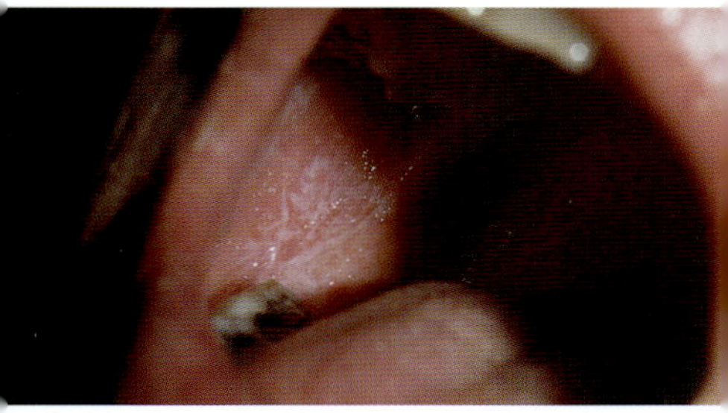

Oral involvement with asymptomatic lacy white thickening of buccal mucosa.

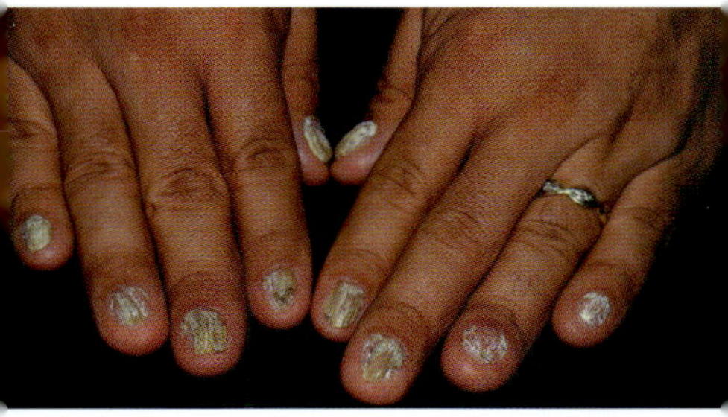

Thickening, narrowing, and crumbling of all 20 fingernails in a child with LP.

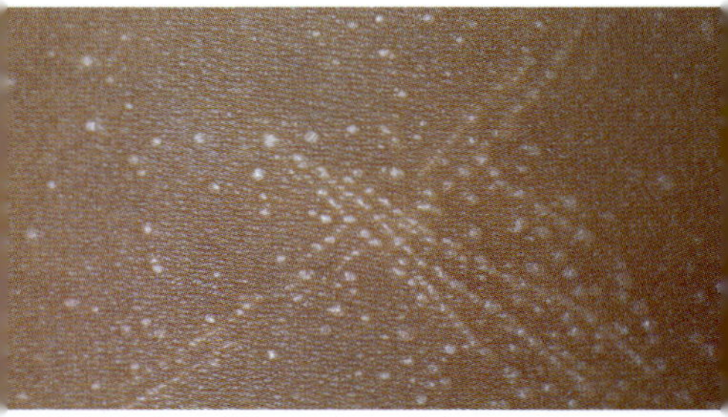

Multiple tiny white papules with isomorphic phenomenon in a child with lichen nitidus.

Lichen planus in some families has an autosomal dominant inheritance pattern. Often, the lesions are so clinically characteristic that the diagnosis is easy. In atypical cases, a skin biopsy may be diagnostic. Certain drug reactions associated with the use of hydrochlorothiazides, quinacrine, chloroquine, or gold can produce a lichen planus-like eruption. These drugs are rarely used in children.

A variant of **lichen planus** is **lichen nitidus** where flat-topped but tiny (<1 mm) papules appear suddenly. In contrast to the severe itching of LP, lichen nitidus usually does not itch. The isomorphic phenomenon is seen. Lichen nitidus has similar pathology to LP but papules are limited to one dermal papilla.

TREATMENT

Because the papules of LP are so itchy, potent topical steroid creams can be used twice daily for 4–8 weeks.

In widespread disease topical preparations may be impractical; oral prednisone 1–2 mg/kg per day may give relief within 2 weeks. Upon withdrawal, LP may recur. Acitretin has been successful in some children with severe LP.

Lichen nitidus can be cleared with super-potent topical steroids.

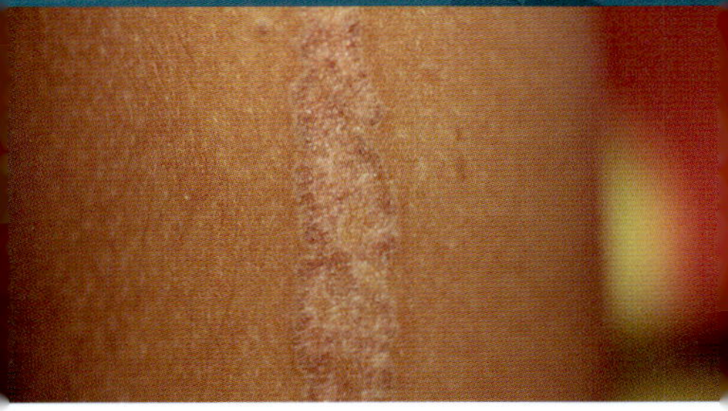

Porokeratosis of Mibelli. Linear scaly plaque with moat-like border in a 9-year-old child.

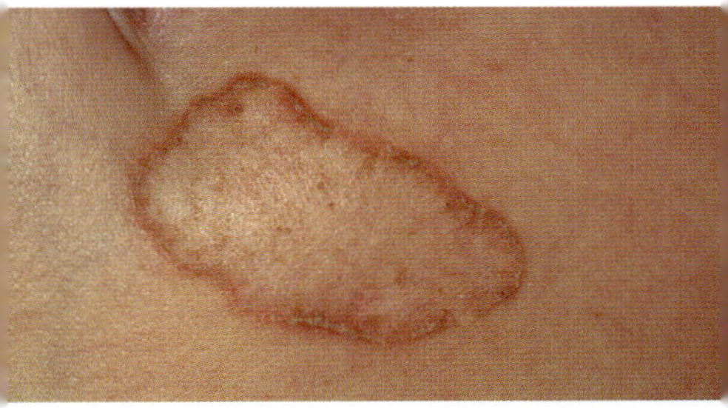

Porokeratosis of Mibelli on the cheek of a boy.

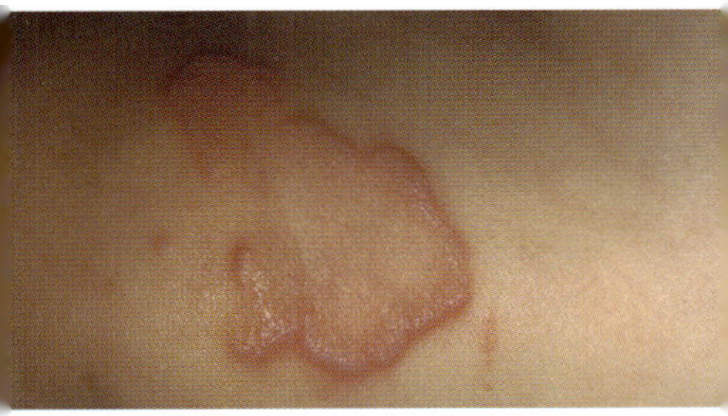

Porokeratosis on the knee of a child.

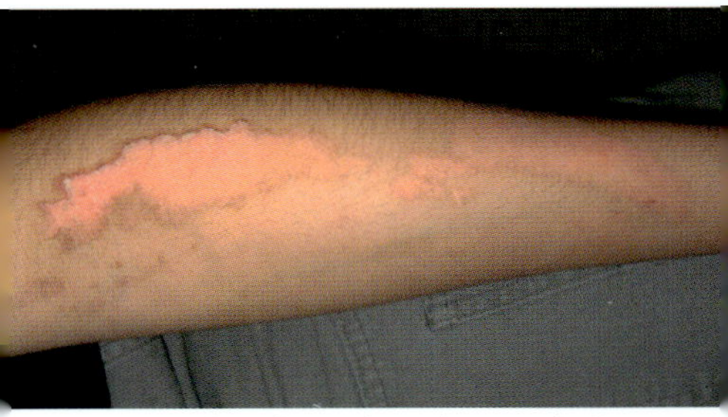

Large area of porokeratosis on the arm of a teen.

CLINICAL FEATURES

Porokeratosis of Mibelli is more common in males and begins in childhood. The primary lesion is a small keratotic papule that enlarges peripherally so that the center becomes depressed, with the edge forming an elevated wall. The central depressed area may be 5–50 mm in diameter and several craters may be present. The configuration of the plaque may be round, oval, or gyrate. The enclosed central area is yellow, gray, or tan, whereas the hyperkeratotic border is dark gray, brown, or black. The most important diagnostic feature of porokeratosis of Mibelli is the appearance of a scaly border in which a double row of scales surmounted by a furrow are observed.

Face, neck, forearms, and hands are commonly involved, but the **knees, buttocks, and feet** may occasionally be affected. Diagnosis is by biopsy of the raised border. Malignant degeneration to squamous cell carcinoma may be observed in long-standing cases. Lesions are usually asymptomatic.

TREATMENT

No treatment is uniformly successful. Liquid nitrogen, carbon dioxide laser, topical retinoids, 5-fluorouracil, imiquimod, salicylic acid, and calcipotriene have been employed with variable success.

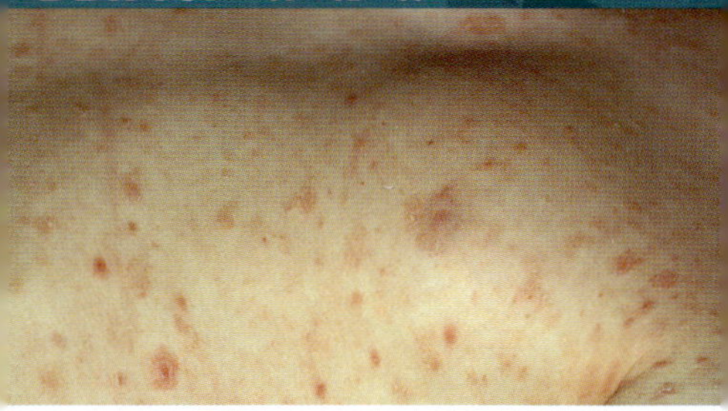

Pityriasis lichenoides acute lesions. Crusted, petechial papules on the trunk of a child.

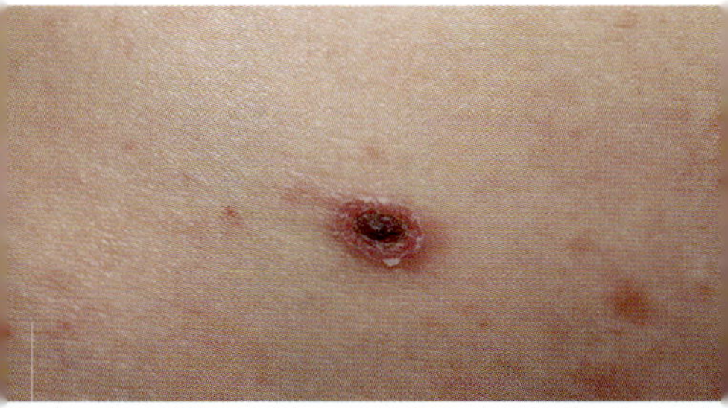

Pityriasis lichenoides acute lesion. Characteristic red papule with central crust.

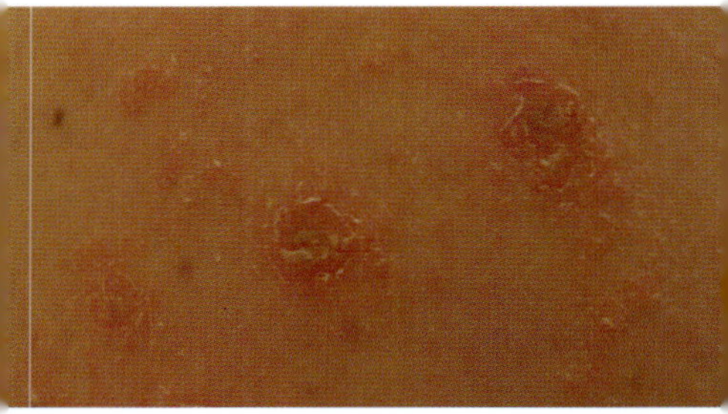

Pityriasis lichenoides. Discrete, oval salmon-colored papules with a thin scale.

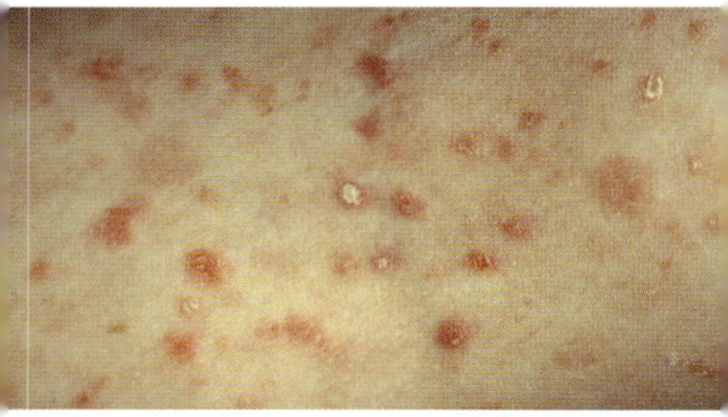

Both acute and chronic lesions on child with pityriasis lichenoides.

Pityriasis lichenoides

DDx ref 66 • 32 • 89

CLINICAL FEATURES

Pityriasis lichenoides has been given multiple names, but it is a single entity with a spectrum of clinical lesions from acute to chronic.

The acute lesions (pityriasis lichenoides et varioliformis acuta, PLEVA; Mucha–Habermann disease) are recurrent crops of red papules 2–4 mm in diameter. The papules have central petechiae and progress to crusting. Lesions of different stages are seen and predominate on the trunk. Individual lesions may last a few weeks. The lesions may heal with central scarring. The acute necrotic lesions may be slightly tender.

The chronic lesions (pityriasis lichenoides chronica, PLC) are salmon-colored oval papules with central clearing. They are fewer in number than acute lesions and individual lesions may last for months. Pruritus is uncommon. Both acute and chronic lesions may be simultaneously found in the same individual. The disease may last for 2–3 years. A very rare and severe acute febrile ulceronecrotic variant may be seen. The ulcerated plaques may be as large as 1 cm and occur on the trunk and upper arms. Arthritis may also be present. Lesions heal with scarring.

TREATMENT

Asymptomatic children with mostly chronic lesions may be treated with skin lubrication alone. Erythromycin, 30–50 mg/kg per day for 1–2 months, has been reported to be effective in some children. Natural sunlight may be of benefit. Narrowband ultraviolet B phototherapy is the treatment of choice for widespread symptomatic disease.

The ulceronecrotic form has been treated with systemic steroids, systemic immunosuppressives, anti-tumor necrosis factor, or anti-T-cell biologic response modifiers.

Dermatomyositis

DDx ref 67 • 72 • 74

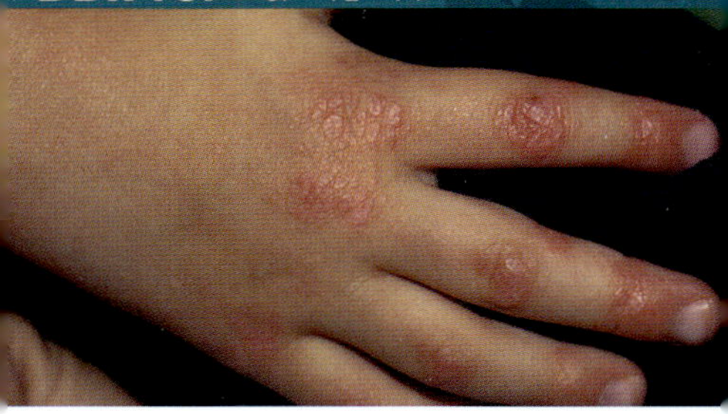

Gottron's papules in childhood dermatomyositis.

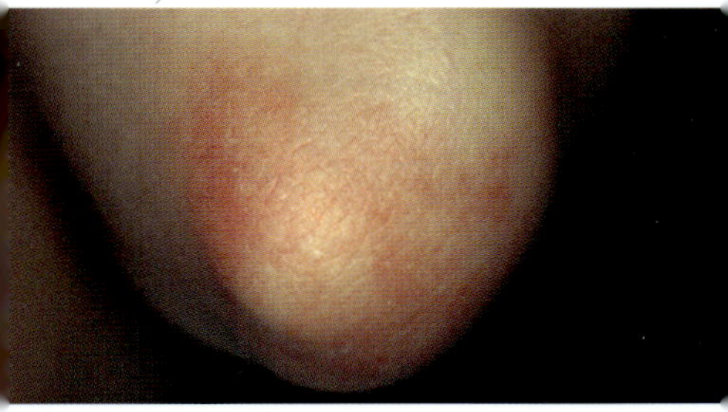

Dermatomyositis. Scaly, rosy-colored plaques over an elbow.

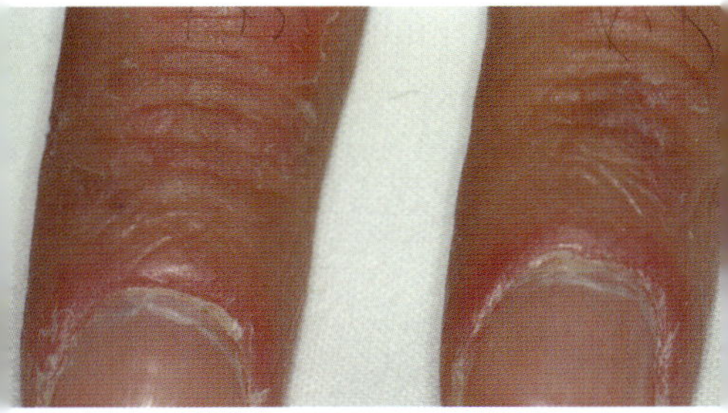

Cuticular telangiectasia in dermatomyositis in an adolescent male.

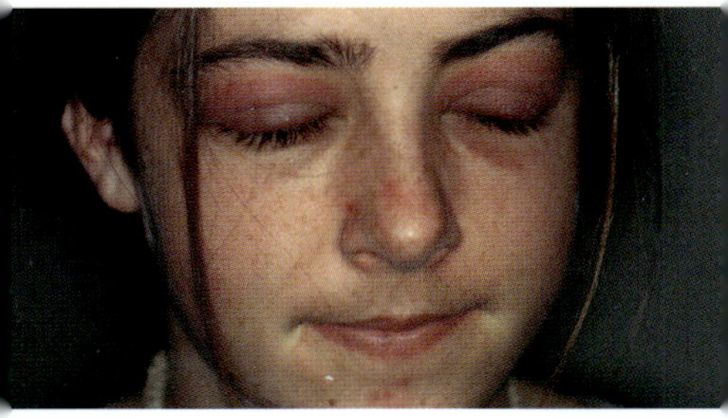

Dermatomyositis. Purple-red discoloration of the eyelids.

Dermatomyositis

DDx ref 67 • 72 • 74

CLINICAL FEATURES

The most common presenting signs in juvenile dermatomyositis are flat-topped purple-red papules over the knuckles (Gottron's papules), a scaly rash over the elbows and knees, periungual erythema and telangiectasia, periorbital edema with a violaceous hue of the eyelids (heliotrope), and malar erythema. A livedo reticularis pattern on the legs may be prominent.

The skin signs may precede, occur simultaneously with, or follow the onset of the muscle weakness. Rarely, minimal or no muscle disease develops.

Children may present with chronic fever, malaise, and anorexia. Proximal muscle weakness with or without pain is most frequently seen. Calcinosis of the skin and muscle develops late in the course of the disease and can be debilitating.

Juvenile dermatomyositis is an autoimmune disease. Both myositis-associated and myositis-specific autoantibodies occur. Diagnosis is clinical and supported by histology of the skin lesions, elevated muscle enzymes, muscle inflammation on magnetic resonance imaging, and abnormal electromyography.

TREATMENT

Systemic steroids, either pulsed, high-dose intravenous, or chronic oral therapy along with weekly methotrexate as a steroid sparing drug, is the primary treatment. Hydroxychloroquine is also often used. Other medications for severe unresponsive disease include intravenous immunoglobulin, mycophenolate mofetil, cyclosporin, cyclophosphamide, and rituximab.

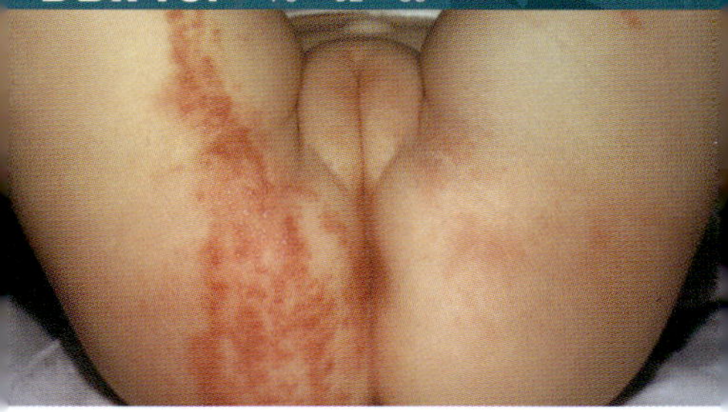

Lichen striatus covering a large portion of a buttock and extending down the leg.

Hypopigmented residual macules in resolving lichen striatus.

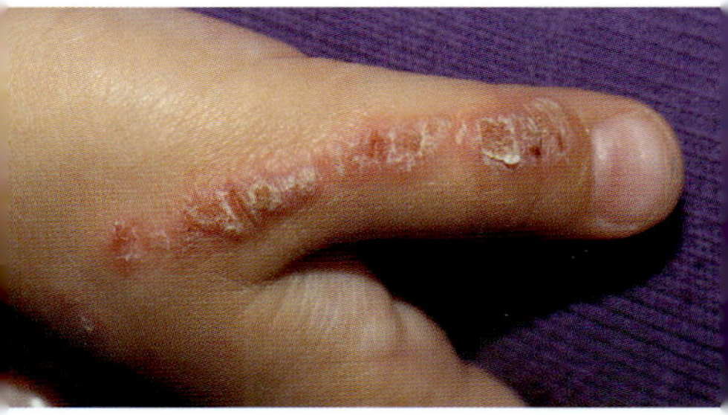

Lichen striatus extending down a digit without nail dystrophy.

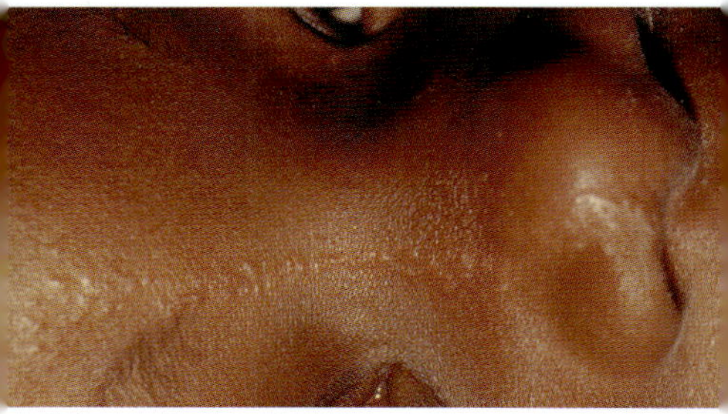

Lichen striatus on the face.

Lichen striatus

DDx ref 75 • 92 • 80

CLINICAL FEATURES

Lichen striatus is a benign, self-limited eruption, consisting of asymmetrical distribution of continuous or discontinuous band(s) of papules following Blaschko's lines.

Blaschko's lines are the curvilinear lines of skin development. Lesions may vary from small hypopigmented papules to very thick lichenified plaques. They characteristically occur on an extremity, but can also involve the face or trunk. If they involve a **digit**, nail dystrophy may be present. It is seen most commonly in the preschool child. Remission in 6–12 months is expected. Most lesions are asymptomatic, but pruritus may occur.

TREATMENT

No treatment hastens resolution. Medium-potency topical steroids may help the pruritus.

Atopic dermatitis (AD)

DDx ref 70 • 71 • 80

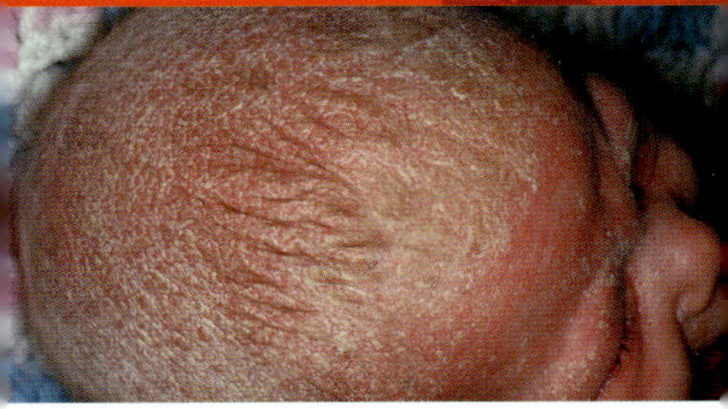

Onset of AD in an infant with a red scaly scalp.

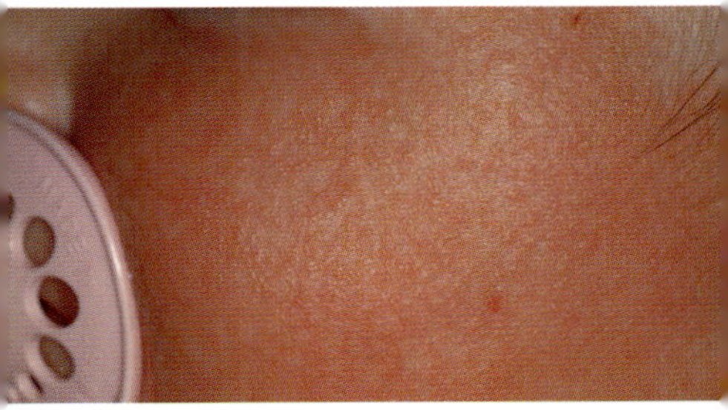

Early redness, fine scale and dryness to cheeks in a baby with AD.

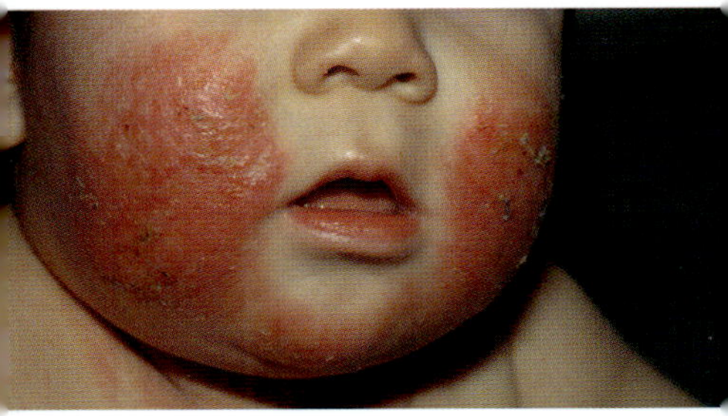

Red, oozing and crusting cheeks of an infant with AD.

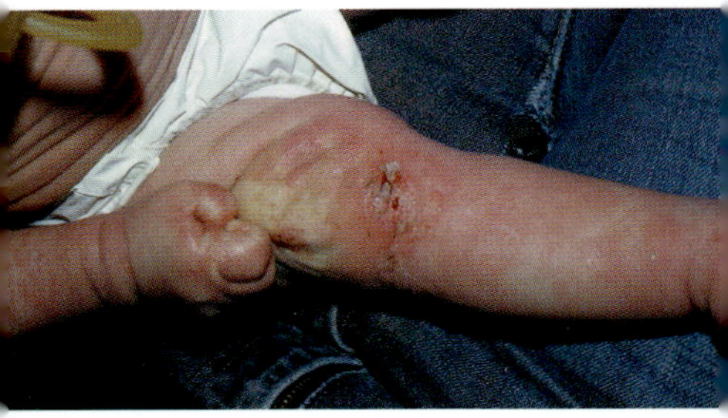

Scratching frenzy in a toddler with AD.

79 Atopic dermatitis (AD)

DDx ref 70 • 71 • 80

CLINICAL FEATURES

The terms 'dermatitis' and 'eczema' are used interchangeably, although eczema was originally used to designate blistering disease. Dermatitis implies inflammation of dermis but eczematous eruptions also have major epidermal involvement with disruption of the skin surface as a major feature. The disruption can be seen clinically as crusting, weeping, scaling, excoriation or fissures, and microscopically as breaks in the epidermal barrier.

Atopic dermatitis is the most common form of childhood dermatitis and affects up to 20% of children. It is inherited, and recent genetic evidence links AD to loss of function polymorphisms or mutations in the filaggrin genes responsible for the integrity of the outer epidermis. This explains the link between **ichthyosis vulgaris** (see DDx ref 70 Ichthyosis) and AD. Functional abnormalities of other epidermal outer envelope genes such as SPINK5 in **Netherton's syndrome** (see DDx ref 70 Ichthyosis) lead to a severe defect in the epidermal barrier and severe AD. The abnormal formation of the epidermal barrier explains the constant finding of dry skin among children with AD.

The first sign of AD is dry skin in the **newborn period**.

In addition to the presence of dry skin, the cardinal signs of AD are onset under 2 years of age, presence of red, disrupted, sensitive skin, and flexural distribution of skin lesions. There has long been a postulated link between AD and asthma or allergic rhinitis. The filaggrin changes also extend to abnormal **nasal mucosal surface and respiratory mucosa**. AD is an inflammatory disease that develops from the outside in because of a faulty epidermal barrier. It is not, as many once believed, due to food allergy.

There are a number of features of AD once thought to be diagnostic, including facial pallor, Denny's wrinkle lines on lower eyelids, intolerance to wool clothing, cataracts, elevated serum IgE levels, and blood eosinophilia. These changes are present sometimes but many children with AD have none of these findings.

Following the dry skin of the newborn period, the first signs of red, itchy skin occur within the **first 6 months**. The pattern is redness, scaling and crusting of the **scalp and face** plus redness on the extensor surface of the extremities.

These changes mimic seborrheic dermatitis. Indeed, many infants diagnosed as seborrheic dermatitis are rediagnosed as AD as the distribution of skin involvement changes. The distribution of the dermatitis changes with age with predominantly flexural changes appearing first in **toddlers**.

The **antecubital** and **popliteal fossae** and the **neck** are the major sites of involvement. As **teen** years approach, flexural involvement spreads to include the **hands and feet**. Itching occurs in paroxysms in AD and the child may have scratching frenzies. Many of the skin changes seen in the itchy child are the result of constant rubbing and scratching of itchy skin seen as lichenification. Lichenification is associated with hypertrophic epidermis that is often hyperpigmented.

ECZEMATOUS DISORDERS (RED WITH DISRUPTION OF SKIN SURFACE)

Atopic dermatitis (AD)

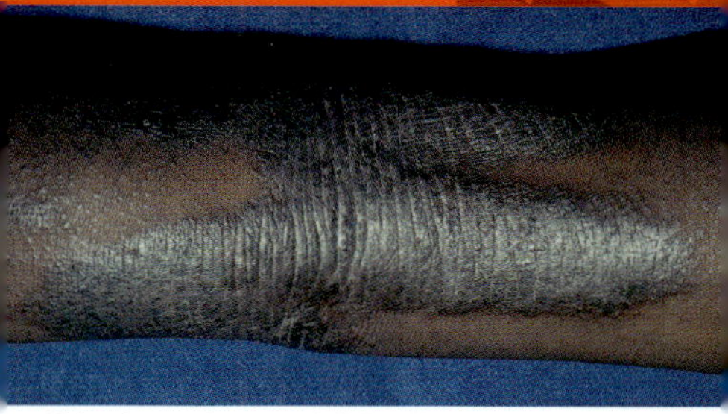

Shiny hyperpigmented, lichenified skin in antecubital fossa of a preteen girl.

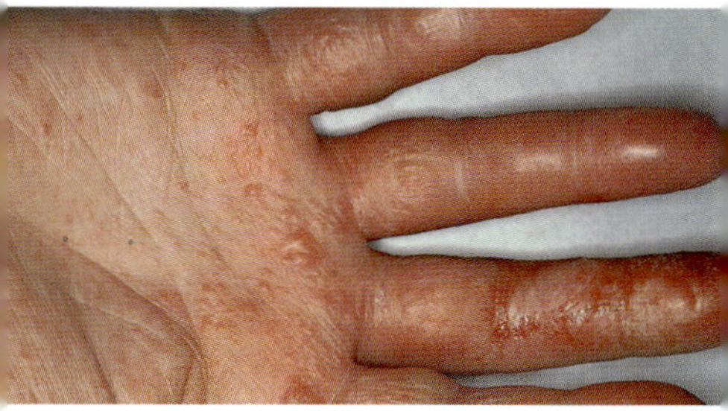

Vesicles and redness of fingers and palm of a preteen with AD.

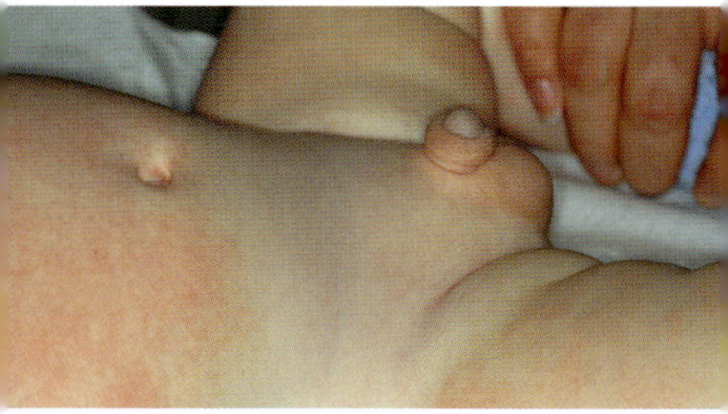

Mild redness and scale of skin, except in the area protected by a diaper, in AD.

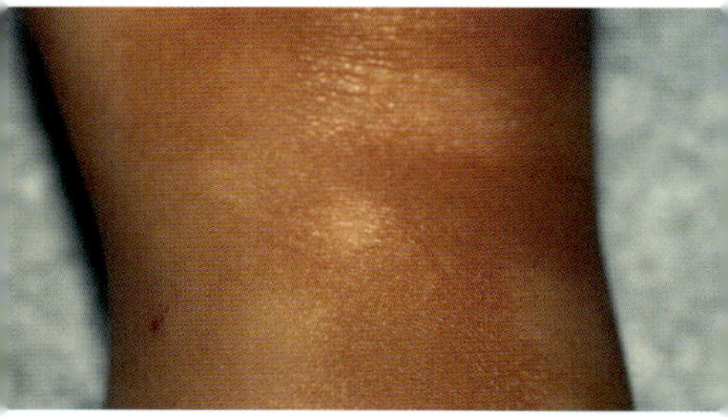

Hypopigmented scaly areas in AD (pityriasis alba).

A shiny skin surface and prominent skin lines are seen in lichenification.

Deep scratching to painful bleeding results in temporary relief from itchiness as pain signals predominate. This leaves the skin with excoriations that may heal with scars.

Chronic mild inflammation may interfere with transfer of pigment from melanocytes to epidermal cells and result in a pale patch with central redness. This is designated pityriasis alba. Thus AD can be both hyperpigmented and hypopigmented. A few untreated children will develop more generalized disease and present with exfoliative erythroderma.

The child with AD is susceptible to bacterial and viral infection secondary to the dermatitis. There is a decrease of epidermal antimicrobial proteins in AD. Three infectious conditions predominate. ***Staphylococcus aureus*** (see DDx ref 28 Furunculosis and Cellulitis) and ***Streptococcus*** (see DDx ref 28 Furunculosis and Cellulitis) produce pustules with moist crusts and regional lymphadenopathy.

Herpes simplex virus produces widespread grouped and satellite vesicles and erosions (eczema herpeticum) (see DDx ref 1 Herpes Simplex). Both may induce fever. Both conditions are usually acquired from an affected family member or close contact.

There are a number of factors that worsen the sensitive skin of AD. These include excessive **drying of skin** as seen in prolonged bathing and excessive soaping.

Sweating aggravates AD and most children are heat intolerant.

Irritating substances applied to the skin surface often induce dermatitis.

Stress and anxiety undoubtedly make the rubbing and scratching worse. It is useful to review the skin care and bathing practices used for the child and determine who is responsible for treatments.

TREATMENT

Care of the child with AD is frustrating as it is a chronic condition that requires consistent daily skin care. Reducing bathing frequency and duration plus twice-daily application of lubricating ointments or creams are the mainstays of long-term therapy.

For red itchy skin the first-line approach should be moderate-potency topical steroid ointments or creams.

Begin with **fluocinolone, mometasone, or triamcinolone** ointment or cream applied twice daily for 2–4 weeks. The amount to apply can be determined by the fingertip unit (FTU). One FTU covers an area of skin covered by two adult palms.

Lichenified skin areas may require longer treatments of 6 weeks to several months. Lower potency topical steroid ointments or creams may be substituted as the lesions heal. Topical tacrolimus may also be used, but it has a black box warning and is not approved for children under 2 years of age.

Atopic dermatitis (AD)

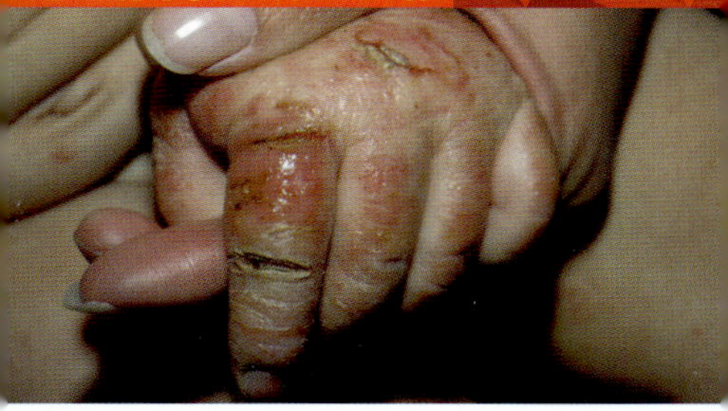

Fissures in skin permit bacterial invasion in AD.

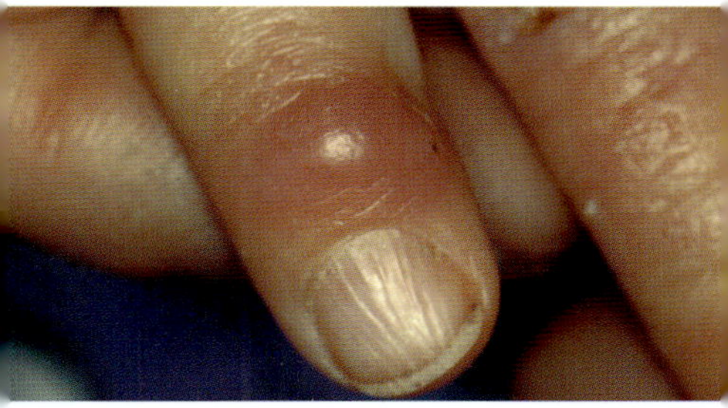

Staphylococcal furuncle on the finger of a child with AD.

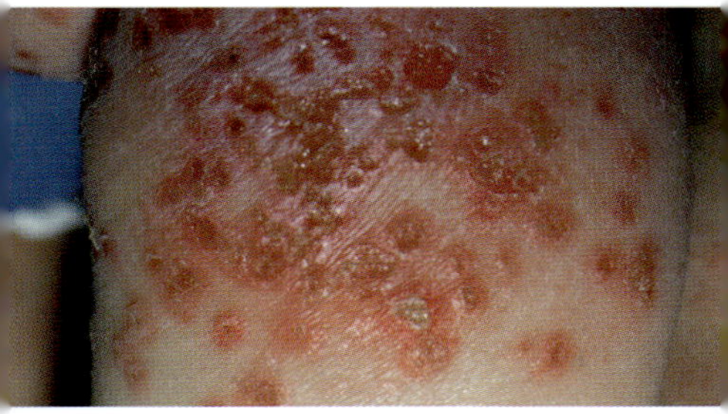

Vesicles and erosions of HSV infecting AD (eczema herpeticum).

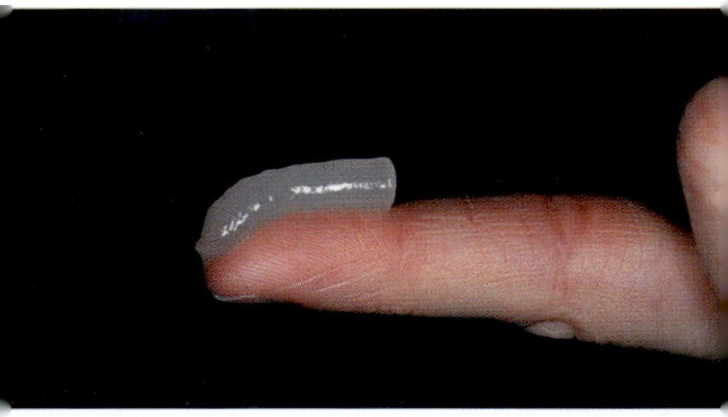

Fingertip unit. Amount of ointment or cream from the distal finger crease to the tip.

Topical pimecrolimus cream equals 2.5% hydrocortisone and can be especially useful in areas of thin skin such as the **face, axillae, or groin** where topical steroids may induce thinning of skin or striae. The ultimate therapeutic goal is to wean the child off topical steroids and substitute with twice-daily lubrications.

Relief of itching If itching is significant, the use of oral antihistamines can be most helpful. A strategy of cetirizine 2.5–10 mg in the morning plus hydroxyzine 1 mg/kg in a single evening dose can be most effective.

Wet dressings For the severely itchy and generally red child, the proper use of wet dressings can provide dramatic relief. The concept is to maintain a **damp skin surface** with the cooling sensation provided by constant evaporation from the skin surface. Thus, temperature-dependent skin sensory nerve signals obfuscate itch nerve signals.

Wet dressings are accomplished by wetting a pair of cotton pajamas and then wringing out until damp. A steroid cream or ointment then can be applied. The child puts on the damp pajamas and covers them with a second dry pair of pajamas. Airtight occlusion must be avoided as evaporation must occur for this to be effective. Thus, no tight bandages or plastic wraps should be used. The clothing is removed after **8 hours**, and the steroid reapplied, the damp dressings restored to initial dampness, and the dry pair reapplied over the damp pair. Wet dressings can be done at home overnight for **3–5 consecutive nights or every 8 hours** at home or in the hospital. Relief of itching is dramatic and limiting access to the skin reduces lichenification and excoriations.

ANTIMICROBIAL TREATMENTS

For bacterial infections cephalexin 25–50 mg/kg per day twice a day for 10–14 days or dicloxacillin 12–25 mg/kg per day for 10–14 days are useful. MRSA may be recovered, but the above antibiotics may clear the infection. Bleach baths once or twice a week are helpful in minimizing recurrence in the child with frequent *Staph. aureus* infection.

Acyclovir 20 mg/kg per day given orally can be most effective in eczema herpeticum. A few affected children may be severely ill and require hospitalization for IV acyclovir and fever control.

Severe disease Children that have been appropriately treated with standard topical steroids, antihistamines, and lubrication and still have severe disease should be referred to a specialist for consideration of narrow band UVB treatment or systemic therapy with an immunosuppressive agent such as methotrexate, mycophenolate mofetil, azathioprine, or cyclosporine.

ECZEMATOUS DISORDERS (RED WITH DISRUPTION OF SKIN SURFACE)

Allergic contact dermatitis (ACD)

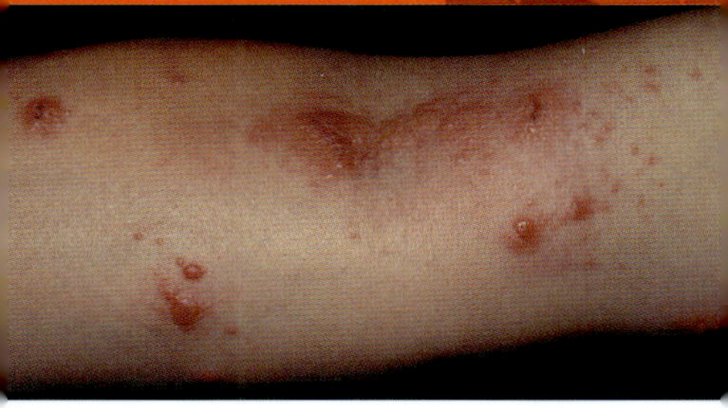

Blistering acute allergic contact dermatitis to poison oak.

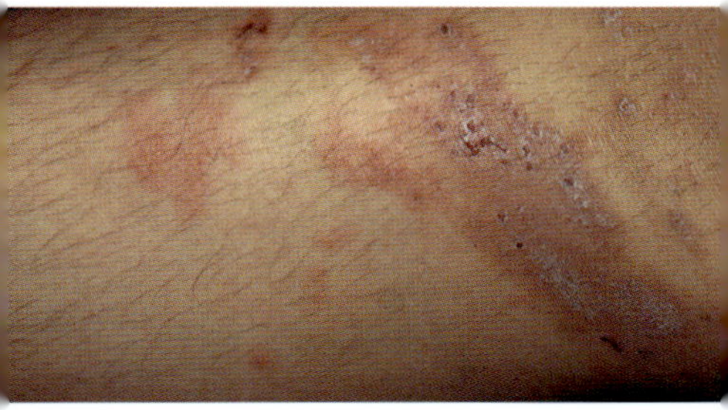

Linear blisters in a teen exposed to poison ivy.

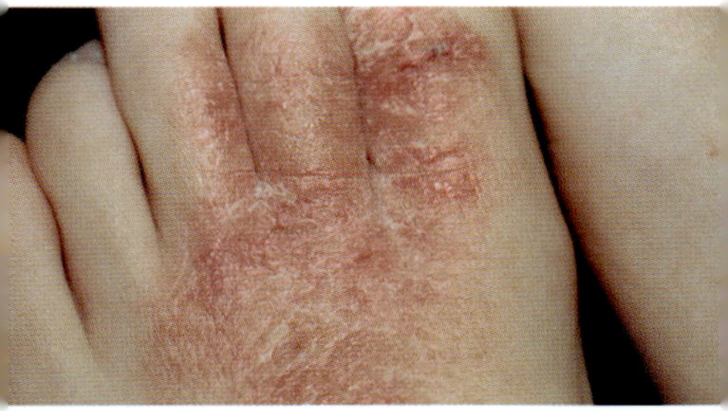

Chronic ACD on tops of the feet due to leather shoes (potassium dichromate).

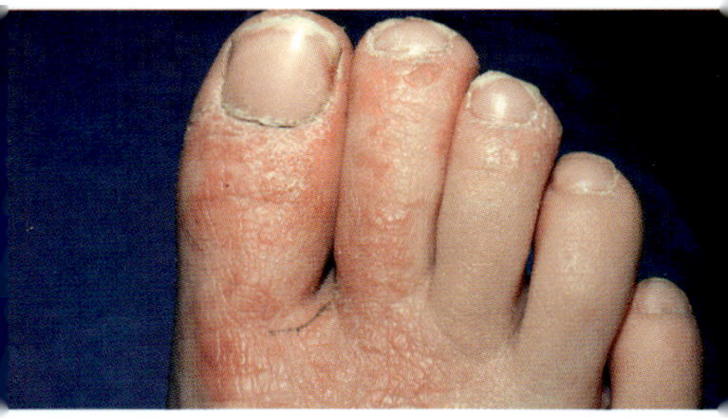

Chronic lichenified ACD on tops of the toes due to shoes (rubber additives).

CLINICAL FEATURES

ACD is a form of T-lymphocyte-mediated immunity, dependent upon allergens that can penetrate intact skin. ACD is common in childhood. By age **5 years**, 10–20% of children have been sensitized to a contact antigen. ACD presents as **blisters and red skin** in patterns determined by the site of contact, especially in **plant dermatitis** where the stem or leaf of poison ivy, sumac, or oak contacts the skin.

In acute blistering ACD the onset follows 8–48 hours after exposure to the plant. In contrast, contact dermatitis to weaker allergens requires repeated contact over weeks to months and presents as red, lichenified, and scaly skin, a **chronic ACD**. Once the dermatitis develops, it persists **3–4 weeks** even when there is no further exposure to the allergen. The distribution of the ACD may provide important clues to the causative allergen. For example, there may be dermatitis limited to the tops of the feet in shoe dermatitis, to the subumbilical skin in nickel allergy from metal snaps on pants or the earlobes in nickel allergy to earrings, on the eyelids and face in cosmetic allergy, in the axilla from deodorants, or on the perioral skin from toothpaste or lip balms.

MOST PREVALENT ALLERGENS IN CHILDHOOD

Plants Poison ivy, oak, sumac.
Metals Nickel, cobalt, gold.
Neomycin and/or bacitracin Antibiotics.
Potassium dichromate Leathers.
Thimerosal Preservative.
Balsam of peru Fragrance.
Formaldehyde, quaterniumn-15 Preservatives in cosmetic products and clothing.
Lanolin Moisturizers.

If there is repeated exposure to the allergen, the dermatitis can spread to **unexposed areas in the so-called id reaction**. ACD occurs in two distinct but interrelated phases. **The sensitization phase** develops upon first exposure to the allergen and requires 5–7 days for processing of the allergen by epidermal Langerhans cells that then carry the antigen to regional lymph nodes for T-lymphocyte sensitization and proliferation. The sensitized lymphocytes enter the circulation and home back to the skin. On the subsequent exposures to the allergen, **the elicitation phase**, T lymphocytes are activated in the skin by the allergen and release inflammatory mediators.

ECZEMATOUS DISORDERS (RED WITH DISRUPTION OF SKIN SURFACE)

Allergic contact dermatitis (ACD)

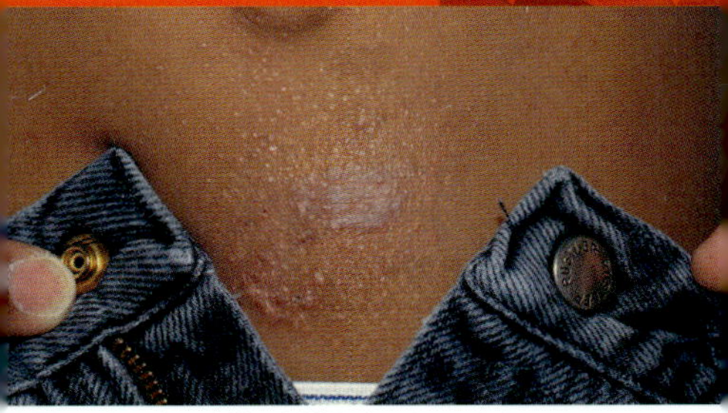

Chronic subumbilical ACD due to metal snaps on pants (nickel).

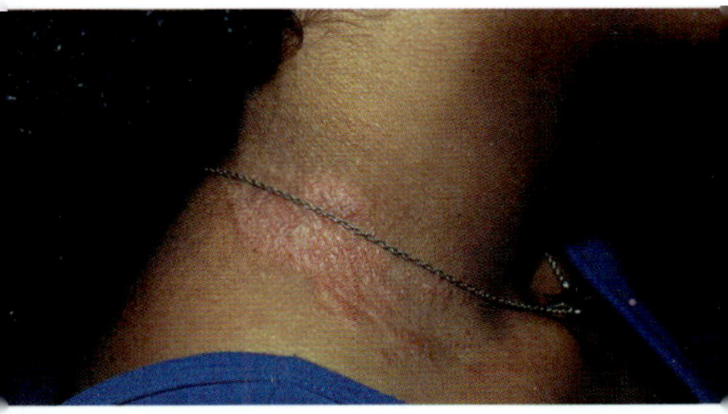

Chronic dermatitis on the neck due to a metal necklace (nickel).

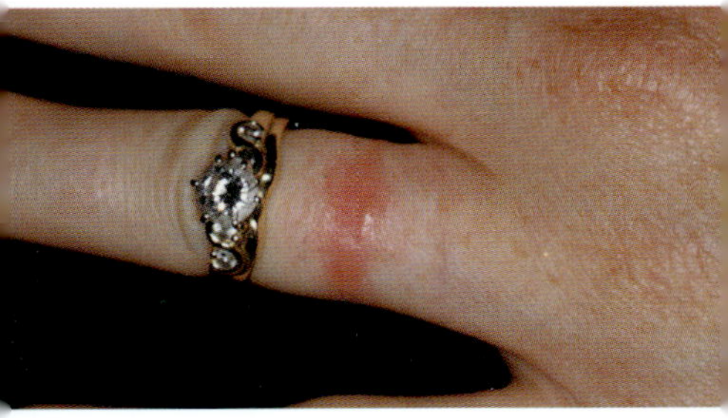

Nickel allergy due to a metal ring.

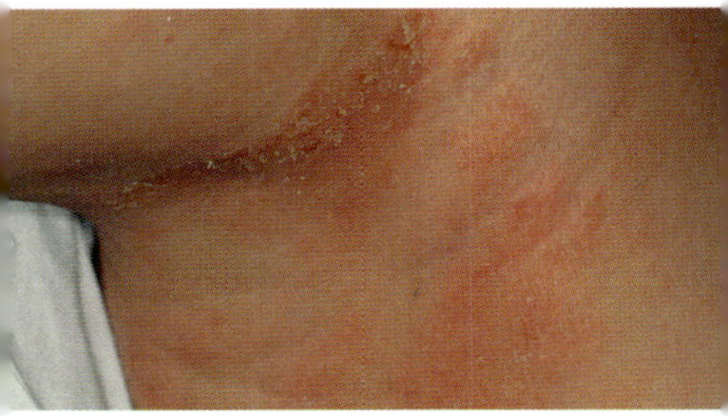

Axillary ACD due to deodorant allergy (formaldehyde).

Treatment If less than 10% of the body is involved, then moderate-potency steroid creams or ointments applied twice daily for 10–14 days will clear the lesions. If lichenified, treatment for 6–8 weeks may be required.

With greater body involvement oral prednisone 1 mg/kg per day for 7–14 days may be required. To identify the cause in chronic ACD, patch testing with the suspected allergen can result in reproduction of the dermatitis, but should be delayed for 3–4 weeks after the dermatitis has improved or cleared.

For acute blistering ACD testing to suspected plants is not indicated, as it might induce a new dermatitis or sensitize a child previously not allergic.

Allergen avoidance is critical, as the allergic sensitivity is long lived, up to 30 years. The history of suspected allergen contact will help guide which allergens to avoid. When the possible allergens are uncertain, patch testing will help pinpoint the allergen(s).

Patch testing reproduces the pathology of ACD by applying the suspected antigens to the skin of the upper back for 48 hours. Antigen concentrations, testing materials, and interpretation of skin reactions have been standardized. Patch testing is useful when the pattern of skin reaction is not predictive. Testing to plant antigens should not be done because of severe reactions. Obvious patterns such as nickel allergy and deodorant allergy do not require patch testing.

ECZEMATOUS DISORDERS (RED WITH DISRUPTION OF SKIN SURFACE)

Diaper dermatitis

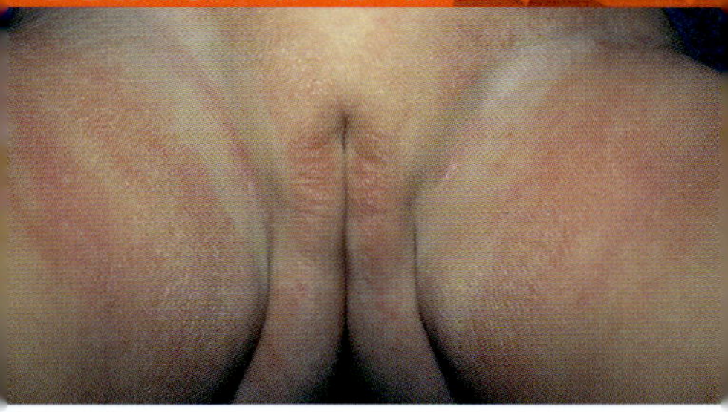

Chafing form of diaper dermatitis in a 9-month-old infant.

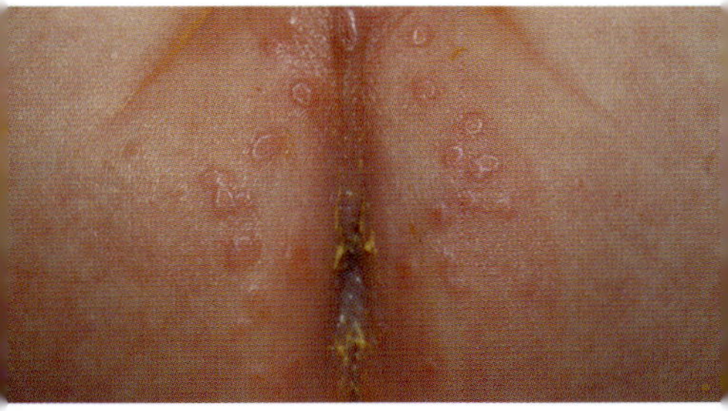

Perianal form of diaper rash secondary to diarrhea.

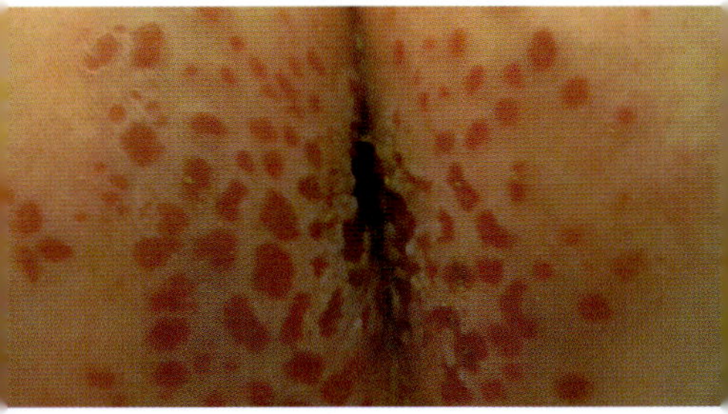

Discrete shallow ulcerative form of diaper dermatitis.

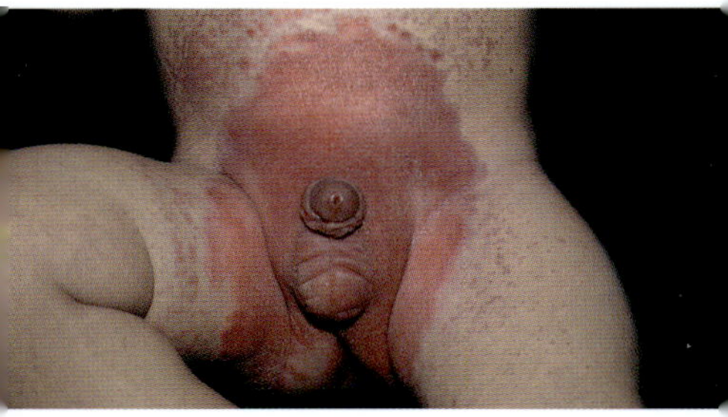

Confluent redness with satellite papules and pustules in diaper rash with *C. albicans* infection.

CLINICAL FEATURES

A rash limited to skin under the diaper is the most common form of childhood irritant contact dermatitis. Some 20% of children will develop some diaper dermatitis during their diaper-wearing years. Four clinical patterns are observed.

The most frequent is **chafing dermatitis** that occurs on the convex surface of the thighs, the buttocks, and the waist areas. It usually begins at 7–12 months of age when the baby's volume of a single urination exceeds diaper capacity.

In the second form the dermatitis is limited to the **perianal skin**.

This pattern is seen with loose stools of newborns or a child who develops diarrhea.

The third form is characterized by discrete shallow ulcerations scattered throughout the diaper area, especially the genitalia.

The final form is seen as beefy-red confluent areas in the inguinal creases and on the genitalia, with satellite oval papules. This is found with ***Candida albicans*** invasion. Any diaper dermatitis that has been present longer than 72 hours is likely to have *C. albicans* superinfection even without the classic pattern with satellite lesions.

Langerhans cell histiocytosis mimics the inguinal crease candidiasis, **psoriasis** mimics candidal infections and **streptococcal perianal cellulitis** mimics perianal diaper dermatitis.

Diaper dermatitis is the result of prolonged contact of urine or feces with skin. Airtight occlusion with plastic diaper covers exaggerates the macerated skin. Frequently, the 'good' baby that sleeps 10–12 hours at night will develop diaper dermatitis, despite having frequent diaper changes during the day. **Overwashing or oversoaping** the diaper area may prolong the rash. A history of diaper change and care routine may be most informative.

TREATMENT

Changing the diaper frequently and removing urine or feces is helpful especially when a change 2 or 3 hours after sleeping is included.

Restricting fluid intake at night just prior to sleep will also reduce the likelihood of prolonged contact with urine. Zinc oxide-containing ointments or pastes applied to the diaper skin after cleansing and drying the skin will help.

Any diaper rash present for more than 72 hours should be treated for *C. albicans* with a topical anti-yeast cream such as nystatin or one of the imidazole creams such as clotrimazole. Topical steroid creams need not be used because of the tendency to produce striae and granuloma gluteale infantum. Frustrated caregivers should be reminded that diaper rash will persist in the baby with diarrhea as long as the diarrhea lasts and that **toilet training** is the ultimate cure.

Intertrigo

81 • 83 • 84

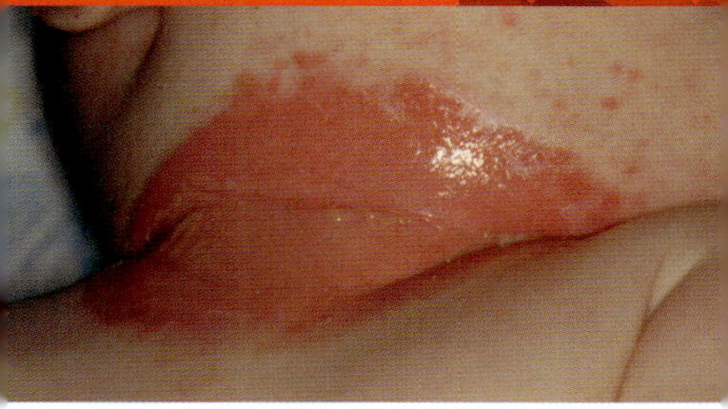

Red, oozing neck skin in a chubby baby with streptococcal intertrigo.

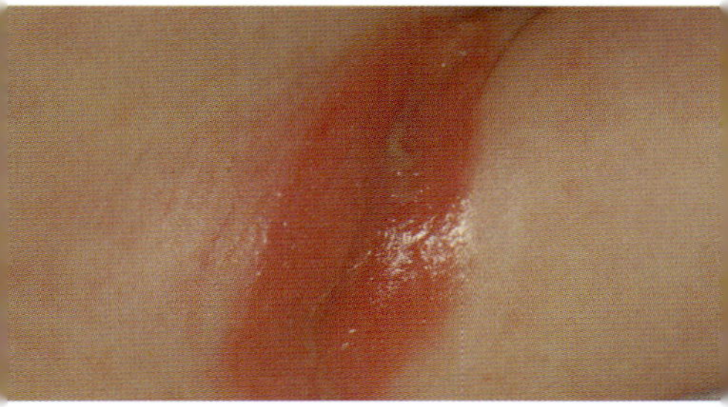

Red, oozing skin of popliteal fossa in an overweight infant with streptococcal intertrigo.

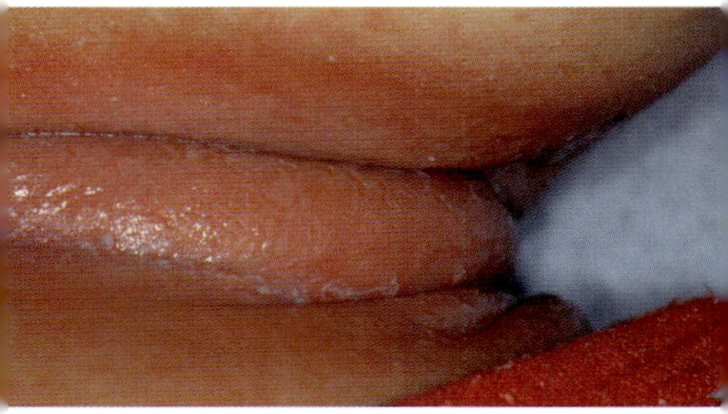

Candidal intertrigo of an infant's neck creases.

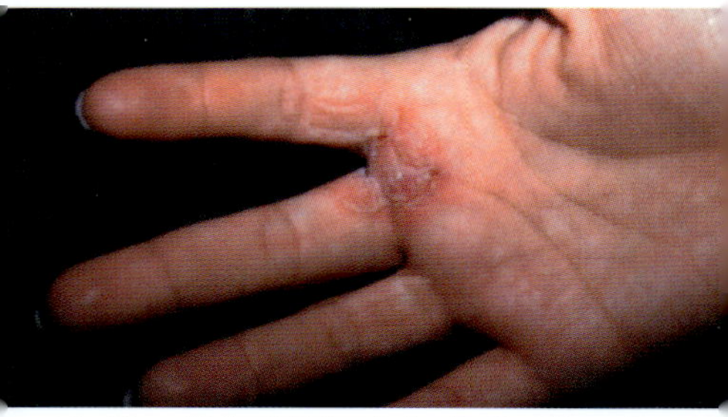

Intertrigo of interdigital web due to *C. albicans* in a teen doing wet work.

82 Intertrigo

DDx ref 81 • 83 • 84

CLINICAL FEATURES

Intertrigo describes redness and oozing in skin folds. The **inguinal area** is usually involved but the **neck, axilla, and interdigital webs** can be involved.

Both bacteria and yeast can produce identical clinical patterns of intertrigo. ***Streptococcus*, *Staphylococcus*, and *C. albicans* infections** are mostly responsible. Prolonged airtight occlusion and wetness predispose to intertrigo.

The chubby baby, or overweight child, or the child who has hands or feet in water for a prolonged time is susceptible to developing intertrigo. The presence of satellite pustules may be a clue to *C. albicans* and the presence of impetigo or ecthyma are clues to bacterial impetigo. A rapid strep test or bacterial culture may help differentiate. Lesions are so inflamed that microscopic examination of skin scrapings for bacteria and yeast are obscured.

TREATMENT

Once infection is established, antimicrobials must be used to clear the condition.

For bacterial intertrigo oral dicloxacillin 15–50 mg/kg per day or oral cephalexin 50–100 mg per day for 10 days may be used. Topical mupirocin for 5 days may also be considered.

For *C. albicans* topical nystatin or an imidazole cream such as clotrimazole cream twice daily may be used for 5–10 days. There is usually no need for oral anti-yeast agents.

Candidiasis

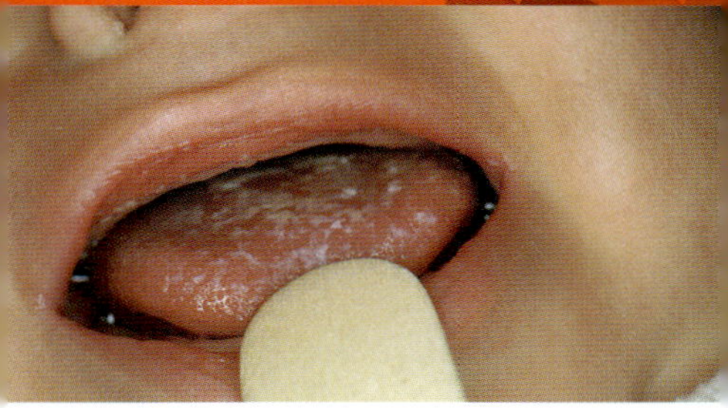

White patches on the tongue in an infant with thrush.

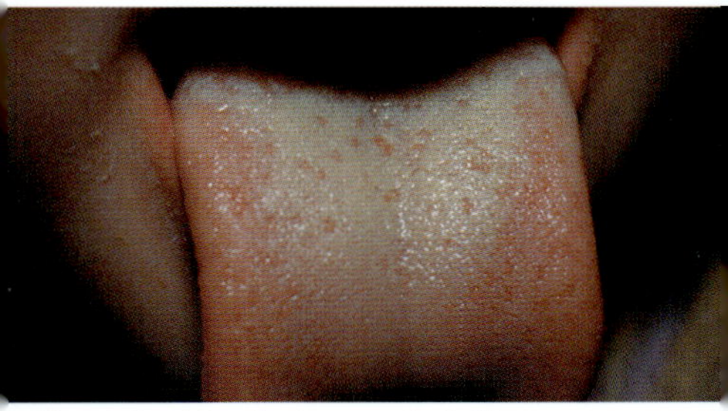

Thrush involving the tongue of a toddler.

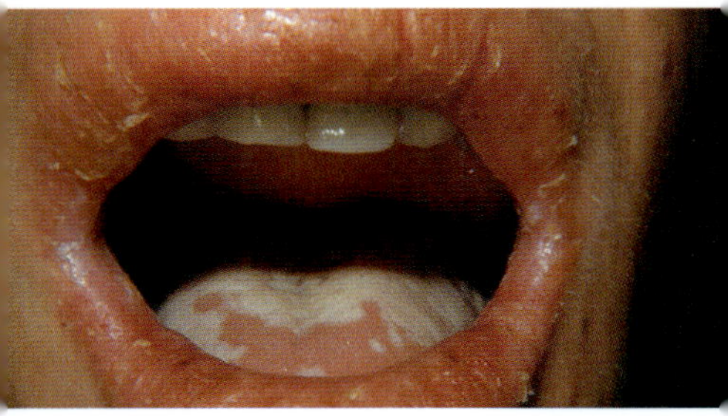

Mucocutaneous candidiasis in immune deficiency. White coated tongue; dry, fissured lips.

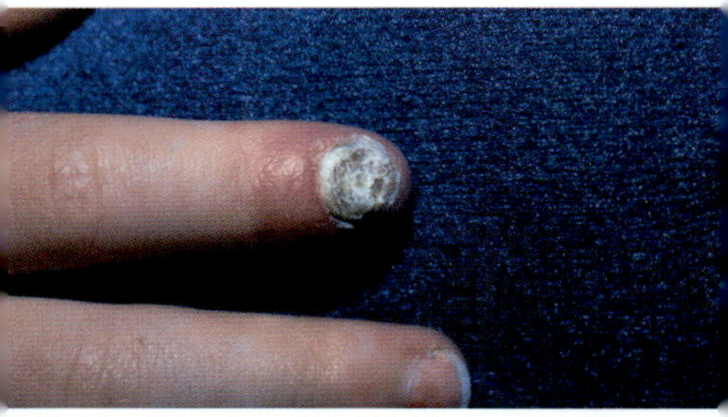

Non-tender, red, swollen distal finger with white crumbly nail in a fingersucker with *Candida* paronychia.

Candidiasis

DDx ref 81 • 82 • 90

CLINICAL FEATURES

In macerated skin, *C. albicans* may invade to establish infection. In different body regions, distinct clinical features are found.

In newborns and infants, white plaques on a red base are seen in the oral cavity, especially the buccal mucosa (thrush). Use of a pacifier may be permissive for oral candidiasis.

In the immunosuppressed or immunodeficient child, the tongue and lips may also be involved. Involvement of the angles of the lips is common (angular cheilitis). *Candida* can invade the skin folds, producing **intertrigo** or **superinfection of diaper dermatitis**. The appearance of satellite red papules or pustules may be a useful clue. Paronychia with red painless swelling of the skin around a thumbnail or fingernail is a common result of thumbsucking.

Congenital candidiasis, which is quite rare, is acquired in utero and presents with red, scaling skin with scattered pustules at birth.

Vulvovaginal candidiasis presents as a thick white discharge with red mucosa. It is seen predominantly in teenage females.

Candidal granulomas are oval red plaques with a thick yellow crust seen on the head and neck of children with defective host defenses. They are accompanied by persistent thrush. Granulomas are quite rare.

Children with HIV infection, long-term glucocorticosteroid treatment, type 1 diabetes mellitus, cancer chemotherapy, or oral contraceptive use are unusually susceptible to candidiasis.

TREATMENT

For infantile thrush, nystatin oral suspension four times daily for 5 days is efficacious.

Older children with thrush and/or angular cheilitis the use of clotrimazole troches may be helpful. Many agents will clear cutaneous candidiasis including nystatin cream, or one of the imidazole creams such as clotrimazole when applied twice a day for 3–5 days. If there are breaks in the skin, the creams may sting. Nystatin ointment will not sting.

Oral therapy is reserved for **children who are immunosuppressed, immune-deficient, or have cancer**. Oral fluconazole or itraconazole 5 mg/kg per day for 21 days is the usual treatment. **Vaginitis** in the adolescent female may be treated with a single 250-mg dose of fluconazole.

84

ECZEMATOUS DISORDERS (RED WITH DISRUPTION OF SKIN SURFACE)

Perianal cellulitis

DDx ref 81 • 83 • 82

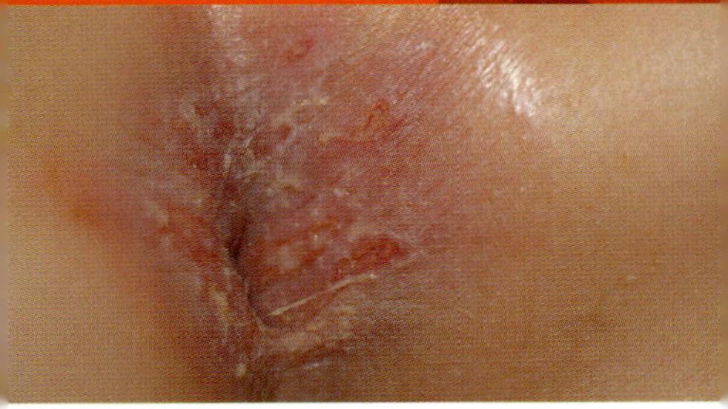

Streptococcal perianal cellulitis. Superficial erosions and erythema of perianal skin.

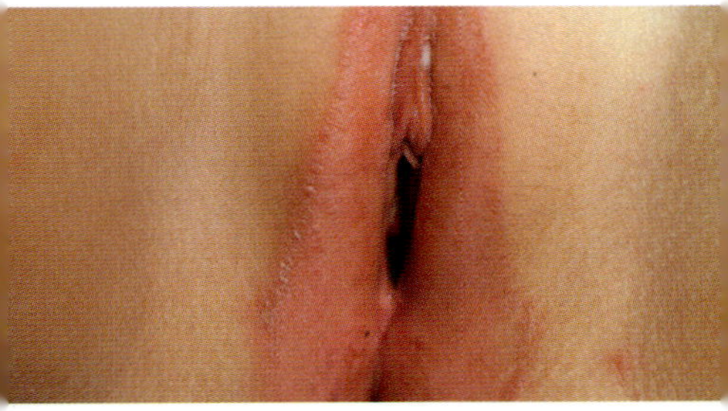

Streptococcal perivaginal cellulitis. Child also had perianal cellulitis.

85

ECZEMATOUS DISORDERS (RED WITH DISRUPTION OF SKIN SURFACE)

Juvenile plantar dermatosis

DDx ref 68 • 80 • 69

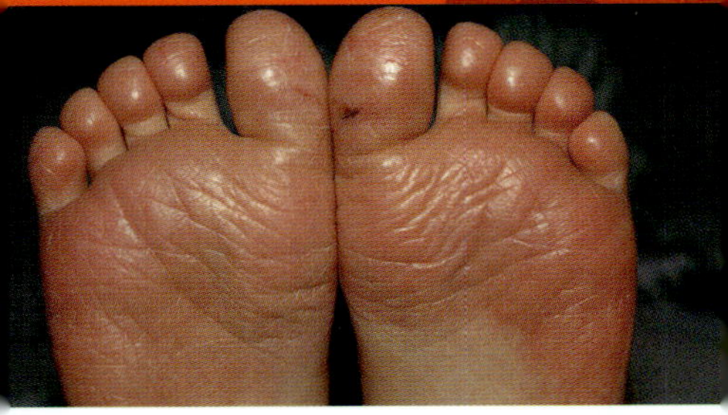

Red, shiny distal soles and toes associated with juvenile plantar dermatosis.

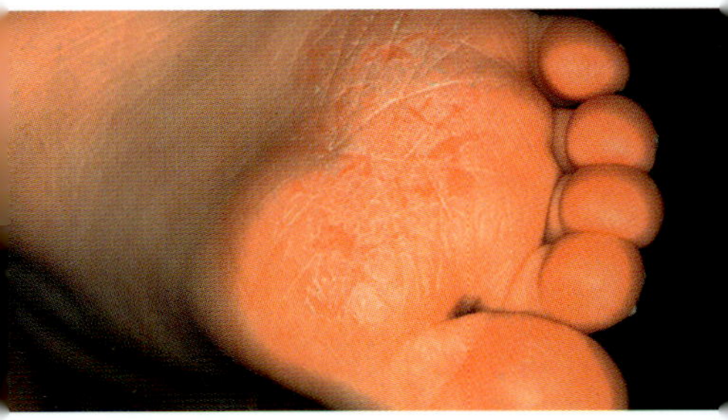

Red, scaly forefoot and toes in juvenile plantar dermatosis.

84 Perianal cellulitis

DDx ref 81 • 83 • 82

CLINICAL FEATURES

Perianal cellulitis presents with tender perirectal erythema and pain on defecation.

Pruritus is common. Superficial erosions and fissures of the perianal skin may be seen. Blood-streaked stools also occur. Lesions may extend beyond the perianal area and involve perivaginal skin.

Infants and toddlers often present with constipation. Perianal cellulitis was historically virtually always caused by **streptococci**, but perianal cellulitis caused by ***Staphylococcus aureus*** is becoming more common. Pustules extending to the buttocks are seen more commonly in staphylococcal disease.

Guttate psoriasis may follow streptococcal perianal cellulitis. Bacterial culture of the perianal area should be performed.

TREATMENT

Traditionally, oral penicillin V 30–60 mg/kg per day or amoxicillin 50 mg/kg per day was the treatment of choice for streptococcal disease, but with the emergence of *S. aureus* being seen in this setting, cephalexin 25–50 mg/kg per day may be a better initial choice, with further therapy dependent on clinical course and culture and sensitivity results.

85 Juvenile plantar dermatosis

DDx ref 68 • 80 • 69

CLINICAL FEATURES

Erythema, fissuring, peeling, and dryness of the weight-bearing surface of the foot are characteristic of juvenile plantar dermatosis.

The great toes are often the first involved, but involvement of the entire forefoot can occur. Involvement is quite symmetric.

Excessive hydration, including sweating followed by rapid drying, leads to cracking of the epidermis and chapping of the skin is frequently seen. Extensive involvement mimics **tinea pedis** (see DDx ref 68 Tinea (Dermatophyte Infections)), which may be excluded by examination of scale with potassium hydroxide and fungal culture. Allergic contact dermatitis usually presents on the dorsum of the foot, not the weight-bearing surface. In persistent eruptions, patch testing may help diagnose atypical allergic contact dermatitis.

TREATMENT

Severe inflammatory involvement may require 1–2 weeks of twice a day medium-potency topical steroid ointments. Application of thick emollients applied 2–3 times a day and always after removal of shoes is often sufficient. Socks should be worn to prevent lubricated feet from slipping on floors. For severe xerosis with minimal inflammation, the feet can be soaked in warm water for 5 minutes before bed and then covered with petrolatum, damp socks and then dry socks, and the child should sleep overnight in these.

86

DDx ref 79 • 68 • 5

ECZEMATOUS DISORDERS (RED WITH DISRUPTION OF SKIN SURFACE)

Nummular dermatitis

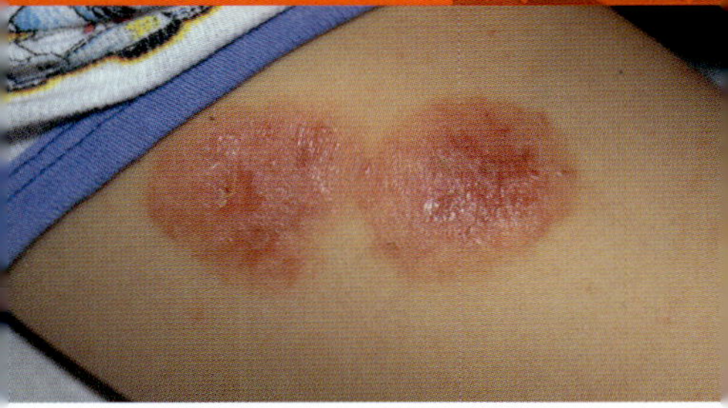

Two oozing coin-shaped areas of nummular dermatitis.

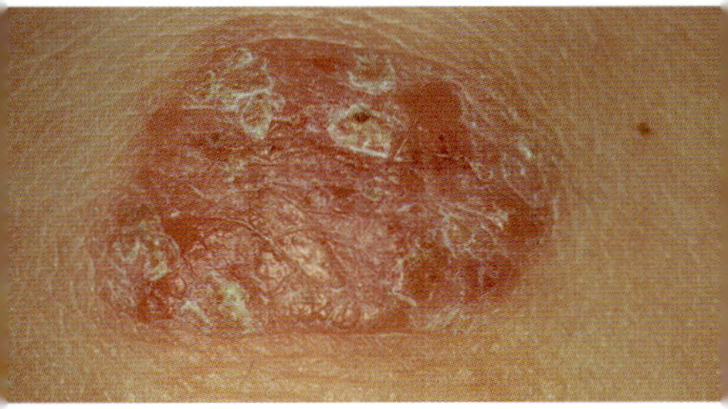

Redness and scale in the dry form of nummular dermatitis that mimics psoriasis.

87

DDx ref 79 • 68 • 89

ECZEMATOUS DISORDERS (RED WITH DISRUPTION OF SKIN SURFACE)

Seborrheic dermatitis

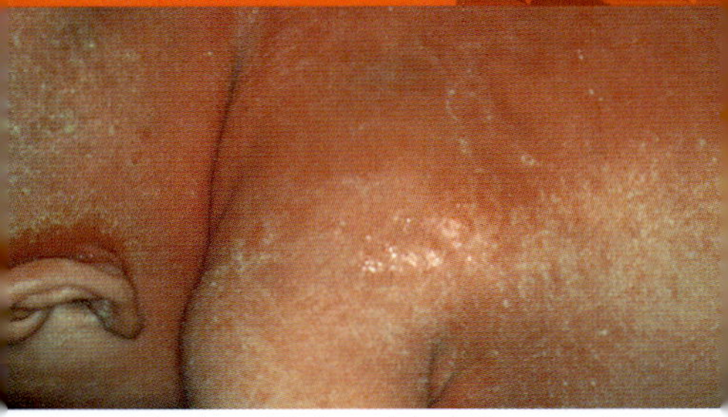

Seborrheic dermatitis in an infant. Greasy scale and erythema in the scalp.

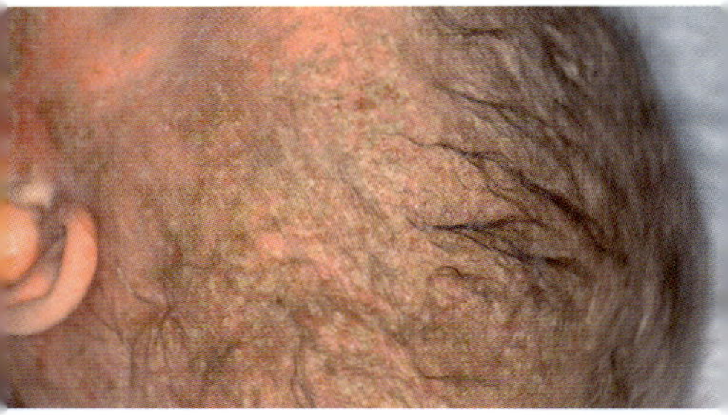

Greasy, yellow scales and redness of the scalp of an infant with seborrheic dermatitis.

86 Nummular dermatitis

DDx ref 79 • 68 • 5

CLINICAL FEATURES

Nummular dermatitis is characterized by coin-shaped plaques most commonly on the extremities and buttocks. Two forms are seen: a wet form with oozing and crusting, and a dry form with erythema and scaling. Both forms are persistent, lasting months if untreated.

Pruritus is often severe, but occasionally is completely absent.

The wet oozing form must be differentiated from impetigo, and **the dry form** from tinea corporis. Most children with nummular dermatitis do not have atopic dermatitis, although some children with atopic dermatitis will have nummular-type lesions as well as the other typical skin changes.

TREATMENT

High-potency topical steroids are required. Lesions are difficult to resolve and treatment must be persistent, often requiring 4–6 weeks for clearing. Antihistamines may be required if pruritus is significant. For severe disease unresponsive to topical therapy, methotrexate may be used for 3–6 months.

87 Seborrheic dermatitis

DDx ref 79 • 68 • 89

CLINICAL FEATURES

Seborrheic dermatitis may be seen in the neonate or the adolescent.

In the neonate, focal or diffuse scaling of the scalp (cradle cap) may be the initial, and at times only, presentation. A greasy, scaly, erythematous dermatitis may involve the face, neck, retroauricular areas, axillae, and diaper area. Pruritus is usually not present. The dermatitis may be patchy or focal, or spread to involve almost the entire body. In extensive cases it mimics atopic dermatitis. In many instances initially called seborrheic dermatitis, the child develops typical flexural dermatitis with time.

In adolescence, seborrheic dermatitis is usually more localized, frequently affecting only the scalp, but also involving the eyelids, retroauricular areas, external auditory canals, nasolabial folds, and flexural areas. Seborrheic dermatitis of the scalp must be differentiated from diffuse scaly tinea capitis due to *Trichophyton tonsurans* by fungal culture. If thick isolated plaques are present, then psoriasis is in the differential. Severe seborrheic dermatitis may be the initial presentation of HIV infection. When associated with failure to thrive and recurrent infections, hereditary immunodeficiencies should be considered. Seborrheic dermatitis with crusted papules and petechiae is seen with Langerhans cell histiocytosis and this presentation requires skin biopsy.

TREATMENT

Low-potency topical steroids applied twice a day are effective.

For infants with severe cradle cap, mineral oil can be applied to the scalp for 5–10 minutes before shampooing with a mild shampoo and then the scale can be gently removed with a soft brush or toothbrush.

Adolescents with chronic scalp involvement will benefit from the use of shampoos containing zinc pyrithione, selenium sulfide, ketoconazole, or tar.

Scabies

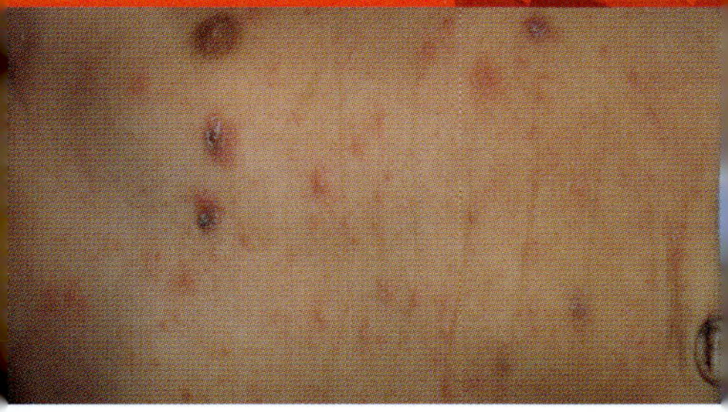

Infant with scabies. Multiple red papules and a few crusted papules on the trunk.

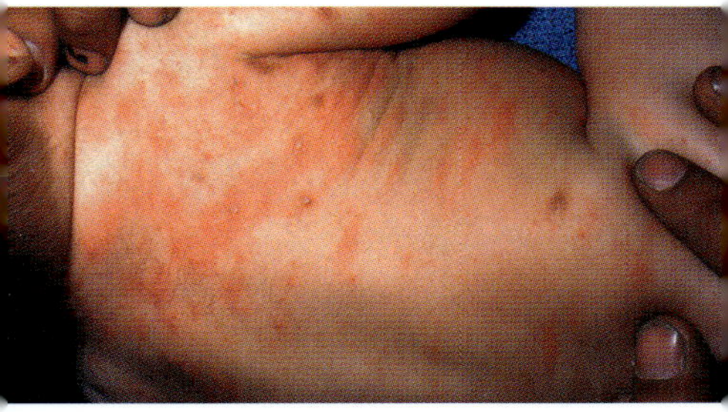

Baby with scabies. Numerous urticated red papules on the back and periaxillary skin.

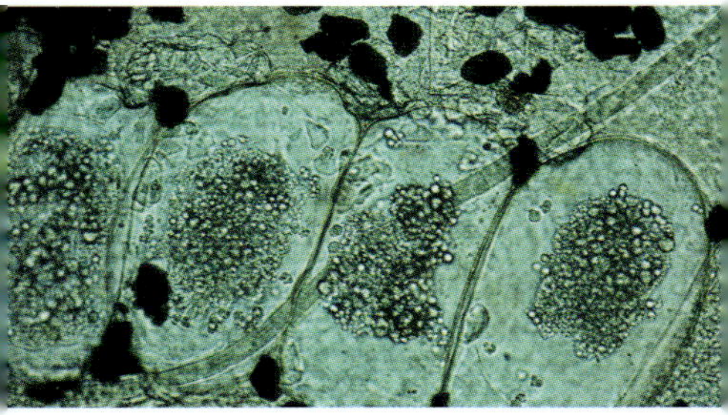

Photomicrograph of skin scraping, depicting oval eggs and dark brown scybala.

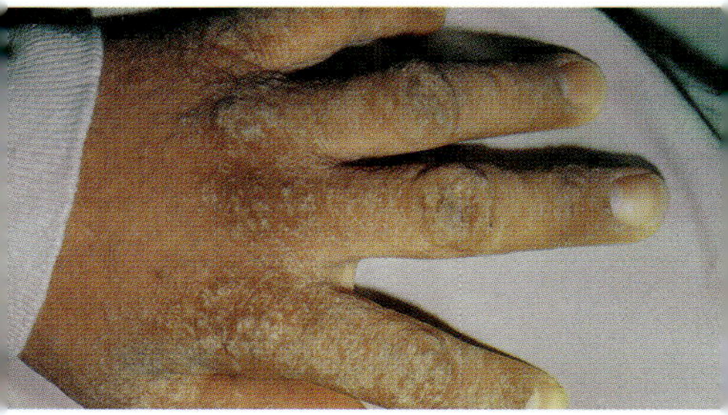

Norwegian scabies. Thick scaling with fissures and multiple mites in a child with Down syndrome.

Scabies

DDx ref 34 • 70 • 89

CLINICAL FEATURES

Scabies is characterized by widespread crusted itchy papules on the trunk, flexural wrist, periaxillary skin, elbows, ankles, feet, and interdigital webs. S-shaped burrows are diagnostic but few in number. Scratching produces eczematous changes that predominate the clinical presentation, especially in babies and toddlers.

Scabies in babies may mimic Langerhans cell histiocytosis, including many histiocytes found in skin biopsies. Babies often have hundreds of mites and widespread eczematous changes; **older children** a dozen or more mites and localized changes. After close examination of the child to locate an unscratched burrow, the burrow should be covered with mineral oil, then scraped with a No.15 blade to obtain the stratum corneum. Microscopic examination of the scraping contents will reveal intact mites, mite parts, eggs, and/or mite feces. Experienced clinicians can also identify mites under dermoscopy. To aid in diagnosis and prevent a possible spread of scabies, evaluation of exposed contacts is useful.

Many adults who carry scabies have little or no itching, only a few skin changes, and may transmit mites to children without realizing they are infested.

In the child unable to scratch, such as the immobilized child and in the child with Down syndrome, scabies infestation induces thick scales on the extremities with thousands of mites present. This presentation is termed **Norwegian scabies** and it can mimic ichthyosis and is most contagious.

The child with Norwegian scabies will have numerous mobile mites in scrapings from thickened scaly skin.

TREATMENT

Topical application of an effective scabicide such as 5% permethrin cream or 1% ivermectin cream left on for 8–14 hours, or the use of oral ivermectin 200 μg/kg in a single oral dose, has a 97% cure rate.

Affected contacts should also be treated. Oral antihistamines may help with itching that lasts 7–10 days, even after successful elimination of mites. A revisit in 2 weeks is recommended. If new lesions are present or if mites are found on skin scrapings, then re-treatment is indicated.

In Norwegian scabies, oral ivermectin may induce peeling of large sheets of thick scale. Scabies epidemics in institutionalized children may be best treated with oral ivermectin.

Langerhans cell histiocytosis

DDx ref 79 • 88 • 87

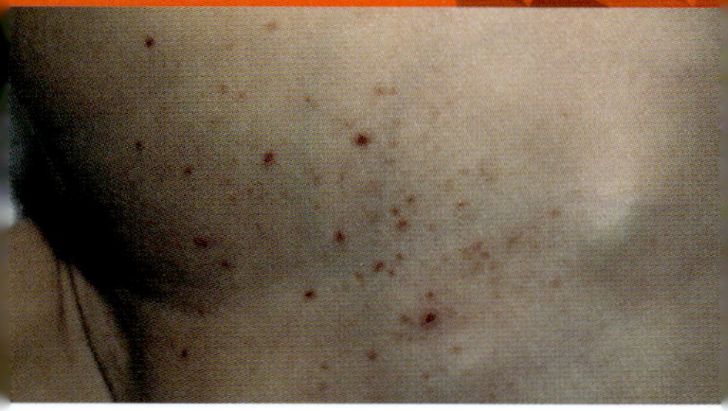

Langerhans cell histiocytosis. Crusted purpuric papules on the lower abdomen.

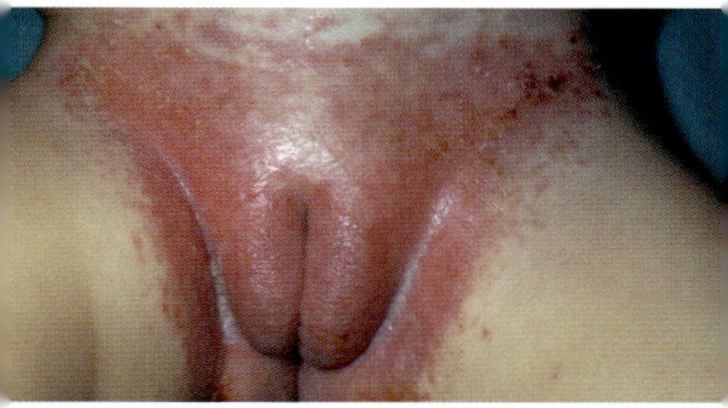

Langerhans cell histiocytosis. Diaper dermatitis-like eruption.

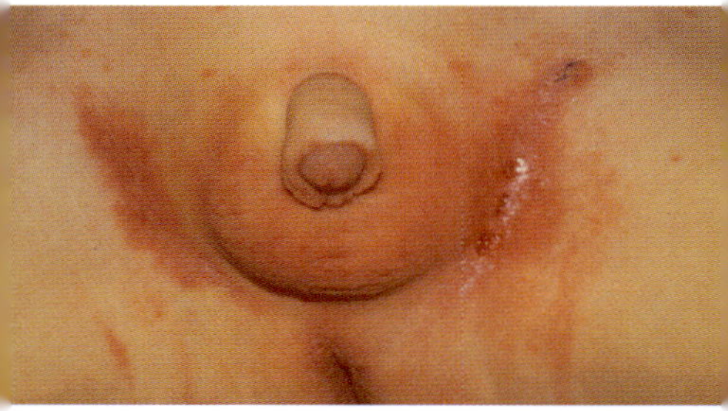

Langerhans cell histiocytosis. Erosions in both inguinal areas in an infant.

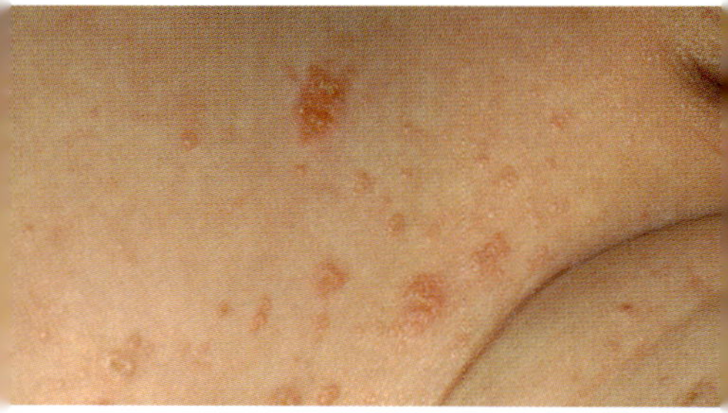

Langerhans cell histiocytosis. Petechial papules and scaly plaques on the trunk.

CLINICAL FEATURES

Langerhans cell histiocytosis may be caused by somatic mutations in BRAF, MAP2K1, and MAP3K1. The cutaneous lesions of Langerhans cell histiocytosis are discrete red, orange, or yellow-brown papules or nodules. A crusted, scaly dermatitis of the scalp, postauricular, perineal, and axillary areas is seen. The presence of red-brown purpuric papules and nodules within or near an area of dermatitis is a clue to the diagnosis. Hepatosplenomegaly and lymphadenopathy may occur. Exophthalmos, oral lesions, otitis media, and pulmonary infiltrates are also seen. Pituitary dysfunction or hypothalamic involvement may lead to diabetes insipidus, growth retardation, and rarely panhypopituitarism. Bone lesions may be present or may be the only site involved, especially in **children older than 5 years**. Bone lesions may be single or multiple and most commonly involve the skull.

Children with severe multisystem disease may present with fever, weight loss, malaise, and irritability. The bone marrow may be involved. Biopsy revealing multiple Langerhans cells is diagnostic. Further evaluation should include complete blood count, liver function tests, coagulation studies, skeletal survey, chest radiograph, and urinalysis.

TREATMENT

Treatment of LCH depends on the extent of disease. Referral to oncology for systemic evaluation to identify the extent and severity of the disease is required. Single-system disease is generally benign and self-resolving.

Multisystem disease requires systemic multi-agent chemotherapy. Response rates to multi-agent chemotherapy are excellent.

ECZEMATOUS DISORDERS (RED WITH DISRUPTION OF SKIN SURFACE)

Acrodermatitis enteropathica

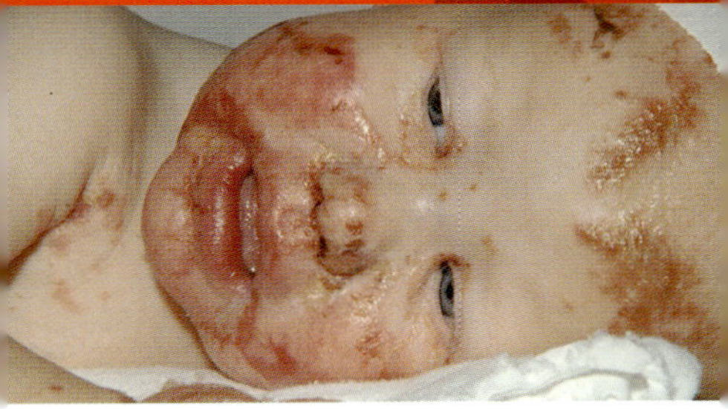

Acrodermatitis enteropathica. Perioral erosions and scalp crusting in an infant.

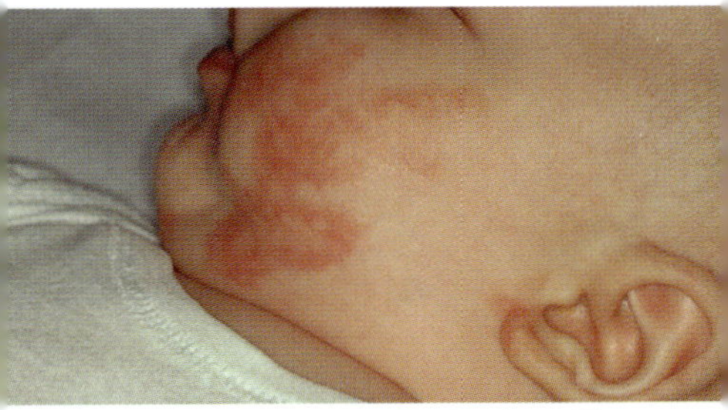

Acrodermatitis enteropathica. Erosive dermatitis on cheeks.

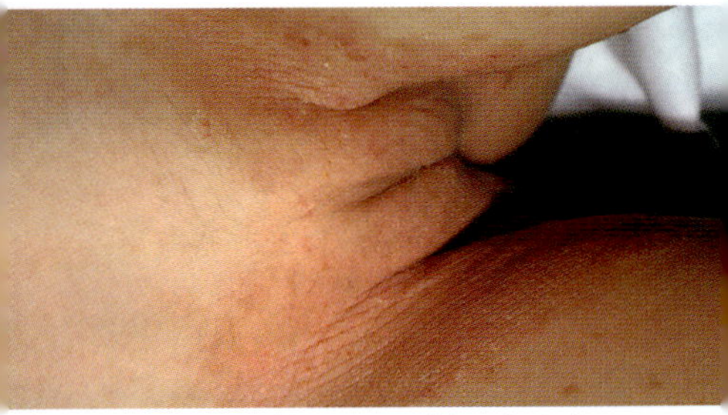

Chronic acrodermatitis enteropathica. Red plaques in the genital area.

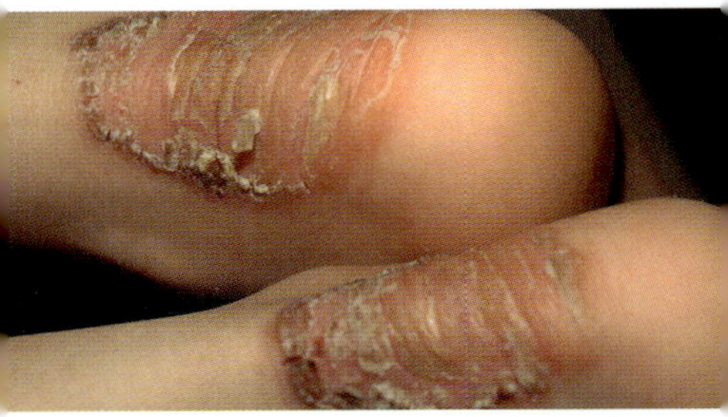

Chronic acrodermatitis enteropathica. Scaly red plaques on the ankles.

Acrodermatitis enteropathica

CLINICAL FEATURES

Acrodermatitis enteropathica (AE) is an autosomal recessive disorder of zinc transport due to abnormalities in the zinc transporter protein SCL394A. Transient AE in breast-fed infants is caused by a mutation in the zinc transporter SCL30A2, which prevents the maternal transport of zinc into breast milk.

Skin lesions are not present at birth, but develop at a few months of age in formula-fed infants or after weaning in breast-fed infants.

Early lesions are vesicular, but rapidly become pustular followed by an erythematous, weeping, oozing, erosive dermatitis. The distal extremities, hands, feet, perioral, and perineal areas are affected. Diarrhea is common and begins a few weeks to months after the onset of the skin disease.

Neurologic abnormalities include irritability and lethargy.

Photophobia, growth retardation, failure to thrive, anemia, and immunosuppression are also seen. Secondary infections with ***Candida albicans*** **and** ***Staphylococcus aureus*** are common.

In chronic disease, the skin lesions become erythematous plaques with silvery scales resembling psoriasis. Diagnosis is made by measuring serum zinc levels. AE from dietary insufficiency of zinc either in premature infants or in developing countries appears clinically identical.

TREATMENT

Oral zinc sulfate 1 mg/kg or more given twice a day results in rapid clinical improvement. Lethargy disappears within 24 hours and the diarrhea and skin disease in 1–2 weeks.

SKIN-COLORED PAPULES AND NODULES WITH A ROUGH SURFACE

Warts

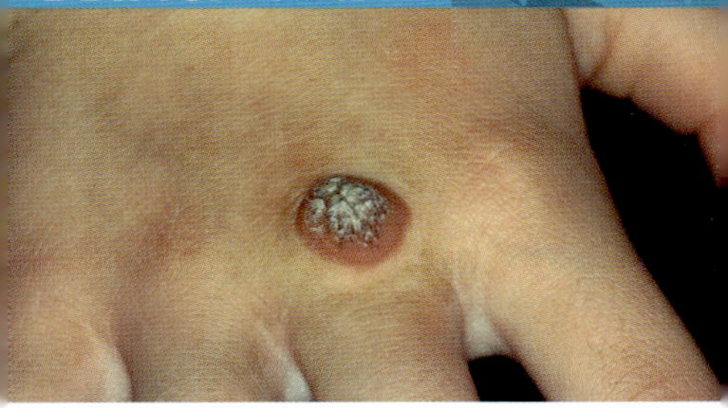

A common wart presents as a verrucous papule on a child's hand.

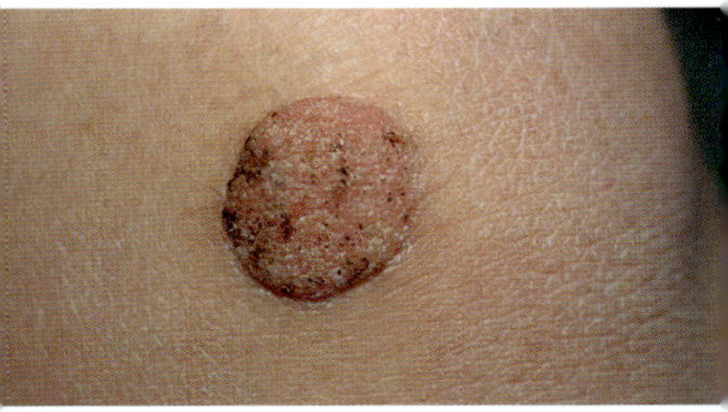

Common wart as a rough-surfaced papule with microbleeding spots from trauma.

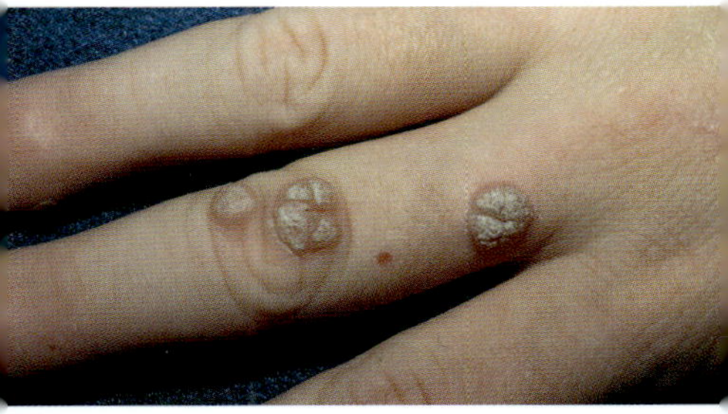

Multiple common warts on a child's hand.

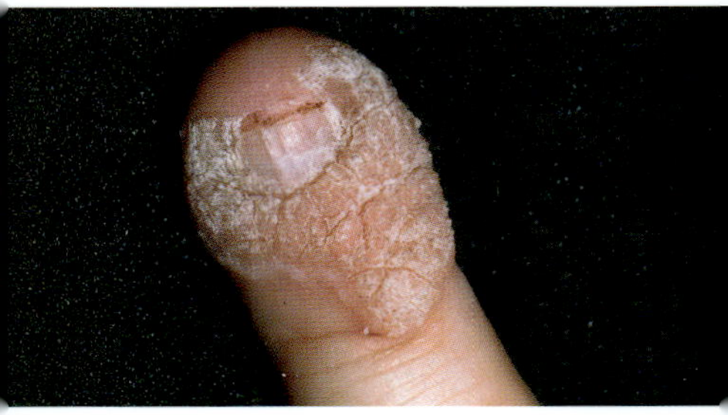

Periungual warts seen as rough-surfaced plaque surrounding a child's fingernail.

Warts

DDx ref 94 • 92 • 93

CLINICAL FEATURES

Warts are epithelial tumors produced by infection with human papillomaviruses (HPV). Different clinical patterns are produced by different HPV types.

Common warts appear as a solitary papule with an irregular, rough (warty) surface, and are frequent in childhood, as 5% of all children will have them with the peak age of 9–10 years. HPV2, HPV4, and HPV29 are responsible for common warts. Periungual warts are a variant of common warts and appear as a plaque with a rough surface surrounding the cuticle of fingers and toes. They are spread by trauma.

Filiform warts appear as spiny projections with a narrow stalk. They are seen on the lips, nose, or eyelids.

Mucosal warts are rare and seen on lips as shiny, rough-surfaced papules. They are associated with HPV13.

Flat warts are flat-topped with a slightly rough feel to the surface, often multiple and skin-colored to light tan. They are mostly on the face or extremities. Flat warts often appear in sites of skin trauma and are due to HPV3 and HPV10 infections.

Plantar warts are found as rough papules or plaques on the weight-bearing surface of the foot. They disrupt the dermal ridges. They frequently are painful and may cause the child to limp. They may group together to form a large 'mosaic wart' plaque. They are due to HPV1, HPV2, HPV4, HPV10, HPV60, HPV63, and HPV65 infection.

Venereal warts (condyloma acuminata) are seen as multiple rough-surfaced papules on genital mucosa and sometimes rough-surface papules and plaques on the adjacent dry perigenital skin. Common warts may sometimes appear on perigenital skin and mimic condyloma. HPV6, HPV11, HPV16, HPV18, HPV42, HPV43, and HPV44 infections are responsible for condylomas. HPV16 and HPV18 are associated with cervical cancer in adults. The moist papules of secondary syphilis may mimic the mucosal condyloma acuminata.

The natural history of any type of wart is highly variable There is a 30% remission rate after 1 year, 65% after 2 years, and 80% after 4 years.

Warts

DDx ref 94 • 92 • 93

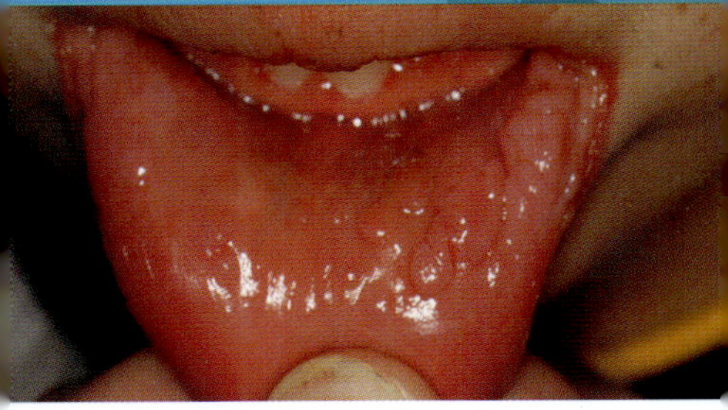

Mucosal warts found as rough papules on a child's inner lower lip.

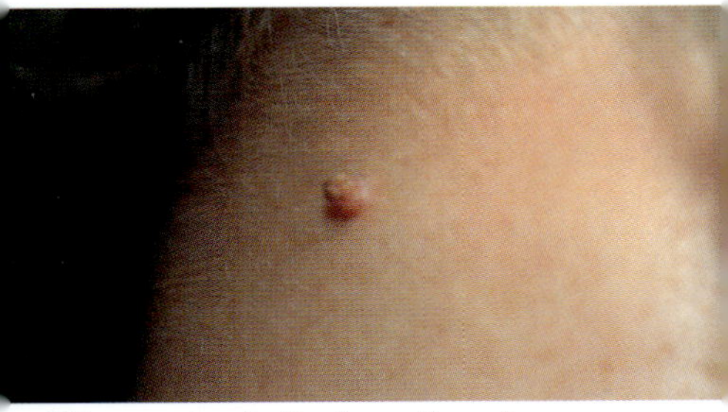

Filiform wart projecting from skin surface on a child's neck.

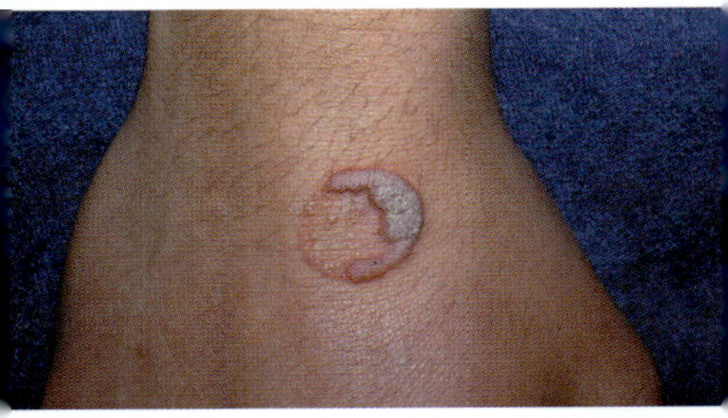

'Fairy ring' of recurrent wart following incomplete cryotherapy.

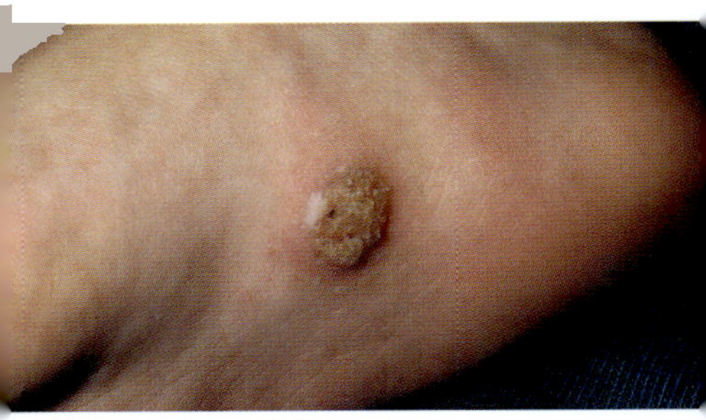

Plantar wart on a child's instep.

TREATMENT

It is unlikely that a single treatment will clear any wart, and, in all therapies, recurrences are commonly seen.

Wart therapy may be cytodestructive, immunologic, antiproliferative, or psychological.

Cryotherapy is the most frequent cytodestructive therapy. Liquid nitrogen spray or cotton swabs dipped in liquid nitrogen are commonly used. Cryosurgery probes are rarely used. The principle is to destroy all the infected epithelial cells. The 'freezing' is applied to the center of the wart until an ice ball is formed with a margin of 1–3 mm of uninvolved skin also turning white. The freeze is maintained 10–30 seconds. An incomplete freeze may result in the reappearance of a rim of warts, the so-called 'fairy ring' warts.

Filiform warts may be treated by dipping forceps in the liquid nitrogen and grasping the narrow base of the filiform wart for 30–45 seconds.

Plantar warts should not be treated with liquid nitrogen because pain may be prolonged with weight bearing. All cryotherapy methods are painful.

Cotton plasters impregnated with 40% salicylic acid are used on plantar warts as well as common warts, especially periungual warts. The plaster is cut to the size of the wart, the paper backing removed, and the gummed side placed against the wart surface. It should be secured by trainer's adhesive tape so the plaster stays in place for 3–5 days. Sweating mobilizes the salicylic acid out of the plaster and into the wart. After the plaster is removed, the child should soak the wart in water for 45 minutes, then rub off the dead white skin. A new plaster is taped in place and the process is repeated for two more changes.

Salicylic acid applicators such as wart stick (40% salicylic acid in wax) or salicylic acid solutions may also be used. The wart stick is applied daily for 3–4 weeks. Salicylic acid solutions are applied with a toothpick as microdrops to the center of the wart. Less potent than plasters, salicylic acid solutions need to be applied once or twice a day for 4–6 weeks. Warts larger than 5 mm will not usually respond to solutions. In all salicylic acid treatments, removal of dead wart tissue every 3–5 days with an emery board may speed up treatment response.

Warts

DDx ref 94 • 92 • 93

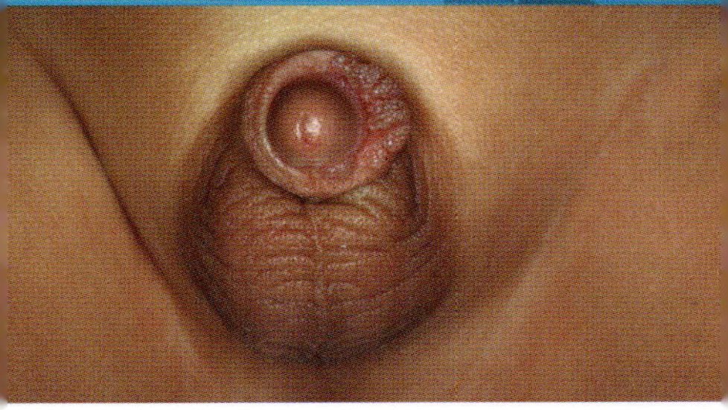

Venereal warts on an infant's foreskin.

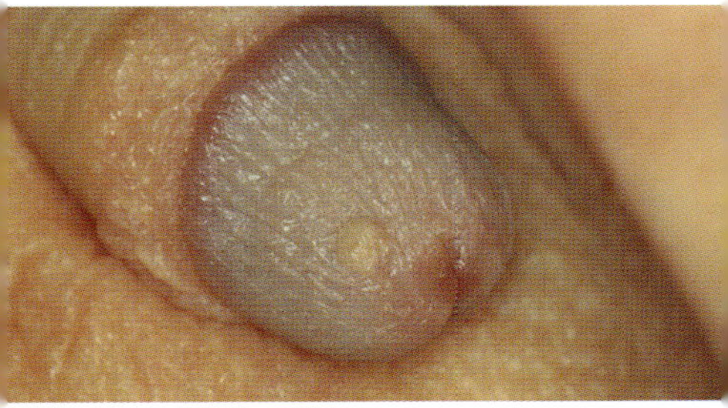

Venereal warts of glans penis in a preschool child.

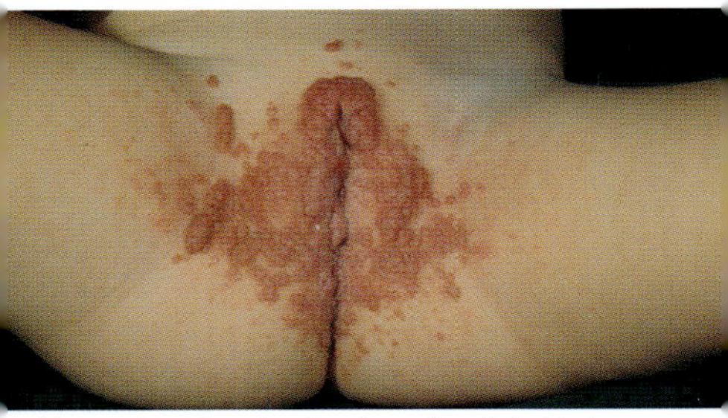

Venereal warts extending to perigenital skin in a female infant.

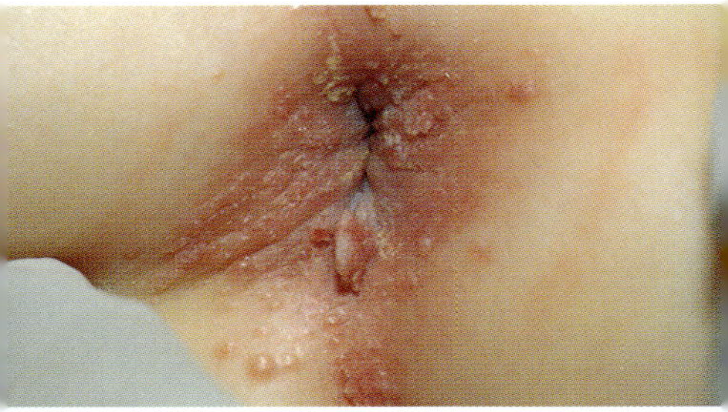

Venereal warts in an infant's anus and perianal skin.

Vascular selective lasers will destroy the feeding blood vessels to the warts with an efficacy rate similar to cryotherapy. Several treatments 2–4 weeks apart are required.

Strong cytodestructive therapies such as the CO_2 laser, electrodessication, and X-ray therapies are not recommended because of side-effects and high recurrence rates. Similarly, surgical removal of warts has a recurrence rate approaching 100% and a surgical scar.

Vesicants such as cantharidin are useful in periungual warts. The solution is applied carefully with a toothpick to the wart surface. A tender blister appears beneath the wart and the wart is sloughed off. The vesicant varies in potency and the blister size is difficult to predict.

Immunologic therapies. *Candida albicans* antigen, 0.3 mL injected weekly into the wart for up to 4 weeks has been effective.

Interferon inducers such as imiquimod applied daily as a 5% cream is painless but requires 1–2 months for a desired result. When the wart becomes red, treatment is discontinued. Cimetidine, an H2 blocking agent, has been used at 30 mg/kg per day for up to 3 months in conjunction with other treatments in children with resistant warts.

Vaccines. There are no effective vaccines for most wart types. The HPV vaccines against HPV6, HPV11, HPV16, and HPV18 may prevent venereal warts in both girls and boys.

Antiproliferative treatments include topical retinoic acid 0.05% cream used once or twice daily for flat warts. It is ineffective in other wart types. Podophyllin is a microtubule inhibitor used for genital and perianal warts. It comes in a 25% solution in alcohol and can be applied carefully, by a healthcare provider, with a toothpick to the warts. It should be washed off in 4 hours to reduce the likelihood of side-effects. It often induces defecation just after application. A commercial preparation for home use is Condylox. It is applied carefully twice daily for 3 days, then reapplied after 4 days of no treatment if the warts have not responded. Podophyllin preparations when overused can cause neurotoxic symptoms, including areflexic coma.

Psychotherapy has the same 'cure' rate as spontaneous regression, which is about 30%.

92

SKIN-COLORED PAPULES AND NODULES WITH A ROUGH SURFACE

Epidermal nevi (ILVEN)

DDx ref 78 • 15 • 91

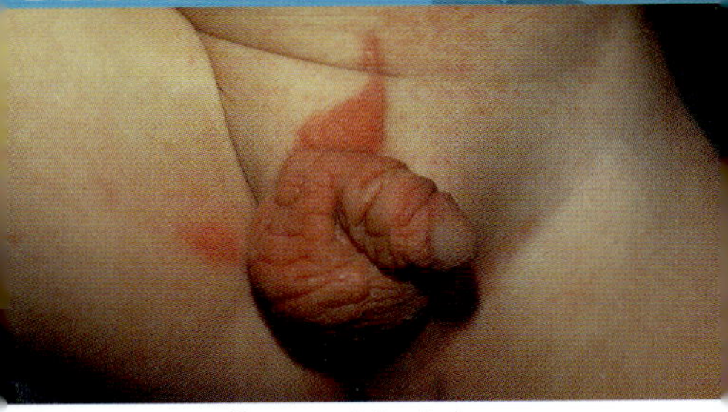

Red, warty, curvilinear, unilateral plaque on a toddler's scrotum, adjacent abdomen, and thigh.

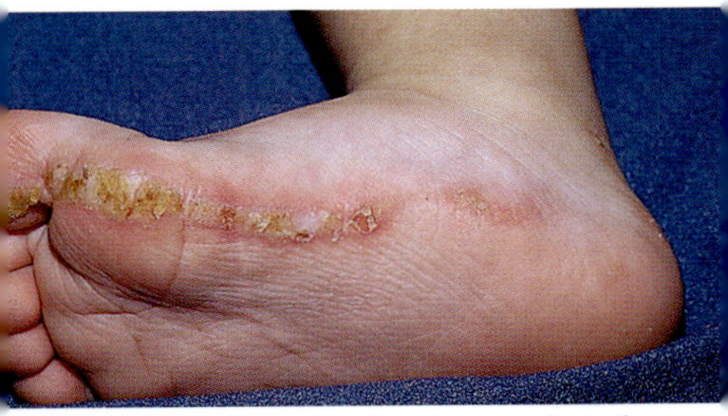

Linear epidermal nevus on the plantar surface of a child's foot.

93

SKIN-COLORED PAPULES AND NODULES WITH A ROUGH SURFACE

Corns and calluses

DDx ref 91 • 94 • 68

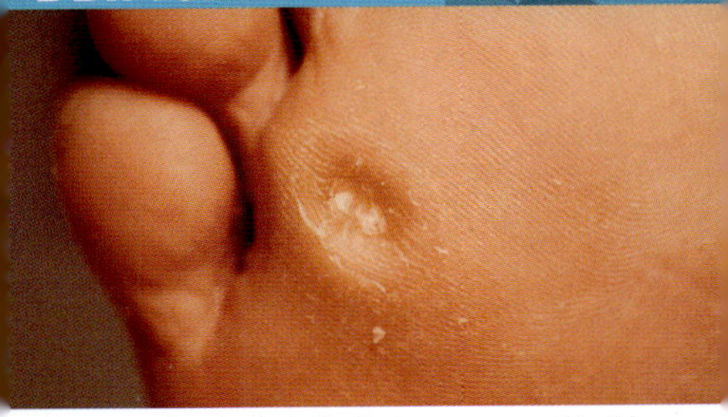

Corn on a teen's foot. Central cores are evident in pared lesion.

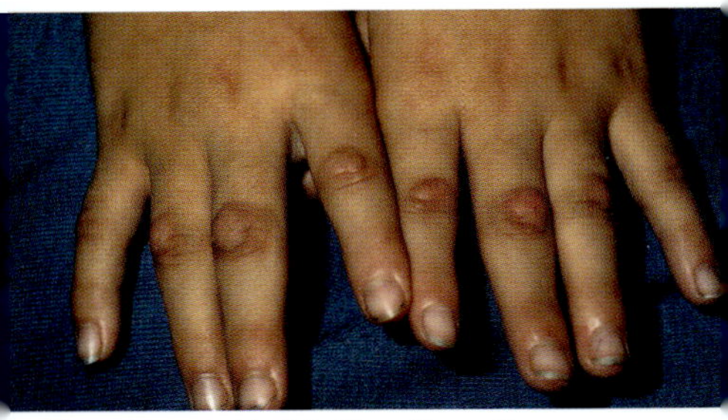

Hyperpigmented isolated knuckle pads.

92

SKIN-COLORED PAPULES AND NODULES WITH A ROUGH SURFACE

Epidermal nevi (ILVEN)

DDx ref 78 • 15 • 91

CLINICAL FEATURES

Epidermal nevi are linear or curvilinear areas of red papules with an irregular, rough surface. The majority of epidermal nevi are present at birth and 95% by age 7 years. Initially, an epidermal nevus may be barely palpable and appear as a confluence of smooth-topped papules. With time, the surface becomes warty.

Most epidermal nevi are small, 2–5 cm in length, but occasionally appear as long unilateral warty streaks covering one half of the body (nevus unius lateris). They are rarely widespread over the entire body (ichthyosis hystrix). Epidermal nevi may be recurrently red and itchy. This is called 'inflammatory linear verrucous epidermal nevus' (ILVEN).

A majority of children with epidermal nevi have no other findings but up to one third will have a variety of associated abnormalities. Skin findings include café-au-lait spots, hypopigmented macules, and congenital pigmented nevi. Skeletal defects, seizure disorders, mental retardation, and ocular anomalies have been associated. All children with epidermal nevi should have a detailed history and physical examination with a careful neurologic and eye examination.

Children with widespread skin involvement have a higher risk of associated abnormalities and should have referral to a children's genetic center or multidiscipline clinic. The skin involvement follows the embryonic skin lines of Blaschko, indicating genetic mosaicism. Affected skin areas may have mutations of the HRAS gene, FGFR 3 or PIK3CA genes. Epidermal nevi with epidermolytic histology may have mutations in keratin 1 or 10 genes.

Small epidermal nevi may be confused with warts; larger lesions with lichen striatus.

TREATMENT

Small lesions may be excised. For the child with widespread skin involvement, topical keratolytics such as retinoid creams may be useful when combined with topical lubrication. Oral retinoids have been helpful in severe involvement.

93

SKIN-COLORED PAPULES AND NODULES WITH A ROUGH SURFACE

Corns and calluses

DDx ref 91 • 94 • 68

CLINICAL FEATURES

Corns and calluses appear as areas of thickened skin that typically appear at sites of skin pressure or friction.

Corns are painful, circumscribed 2–5-mm thickenings that mimic plantar warts. They have a central core that interrupts dermal ridges when pared down. Corns are usually related to ill-fitting footwear.

Calluses are diffuse thickenings of plantar, palmar, or knuckle surfaces related to skin trauma.

Knuckle pads are often seen as isolated findings, in keratin 9 mutations or in compulsive rubbing of the knuckles. Genetic pads are associated with diffuse palmar thickening.

Epidermolysis bullosa simplex may mimic palmar or plantar calluses. A history of blisters will help differentiate.

TREATMENT

For corns, shaving off the excess stratum corneum and covering with a 40% salicylic acid plaster for 3–7 days will often result in improvement. Changing footwear will prevent recurrences.

For calluses, use of salicylic acid plasters will help.

Molluscum contagiosum

DDx ref 91 • 95 • 74

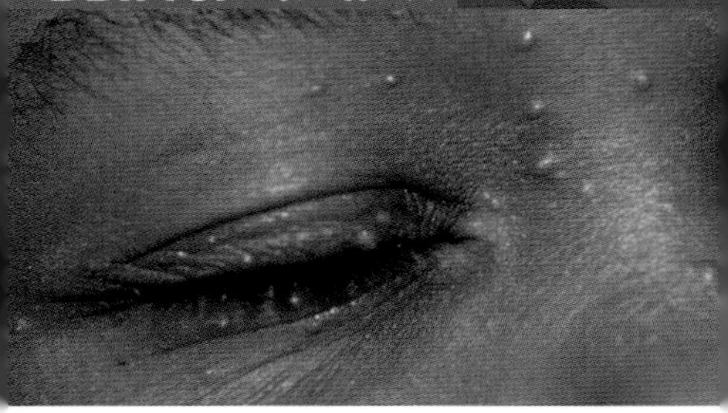

Multiple umbilicated papules of molluscum on the face of an infant.

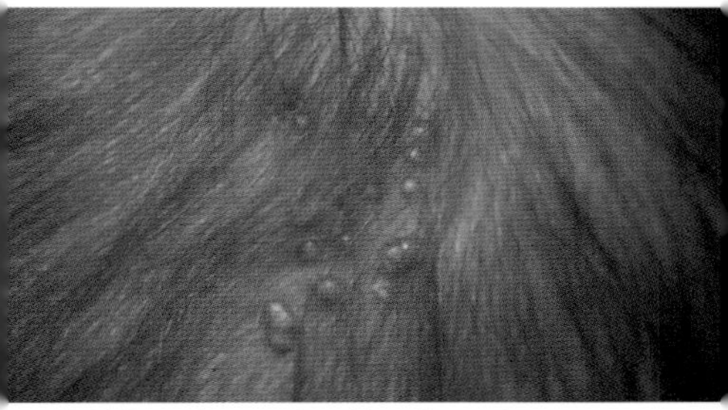

Multiple molluscum involving the scalp.

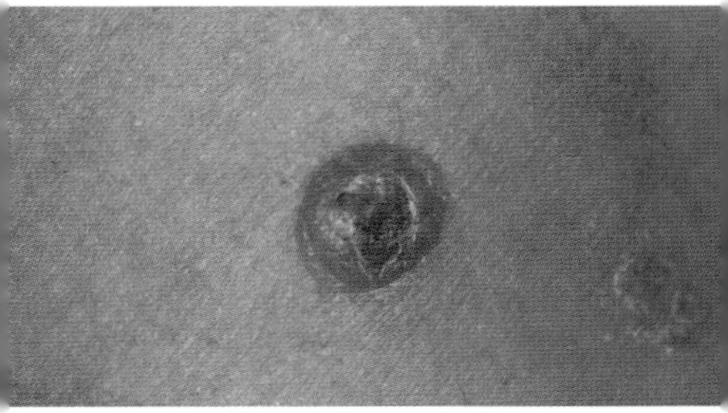

Giant umbilicated molluscum in an HIV-positive child.

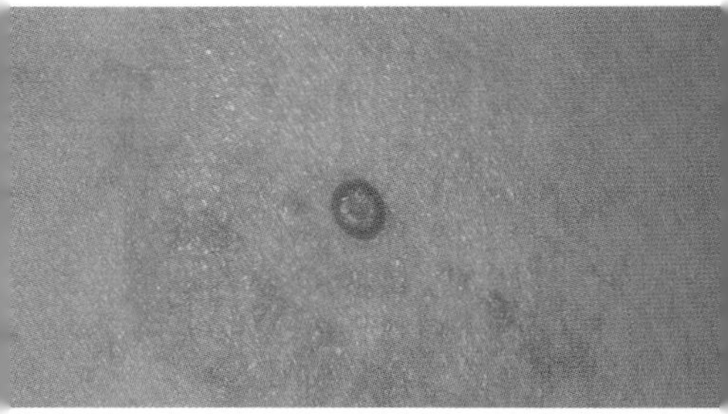

Red, dry skin surrounding umbilicated papule in molluscum dermatitis.

Molluscum contagiosum

DDx ref 91 • 95 • 74

CLINICAL FEATURES

Molluscum are white to yellow-white discrete 1–6-mm papules with larger lesions having a central umbilication. They may be seen anywhere on the body and frequently on the face and trunk. The papules may extrude their contents through the central umbilication. Uncommonly, papules of ≥15 mm are seen. Eczematous changes surrounding individual molluscum papules are seen as 'molluscum dermatitis'. As mollusca resolve, they may appear to be pustular and be painful.

In the child with atopic dermatitis, dozens to hundreds of mollusca can be seen. Genital mollusca can be found in **sexually active teens**.

In immune suppressed children or those with HIV infection, numerous and atypically large mollusca may be noted. Molluscum is caused by a poxvirus and three viruses (MCV 1, 2, and 3) have been identified.

MCV 1 is associated with the common childhood molluscum and **MCV 2 and 3** with genital involvement. The viruses evade cellular interferon action by encoding a false chemokine receptor. The incubation period is 2–7 weeks, and untreated molluscum can persist for 1–5 years.

Molluscum papules can be mistaken for blisters (they are solid), juvenile xanthogranulomas, or warts.

TREATMENT

50% of molluscum will resolve within 1 year For those who desire treatment, if only a few papules are present, removal by curette or needle may be curative, but painful even with the prior use of topical anesthetics. Another strategy useful when a few lesions are present is to use one application of a microdrop of cantharidin to each molluscum, covering with a bandage then washing off in 4–6 hours. The disadvantage is that giant blisters can ensue.

If many mollusca are present, the use of an interferon inducing cream (imiquimod 5%) applied daily to twice daily is preferred. Individual mollusca are treated until they become red. Injection into the molluscum 0.3 mL of *Candida albicans* antigen every 4 weeks for 2–3 treatments is also effective. Oral cimetidine for 6 weeks has been claimed to be successful.

New mollusca may appear after any type of treatment, as incipient infected sites may be difficult to detect.

Pustular mollusca do not require antibiotics.

Milia and sebaceous hyperplasia

DDx ref 96 • 102 • 98

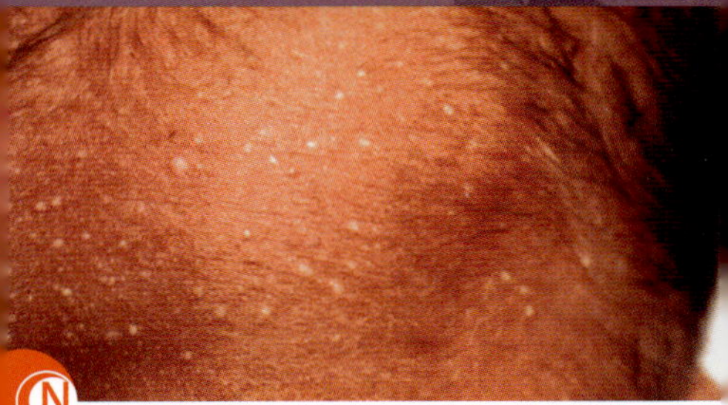

N Neonatal milia as tiny whitish-yellow papules on the forehead.

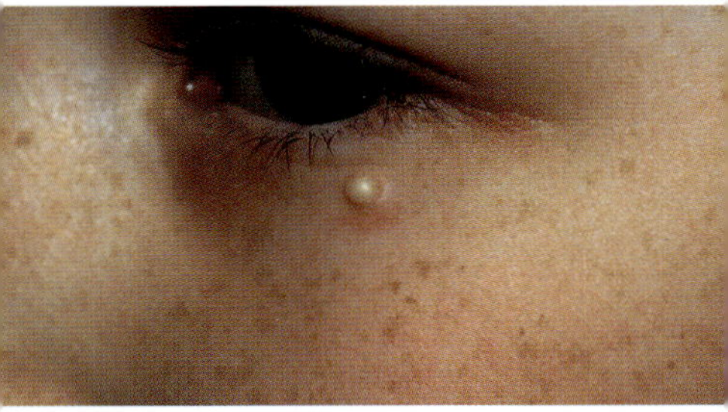

Milia on the cheek of an older child.

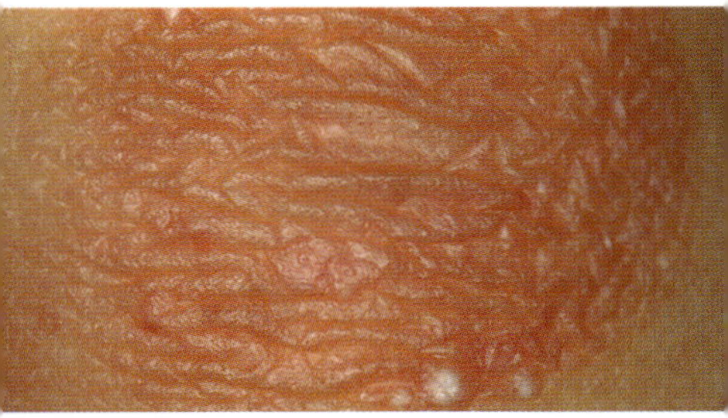

White milia entrapped in a scar of a child with recessive epidermolysis bullosa.

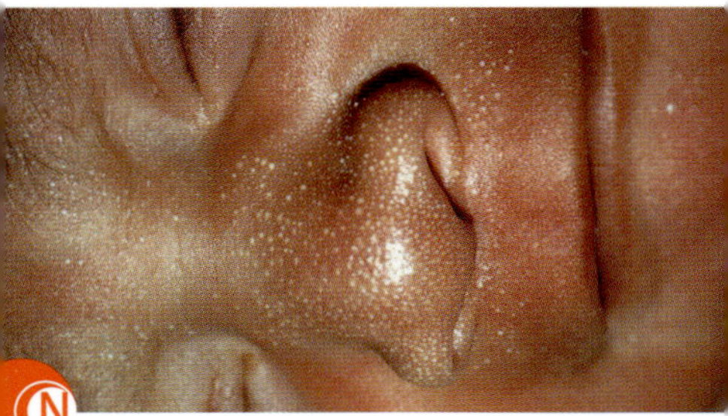

N Neonatal sebaceous gland hyperplasia on the nose and perinasal skin.

Milia and sebaceous hyperplasia

DDx ref 96 • 102 • 98

CLINICAL FEATURES

Both milia and sebaceous hyperplasia are seen as numerous skin-colored to yellow tiny 1-mm smooth-surfaced papules.

Milia are seen over the forehead, cheeks, and nose of newborns and infants. On the palate they are called Epstein's pearls; 60% of **newborns** have oral mucosal milia and 40% on the skin. Neonatal milia are epidermal rests.

Milia are also seen in **older children** on the facial skin and appear to be becoming more common. They are occasionally seen within scars of normal children and frequently in scarring forms of epidermolysis bullosa. Milia are filled with keratin and often spontaneously extrude their contents.

Sebaceous hyperplasia papules may have a yellow or yellow-white discoloration.

They are restricted to pilosebaceous openings and are also found on the nose, cheeks, and forehead in 50% of **newborns**. They are believed to be part of the miniature puberty of the newborn due to maternal androgens.

They spontaneously regress by **4–6 months of age**.

TREATMENT

Since neonatal milia and sebaceous hyperplasia resolve without sequelae, no intervention is necessary.

In the older child, use of a small needle or comedone extractor to remove the contents may be considered.

SKIN-COLORED PAPULES AND NODULES WITH A SMOOTH SURFACE

Epidermal cysts

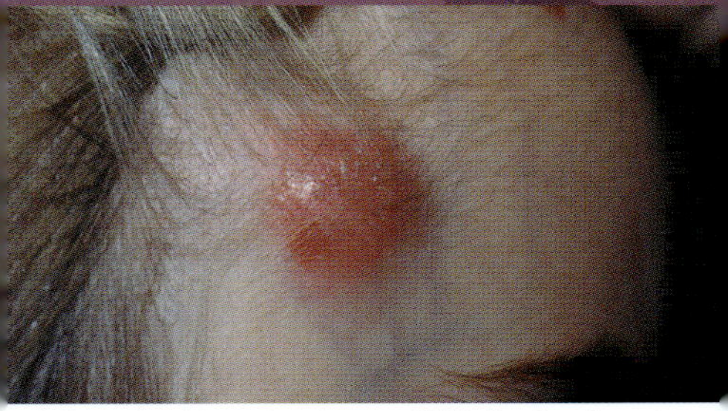

Inflamed epidermal cyst on a child's forehead.

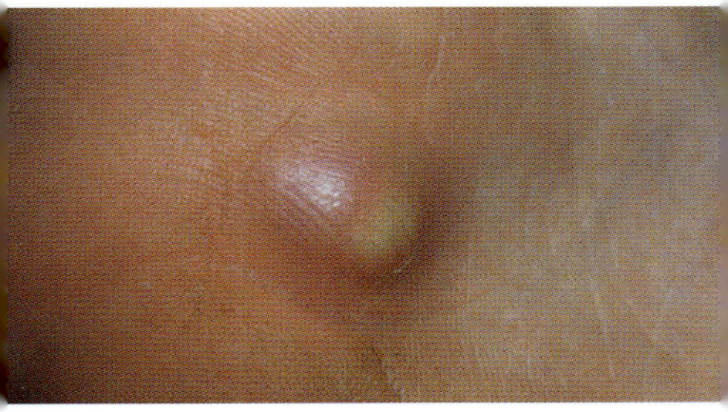

Epidermal cyst on the plantar surface of a child's foot.

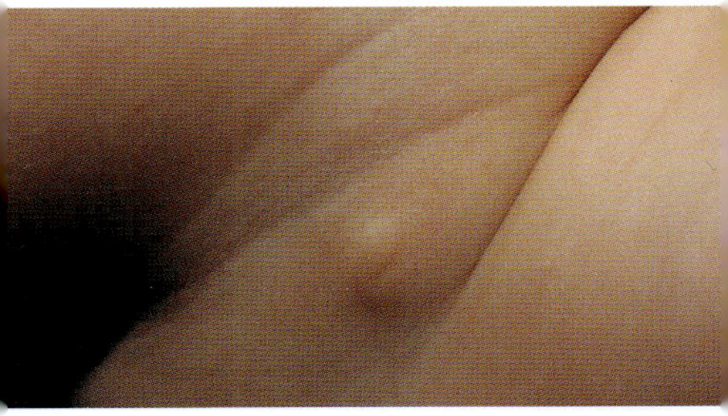

Branchial cleft cyst on lateral neck of a child.

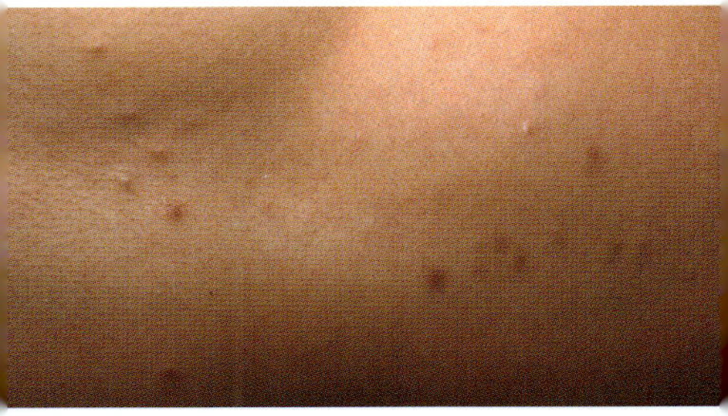

Multiple eruptive vellus hair cysts on an 8-year-old boy.

Epidermal cysts

CLINICAL FEATURES

Epidermal cysts are slow-growing, smooth-surfaced, round 1–15-cm nodules that appear at **any age in childhood**. Epidermal cysts are lined with epithelium and filled with keratins. They are usually found on the upper body but can be seen anywhere on the skin, including the palms and soles. If multiple cysts are present, one should consider genetic syndromes such as **Gardner's syndrome**, an autosomal dominant condition due to mutations in the APC gene. Gardner's syndrome is associated with adenomatous polyps of the colon, some of which eventuate into colorectal cancer. If epidermal cysts are red and tender, bacterial infection should be considered.

Branchial cleft cysts are specialized epidermal cysts that develop on the lateral neck. They are remnants of branchial clefts and represent defects of embryonic closure.

Midline epidermal cysts on the nose should bring concern for possible intracranial connections.

Eruptive vellus hairs cysts are specialized epidermal cysts seen as five or more smooth, skin-colored, 2–5-mm papules over the mid-upper abdomen and lower mid-chest. They begin between 5 and 12 years of age. Vellus hair cysts contain coiled vellus hairs in addition to keratins in the cyst cavity.

TREATMENT

Generally, no treatment is necessary for **asymptomatic epidermal cysts**. If infected, oral antibiotics may be required, and incision and drainage considered. Excision to improve the appearance of a noninfected epidermal cyst may be done.

Midline nasal cysts should first have imaging before any intervention is considered.

Branchial cleft cysts require complete excision and may have connections with deep structures. Patients should be referred to an experienced pediatric otolaryngologist for treatment.

SKIN-COLORED PAPULES AND NODULES WITH A SMOOTH SURFACE

Dermoid cysts

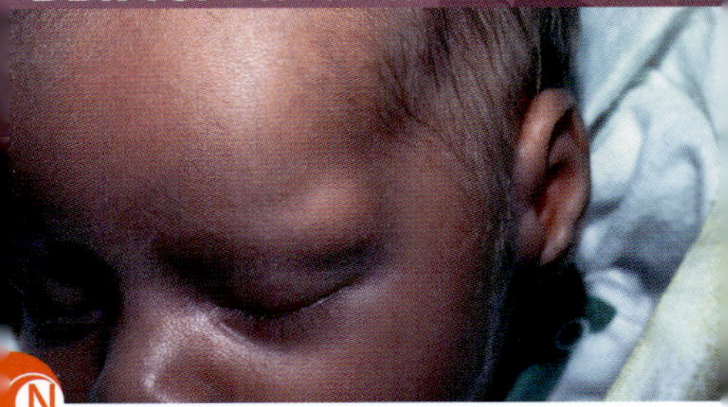

Cystic nodule on lateral eyebrow of a newborn.

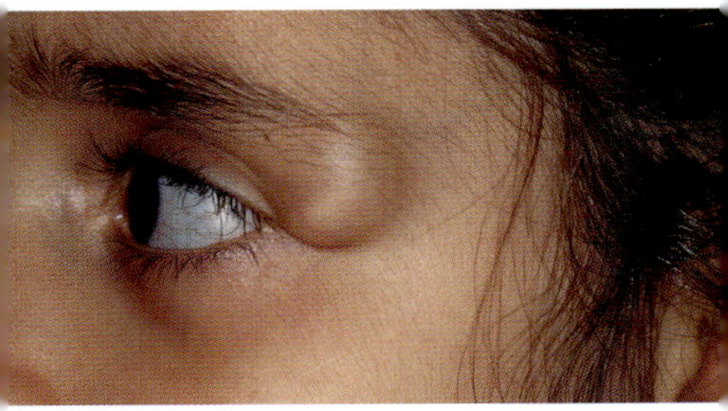

Persistence of dermoid cyst on lateral eyebrow of an 11-year-old girl.

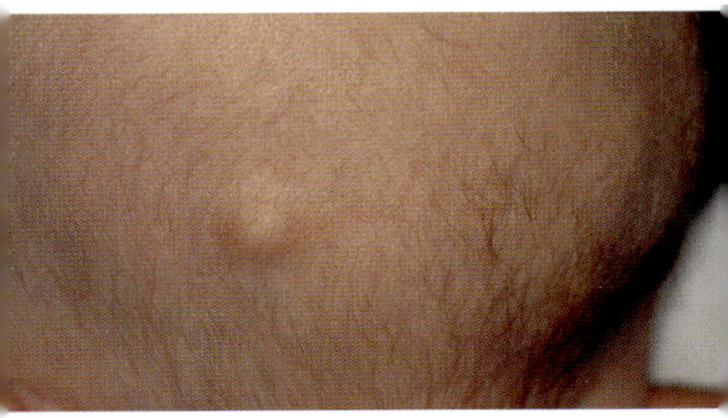

Dermoid cyst on occipital scalp of an infant.

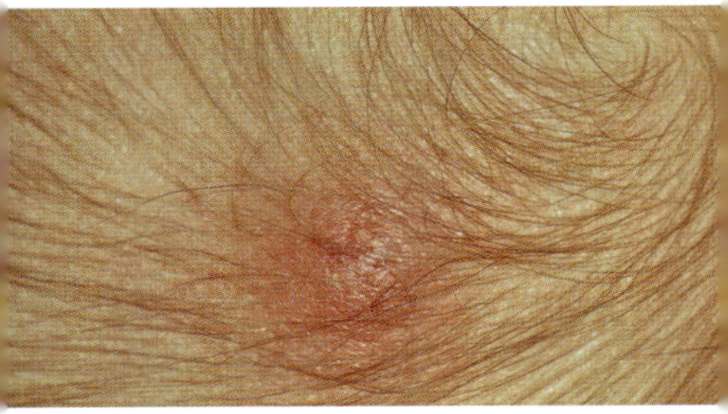

Inflamed dermoid cyst on an infant's scalp after the family attempted to open it.

97 Dermoid cysts

DDx ref 96 • 95 • 98

CLINICAL FEATURES

Dermoid cysts are seen as 1–10-cm smooth-surfaced, skin-colored nodules on the scalp or lateral eyebrow. They are often present in the **newborn period** and continue to grow slowly.

In addition to keratins in the cyst cavity, hair, sebaceous, or sweat structures may be found. Dermoid cysts represent sequestration of skin along the lines of embryologic closure. They rarely spontaneously resolve but almost all will persist. Midline dermoid cysts should be imaged prior to excision, to determine if they have any deeper connections.

TREATMENT

No treatment is usually necessary unless surgery for cosmetic concerns is considered.

SKIN-COLORED PAPULES AND NODULES WITH A SMOOTH SURFACE

Pilomatricoma and trichoepithelioma

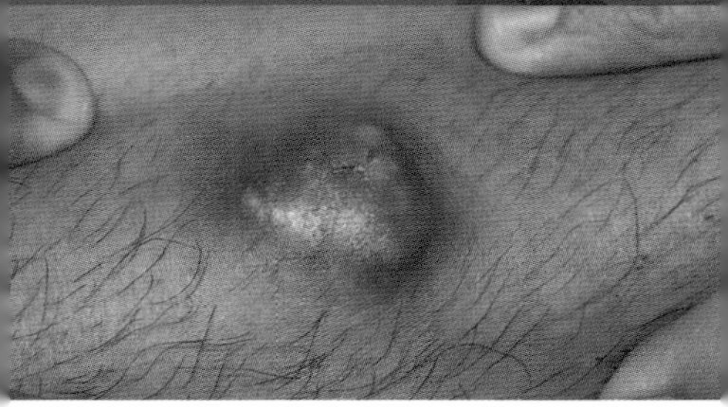

Large multilobulated pilomatricoma on the thigh of a teenage boy.

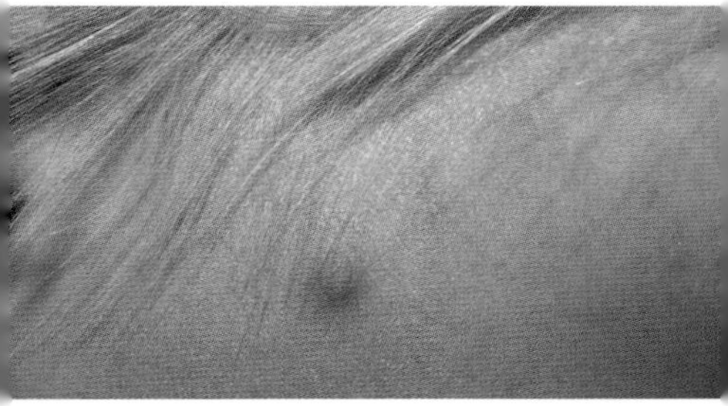

Calcified pilomatricoma appearing as a tender bluish papule on a girl's cheek.

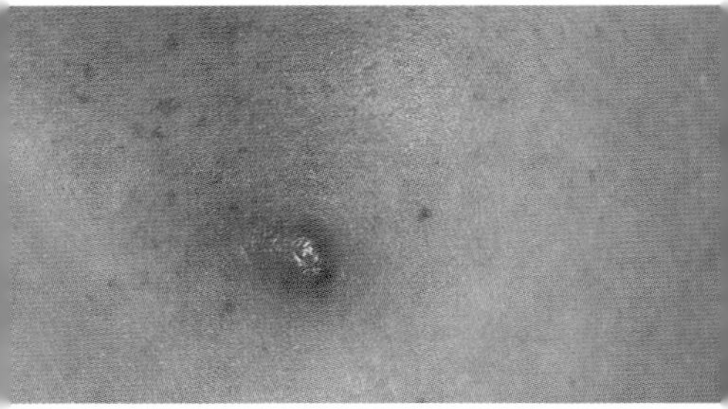

Inflamed pilomatricoma on a child's cheek.

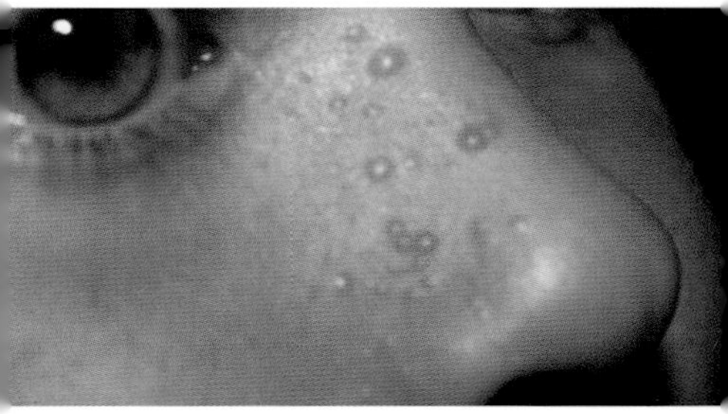

Trichoepithelioma. Multiple skin-colored smooth papules on a child's nose.

CLINICAL FEATURES

Pilomatricomas are solitary, smooth-surfaced, skin-colored, multi-lobulated 2–5-mm nodules seen on the cheeks and extremities of children. They often are tender, especially when compressed. The overlying surface is at first skin-colored but may become bluish or red. Large pilomatricomas will have yellowish coloration. Pilomatricomas are very common in **childhood**, accounting for 10% of all skin nodules. Pilomatricomas are benign hyperplasias of the hair matrix that frequently calcify. Mutations in beta-catenin have been linked to multiple pilomatricomas and myotonic dystrophy. Multiple pilomatricomas may be seen in association with Gardner's syndrome.

Trichoepitheliomas are 1–3-mm smooth-surfaced, skin-colored papules that appear on the mid-face skin of children. Occasionally, they are seen in other locations such as the scalp, upper trunk, and neck.

Multiple trichoepitheliomas may be associated with large scalp tumors called 'cylindromas'. Trichoepitheliomas are benign hamartomas of hair follicles.

Multiple trichoepitheliomas are inherited as an autosomal dominant trait and caused by mutations in the CYLD gene.

TREATMENT

Pilomatricomas may be removed by surgical excision.

Trichoepitheliomas may also be surgically excised, but when many are present, this may be impractical. Imiquimod 5% cream applied daily may cause some lesions to regress and control the growth of others. Carbon dioxide laser has also been successfully used to treat multiple lesions.

Granuloma annulare

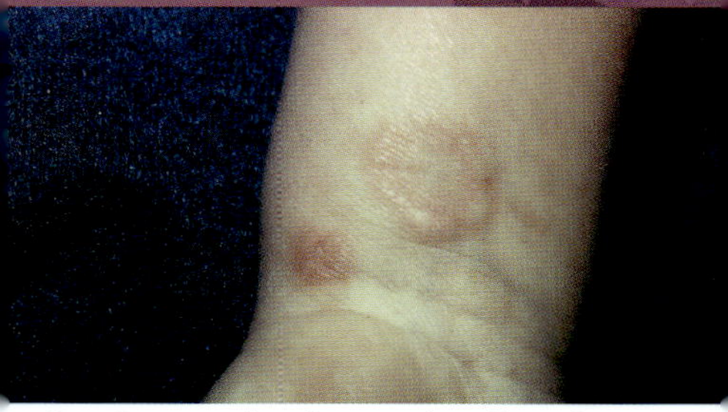

Granuloma annulare. Large and small annular plaques on the ventral surface of the arm.

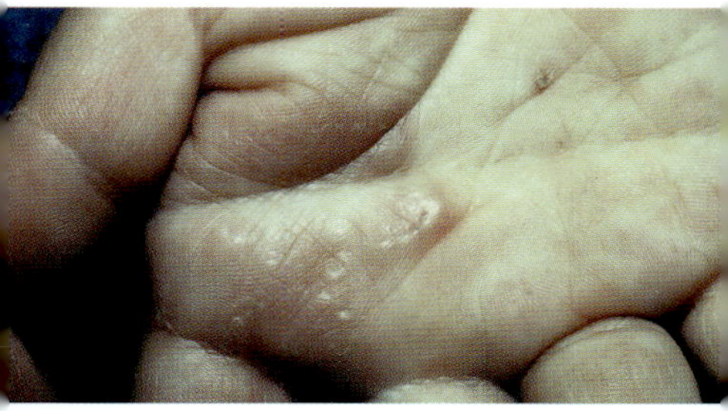

Granuloma annulare. Annular papules on the palm.

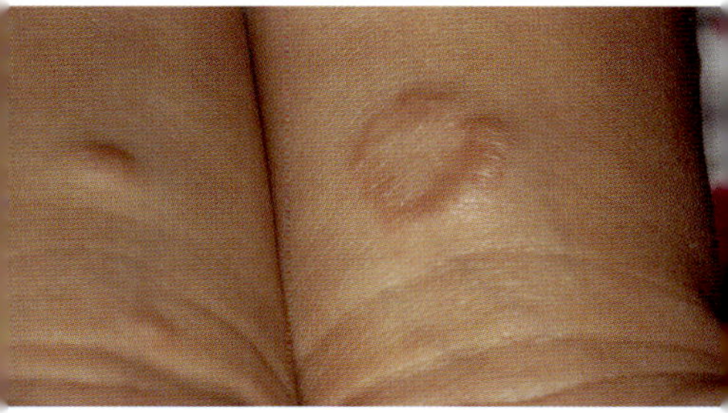

Annular lesion on one wrist with a solitary nodule of granuloma annulare on the other.

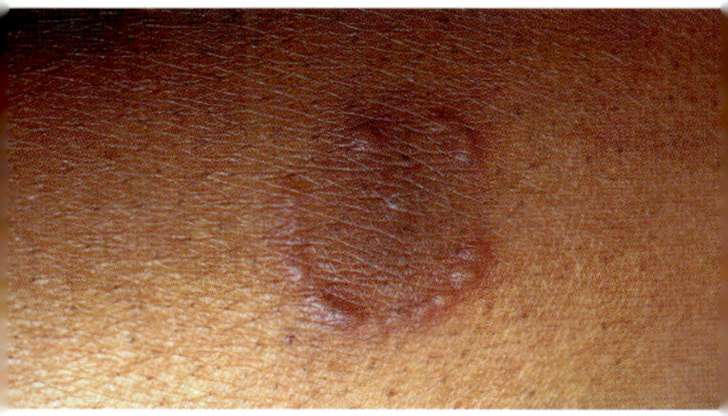

Granuloma annulare. Annular pink papules with dusky violaceous center.

Granuloma annulare

DDx ref 68 • 35 • 86

CLINICAL FEATURES

Small, firm papules or nodules that coalesce to form a circle or semicircle are characteristic of granuloma annulare. They may be skin-colored, but more often they have a dusky violaceous hue. The lesions occur predominantly on the acral areas, on the digits, ankles, and wrists. Half of the children will have only one lesion. Lesions vary in size from 1 to 8 cm, with the smaller lesions being seen on the digits.

A subcutaneous form is also seen. The predominant sites for subcutaneous granuloma annulare are the scalp and tibia. Subcutaneous granuloma annulare presents as firm, non-tender, skin-colored nodules that are fixed to the bone. Subcutaneous granuloma annulare of the scalp may be misdiagnosed clinically as a malignancy.

The disseminated papular form of granuloma annulare is rare in children. Granuloma annulare is often mistaken for ringworm, but the lack of epidermal change and absence of scale as well as the ring of dermal papules differentiates the two.

Subcutaneous granuloma annulare mimics rheumatoid nodules clinically and they are also histologically similar. The pathogenesis is unknown.

TREATMENT

Granuloma annulare is a spontaneously resolving entity, therefore treatment is not necessary. Half of the affected children will be clear within 2 years. Rarely, a large lesion on the foot will interfere with wearing shoes and may be treated with intralesional corticosteroids, 5 mg/mL.

100 DDx ref

SKIN-COLORED PAPULES AND NODULES WITH A SMOOTH SURFACE

Neurofibroma and lipomas

58 • 55 • 96

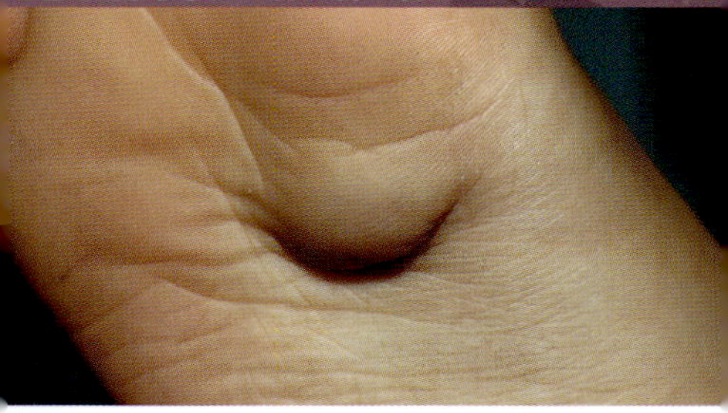

Neurofibroma. Soft, skin-colored nodule on the mid-plantar skin of a child.

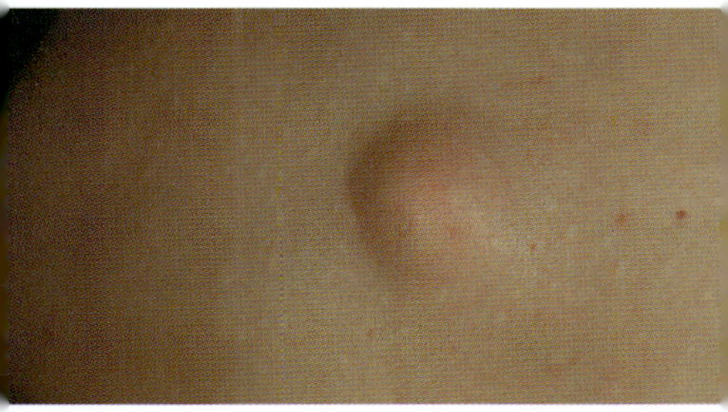

Lipoma. Soft, subcutaneous nodule unattached to the overlying skin.

101 DDx ref

SKIN-COLORED PAPULES AND NODULES WITH A SMOOTH SURFACE

Piezogenic papules

99 • 100 • 38

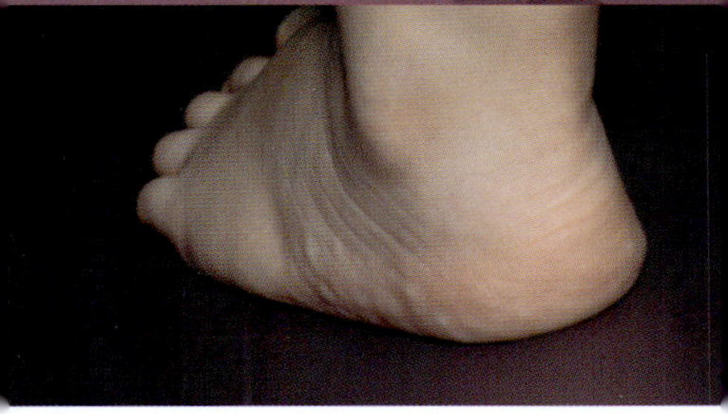

Piezogenic foot papules induced by pressure on the heel.

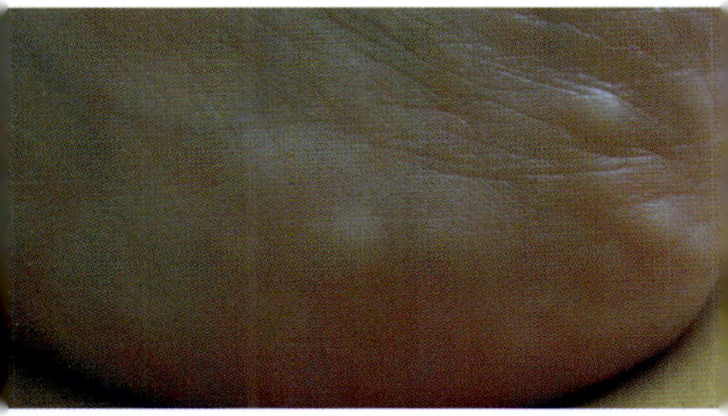

Smooth-surfaced papules that appear on a child's heel upon standing.

100

SKIN-COLORED PAPULES AND NODULES WITH A SMOOTH SURFACE

Neurofibroma and lipomas

DDx ref 58 • 55 • 96

CLINICAL FEATURES

Neurofibromas are soft, easily inverted, skin-colored to brown papules or nodules that may occur anywhere on the skin. A large plaque-like neurofibroma (plexiform neurofibroma) is occasionally seen.

Cutaneous neurofibromas may occur as solitary lesions or may be associated with neurofibromatosis (see topic 118).

Solitary lesions when present early in life, may precede the other features of neurofibromatosis. Usually, café-au-lait macules occur first, then neurofibromas later in childhood.

Lipomas are soft, subcutaneous nodules unattached to the overlying skin. They usually do not occur until adolescence. The neck, upper chest, and arms are the predominant locations. The **angiolipoma** variant of lipoma may be painful.

TREATMENT

Surgical excision is the only treatment option, but should be used judiciously.

101

SKIN-COLORED PAPULES AND NODULES WITH A SMOOTH SURFACE

Piezogenic papules

DDx ref 99 • 100 • 38

CLINICAL FEATURES

Piezogenic papules are common, rarely painful papules that occur most often on the **feet**. They may occasionally be seen on the **wrist**.

The lesions represent herniation of subcutaneous fat into the connective tissue.

The herniations are seen when pressure is applied to the heel, as on standing.

TREATMENT

Treatment is usually unnecessary, but painful lesions may be excised or treated with orthopedic padding (heel cups) or compression stockings.

102

SKIN-COLORED PAPULES AND NODULES WITH A SMOOTH SURFACE

Sweat gland tumors

DDx ref 98 • 95 • 94

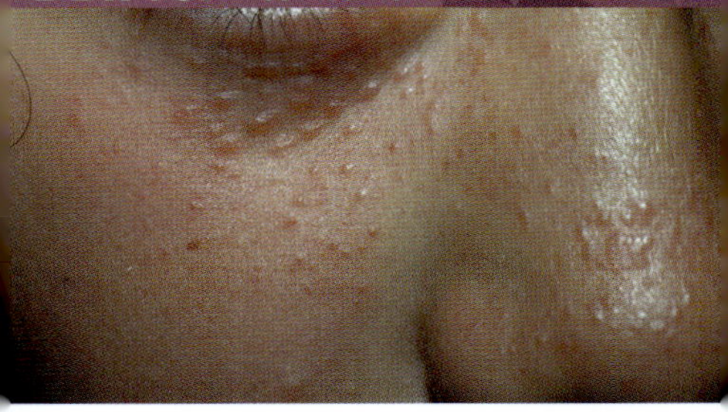

Syringomas. Multiple skin-colored papules on the face and lower eyelid.

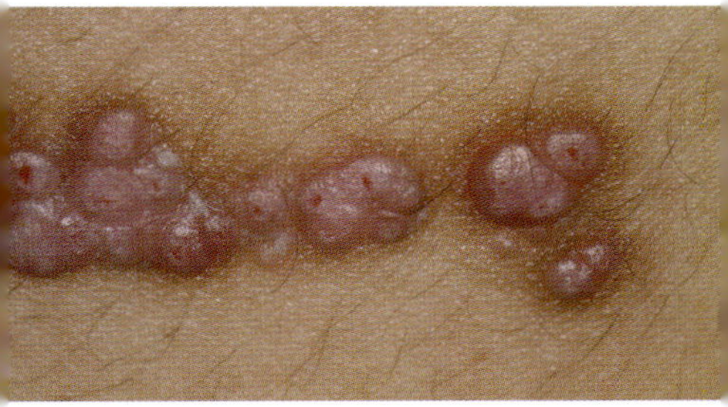

Syringocystadenoma papilliferum arising within a nevus sebaceous.

103

SKIN-COLORED PAPULES AND NODULES WITH A SMOOTH SURFACE

Gianotti–Crosti syndrome

DDx ref 91 • 94 • 31

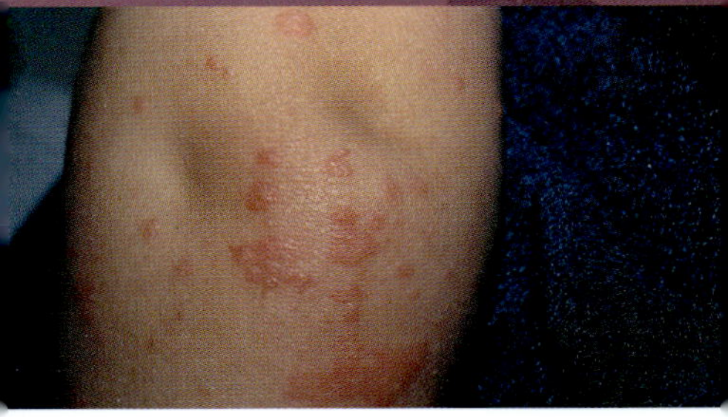

Grouped and linear papules around the elbow in a child with EBV-related Gianotti–Crosti syndrome.

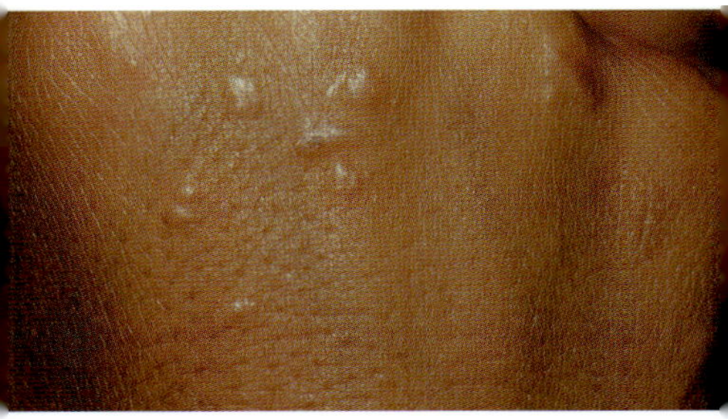

Gianotti–Crosti syndrome. Skin-colored flat-topped papules on the back of the hand.

102 Sweat gland tumors

DDx ref 98 • 95 • 94

CLINICAL FEATURES

Sweat gland tumors in childhood are rare. They may be seen as solitary or multiple lesions.

Syringomas appear at puberty as 1–2-mm skin-colored to yellowish soft papules. They occur on the eyelids, cheeks, axillae, abdomen, and vulva. They are more common in girls and in children with Down syndrome. Most often, lesions are limited to the eyelids. There is an eruptive autosomal dominant form, but the gene defect has not been isolated.

Syringocystadenoma papilliferum are seen as pink papules most commonly arising in sebaceous nevi in adolescence. At times, they will drain and crust.

TREATMENT

Treatment of choice for solitary lesions is surgical excision. Multiple lesions are difficult to treat, but carbon dioxide laser has been employed.

103 Gianotti–Crosti syndrome

DDx ref 91 • 94 • 31

CLINICAL FEATURES

Gianotti–Crosti syndrome (papular acrodermatitis) is characterized by groups of flat-topped papules in acral areas. They may be erythematous or skin-colored. The lesions can vary markedly in size between affected individuals, but are relatively monomorphic in a given child. Involvement of the cheeks, buttocks, and limb with prominence over the hands, elbow, and knees is usual, but the eruption may be more widespread. The trunk may occasionally be involved, but the scalp and mucous membranes are spared. The degree of pruritus is quite variable. The eruption was initially described in relationship to the hepatitis B virus in Italy, but in the USA, infection with EBV predominates, although many other viruses and immunizations have been associated. In some cases, the rash is preceded by low-grade fever and mild upper respiratory tract symptoms. Generalized lymphadenopathy and hepatosplenomegaly are rare. The eruption is chronic, lasting 2–8 weeks.

TREATMENT

The lesions resolve spontaneously and treatment does not alter time to resolution. Antihistamines and mid-potency topical steroids may help with pruritus.

Post-inflammatory hypopigmentation and pityriasis alba

105 • 107 • 108

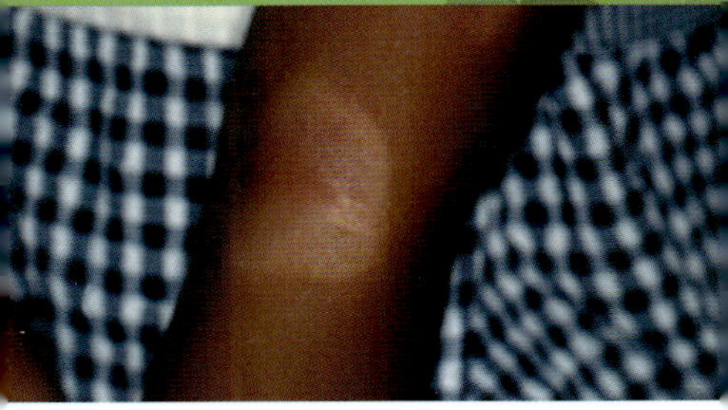

Blotchy post-inflammatory hypopigmentation after treatment for atopic dermatitis.

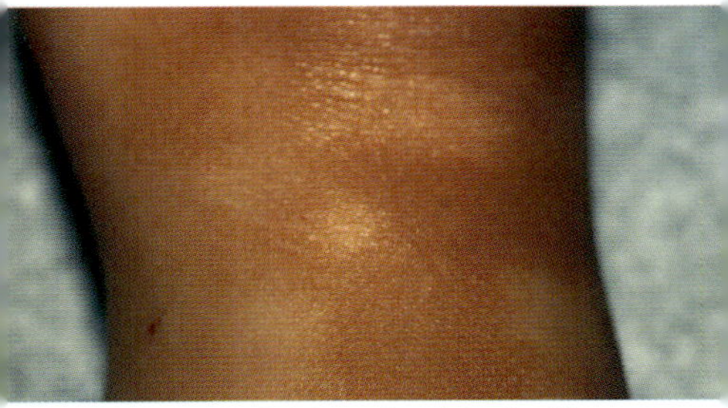

Hypopigmented, slightly scaly patch of mild dermatitis referred to as 'pityriasis alba'.

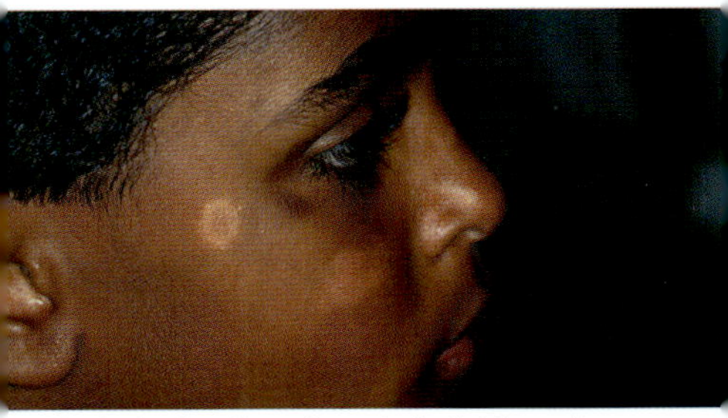

Pityriasis alba. Hypopigmented, slightly scaly, plaques with indistinct borders on a child's face.

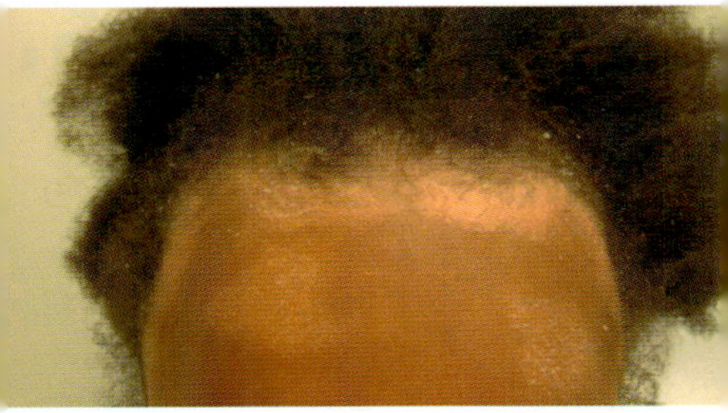

Inflammatory hypopigmentation along frontal hairline and forehead.

CLINICAL FEATURES

Post-inflammatory hypopigmentation may be seen after any inflammatory skin condition. In childhood, it is most commonly seen following resolution of plaques of atopic dermatitis. It may be seen along with areas of post-inflammatory hyperpigmentation. The hypopigmentation is most obvious in dark-skinned children. The normal pigmentation returns several months after the resolution of the inflammatory disorder.

Pityriasis alba is characterized by multiple, oval, scaly, flat, hypopigmented plaques on the face, extensor surface of the arms, and upper trunk. The lesions range from a few millimeters to 5 cm in diameter and multiples may be seen. Pruritus is rare. It is also more obvious in dark-skinned children and in the summer when the rest of the skin tans and these lesions remain light. As opposed to vitiligo, it is not totally depigmented and the borders of the lesions are indistinct. The lesions usually resolve spontaneously and may recur intermittently throughout childhood and adolescence.

In both conditions, inflammatory injury to melanocytes results in decreased pigment production and transfer.

TREATMENT

Bland lubrication will often suffice. Low-potency topical steroids twice a day for 2 weeks or topical tacrolimus are often prescribed. Normal color will not return within the 2-week period of treatment.

WHITE LESIONS

Vitiligo

104 • 106 • 115

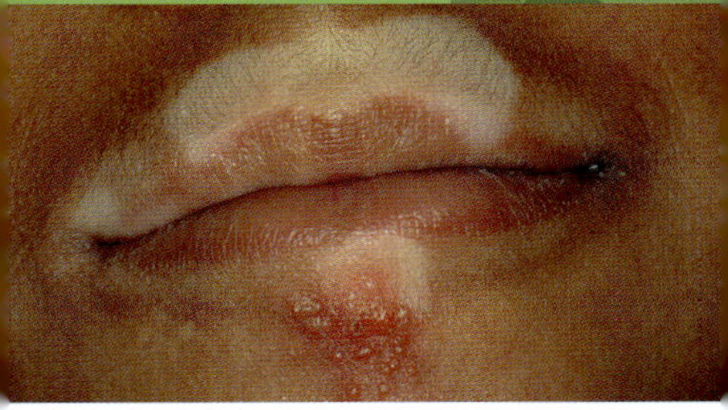

Generalized vitiligo. Symmetrical involvement of the lips. Note the distinct borders.

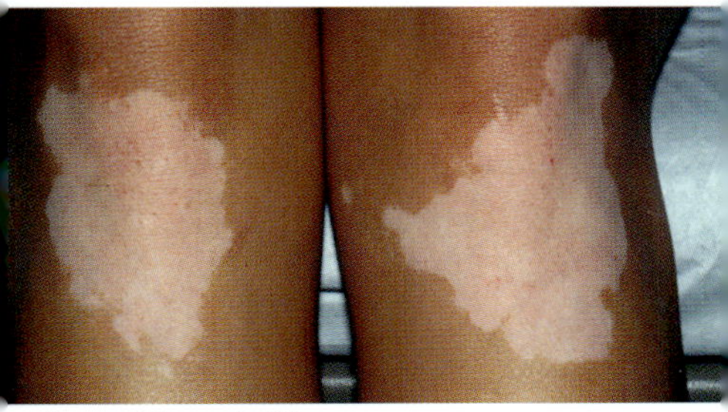

Symmetric acral vitiligo.

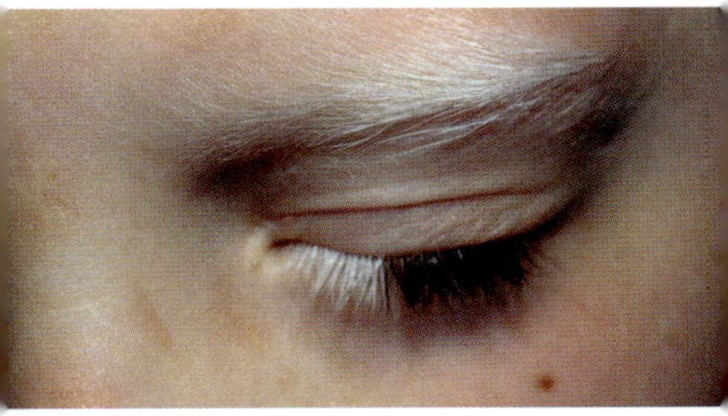

Vitiligo of the eyelashes and eyebrows.

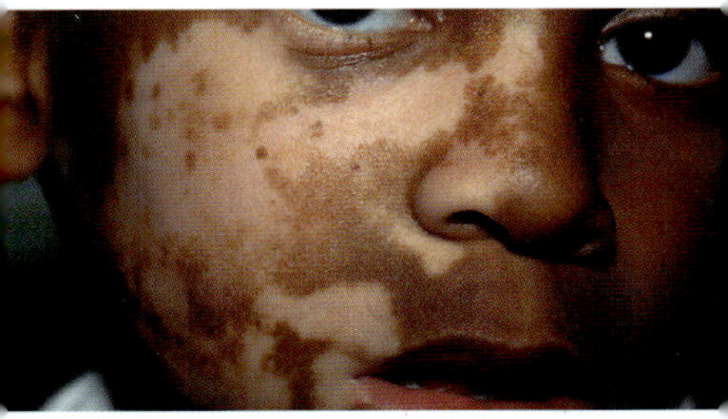

Rapidly progressing segmental vitiligo.

CLINICAL FEATURES

Vitiligo is an acquired patchy depigmentation of the skin secondary to localized destruction of melanocytes. It occurs in 1–2% of the population worldwide. The patches are completely depigmented with distinct borders.

In dark-skinned children early in the course of lesional development before total melanocyte destruction, hypopigmented skin can be found in between the depigmented and normal skin (trichrome vitiligo). Hair within a patch of vitiligo is often depigmented. Of the cases of vitiligo, 50% begin before the age of 18 years. Vitiligo may either be generalized or segmental.

Generalized vitiligo begins acrally and is remarkably symmetrical. The extensor surfaces of extremities, the face, and neck are the most common areas involved. Generalized vitiligo is slowly progressive, although most children will have <20% of the body surface affected. Generalized vitiligo is not one disease, but a common endpoint of melanocyte destruction. Generalized vitiligo is the most common form of vitiligo seen in children and is associated with multiple other autoimmune disorders, most commonly hypothyroidism.

Segmental vitiligo affects only one part of the child's body. Segmental vitiligo spreads rapidly within the involved area and then stabilizes, usually within 1 year. Segmental vitiligo is not associated with autoimmune diseases.

TREATMENT

In children with minimal disease in cosmetically unimportant areas, therapy is not necessary since it does not alter long-term prognosis. The family must be counseled on the need for rigorous sun protection to the affected areas.

For children with <20% of the body surface involved and wishing therapy, the first-line of treatment is topical therapy. Topical steroids have been used for decades. Potent topical steroids are as effective as superpotent topical steroids and have less risk of side-effects. The topical immunomodulators (pimecrolimus and tacrolimus) are also used and are preferred for the treatment of facial vitiligo. Topical calcipotriol has also been used, but needs further study.

If >25% of the body surface is involved or topical therapy has been ineffective and the child desires further treatment, phototherapy may be employed. Narrowband UVB (UVB 311 nm) is the treatment of choice. Narrowband UVB therapy is safe and more effective than topical therapy, but is very time consuming. Home units may be obtained to minimize travel time. The 308 nm excimer laser is useful for localized areas not responsive to other modalities.

In chronic vitiligo, treatment unresponsive, stable vitiligo melanocyte transplantation may be considered. Repigmentation in vitiligo is a slow process taking many months to years and 100% repigmentation should not be expected. With every treatment modality, the face repigments better than any other area, but areas of vitiligo located on skin without hair follicles will not repigment.

106 WHITE LESIONS

Piebaldism

DDx ref 105 • 104 • 112

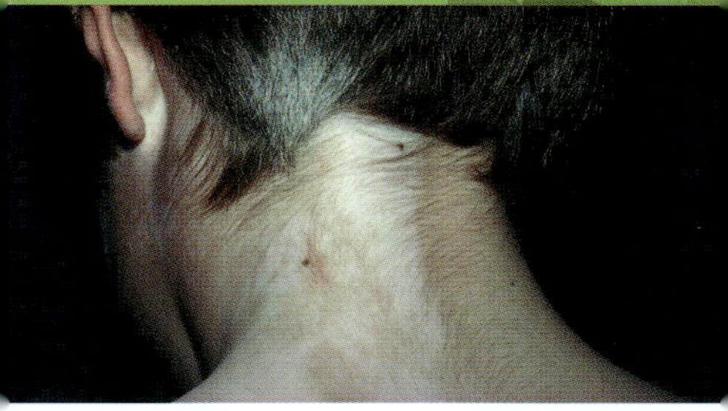

Piebaldism. Segmental white patch on posterior neck and white scalp hair present since birth.

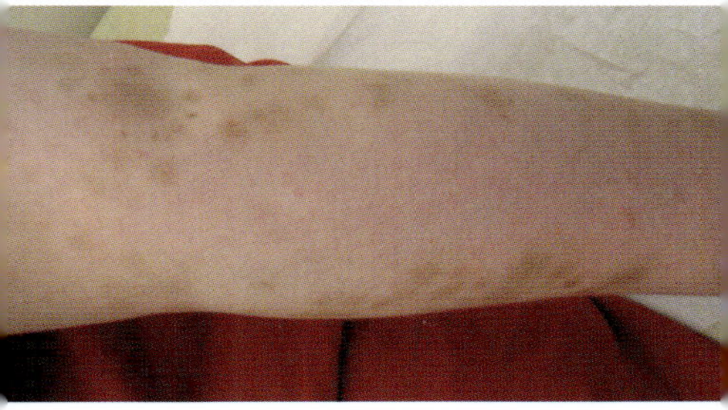

Piebaldism. Depigmented patch on the left arm.

107 WHITE LESIONS

Ash leaf macules

DDx ref 105 • 104 • 114

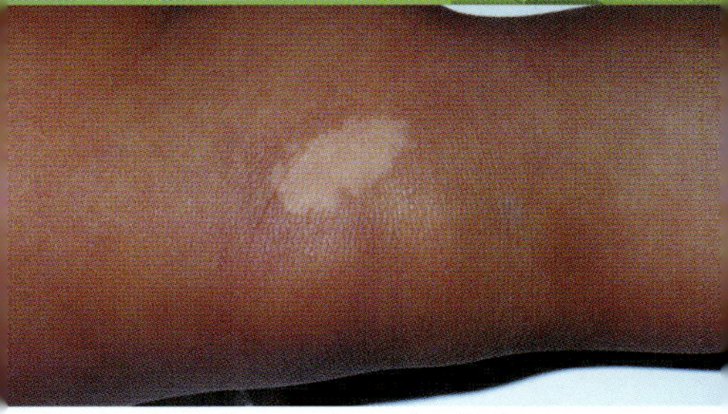

Ash leaf hypopigmented macule of tuberous sclerosis.

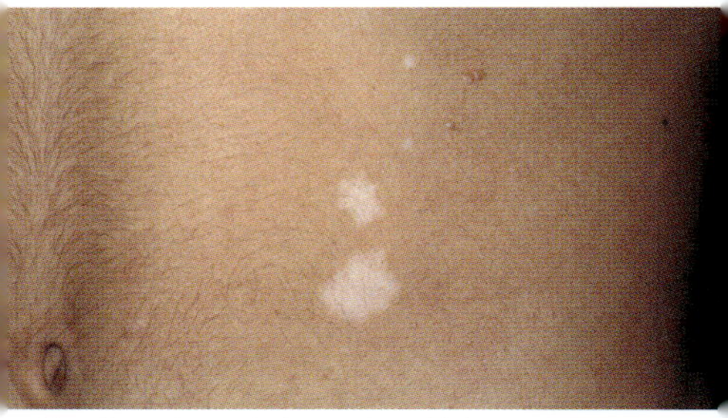

Two hypopigmented macules of tuberous sclerosis. Note the different shapes.

106 WHITE LESIONS

Piebaldism

DDx ref 105 • 104 • 112

CLINICAL FEATURES

Piebaldism describes depigmented areas of skin present from birth. A white hair or hairs in the affected area is a useful clue. Piebaldism is an autosomal dominant condition.

At birth, piebaldism may be difficult to detect without the use of a Wood's lamp that accentuates the color difference. The depigmented areas may be large and block-like on the trunk. Areas of hyperpigmentation may be found within and surrounding the areas of depigmentation. The majority of children with piebaldism have mutations of the c-kit gene or uncommonly, the WS SNA12 gene. Also with depigmented patches at birth is Waardenburg syndrome that features a white forelock, different-colored irises in each eye, and dystopia canthorum.

There are four types of Waardenburg: type I having the typical features; type II lacking dystopia canthorum but with deafness; type III having musculoskeletal abnormalities; and type IV having associated Hirschsprung disease of the colon. All are autosomal dominant except the recessive type IV.

Waardenburg I and III children have mutations in the PAX3 gene; type II in the WS2A MITF, WS2D SNA12 genes, and type IV in EDN3, EDNRB or SOX10 genes.

TREATMENT

There is no treatment to repigment areas of piebaldism. If Waardenburg syndrome is suspected, referral to hearing and other specialists may be of benefit.

107 WHITE LESIONS

Ash leaf macules

DDx ref 105 • 104 • 114

CLINICAL FEATURES

Ash leaf macules are lance-ovate-shaped hypopigmented macules, which resemble the leaves of the eastern mountain ash tree. They are seen in normal infants and are a diagnostic criterion for tuberous sclerosis. Not all hypopigmented macules are ash leaf–shaped. They may be polygonal or confetti-like. Hypopigmented macules are difficult to see in light-skinned children and should be examined in a dark room with a Wood's lamp to accentuate the areas of hypopigmentation.

TSC is autosomal dominant, caused by mutations in the genes coding for hamartin (TSC1) or tuberin (TSC2). TSC may be diagnosed either by gene testing or by diagnostic criteria. Two major features or one major feature plus two minor features is diagnostic. Three or more hypopigmented macules are one of the major features and confetti-like macules are a minor feature. Other major features on the skin in TSC include the shagreen patch (connective tissue nevus), facial angiofibromas, fibrous forehead plaque, and non-traumatic ungual and periungual fibromas. CNS disease, including infantile seizures and mental retardation may be severe, as may be the renal involvement.

TREATMENT

Treatment of the hypopigmented lesions, shagreen patch, and fibrous forehead plaque is unnecessary.

Facial angiofibromas, if small, will respond to pulsed dye laser treatment. Larger, thicker facial angiofibroma lesions will require treatment with a carbon dioxide laser or use of the oral mTOR inhibitor rapamycin.

Ungual and periungual fibromas require surgical excision.

WHITE LESIONS

Tinea versicolor

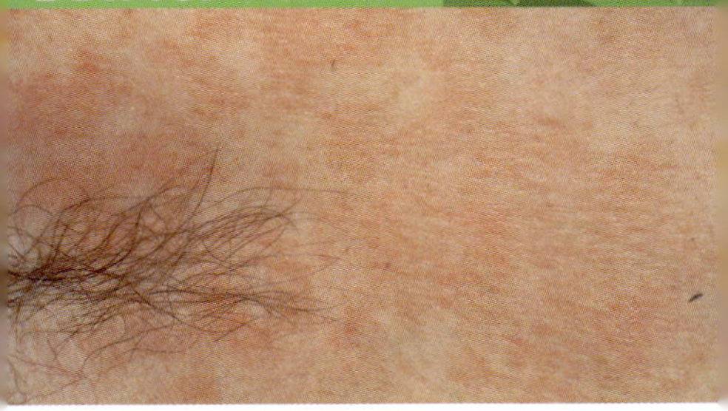

Multiple tan macules with a fine scale over the chest of an adolescent with tinea versicolor.

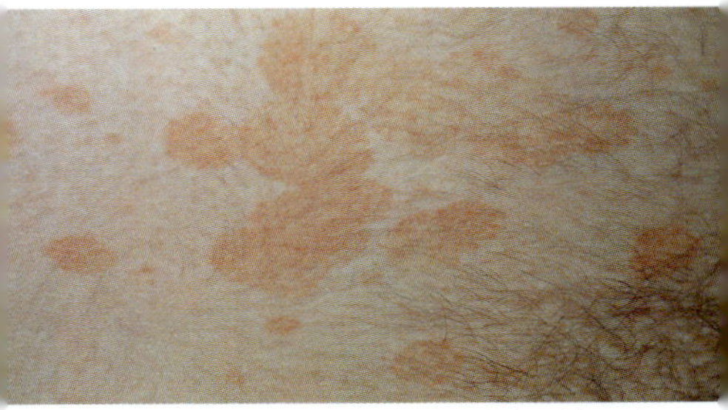

Tan macules of tinea versicolor in a light-skinned child.

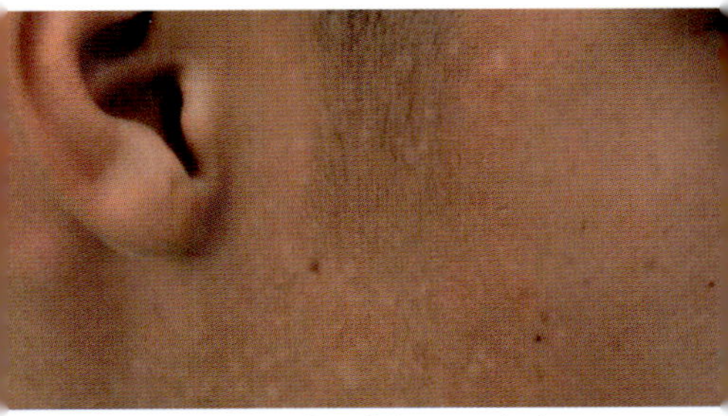

Hypopigmented macules of tinea versicolor on a child's face and neck.

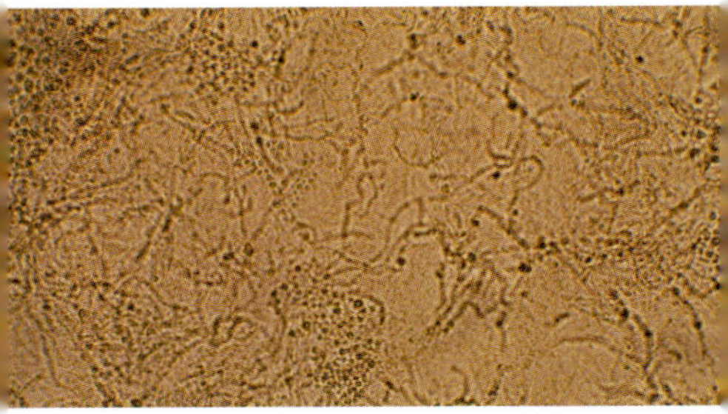

Photomicrograph of KOH examination of tinea versicolor. Multiple short hyphae and spores are seen.

Tinea versicolor

DDx ref 104 • 105 • 74

CLINICAL FEATURES

The lesions of tinea versicolor vary widely in color.

In light-skinned individuals, they are typically reddish brown.

In dark-skinned individuals, they are more often hypopigmented. Multiple oval macules with a fine scale are seen on the neck, chest, upper back, shoulders, face, and upper arms of adolescents. Occasionally the lesions become confluent, forming large plaques. The lesions tend to be persistent.

KOH examination of scrapings reveals numerous short, curved hyphae and circular spores, the so-called 'macaroni and meatballs' appearance.

The cause is a yeast organism, *Malassezia globosa*. Tinea versicolor must be differentiated from seborrheic dermatitis, contact dermatitis, tinea corporis, pityriasis alba, post-inflammatory hypopigmentation, and confluent and reticulated papillomatosis.

TREATMENT

Multiple treatment modalities have been employed.

For small areas of involvement, topical imidazole creams applied twice a day for 2–4 weeks are effective. Topical nystatin is not effective.

For adolescents with large areas of involvement, selenium sulfide 2.5% applied overnight for 1 week and then weekly for 4 weeks is the treatment of choice. Skin irritation is the main side-effect. Oral fluconazole 400 mg given twice 7 days apart is also a convenient therapy. No matter what forms of treatment are used, recurrence is common.

109 WHITE LESIONS

Lichen sclerosis

DDx ref 105 • 111 • 74

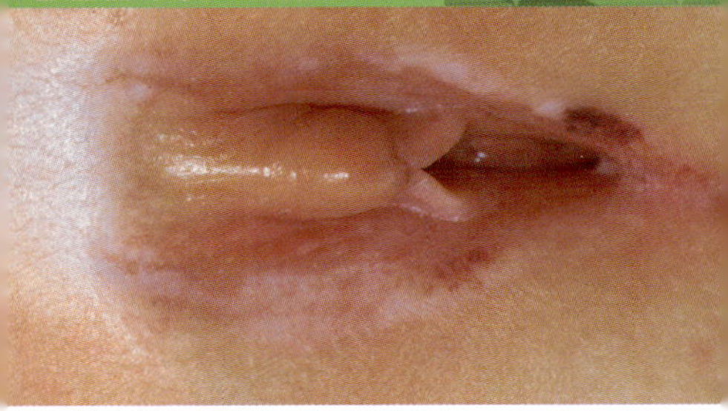

Lichen sclerosis of a child's vulva.

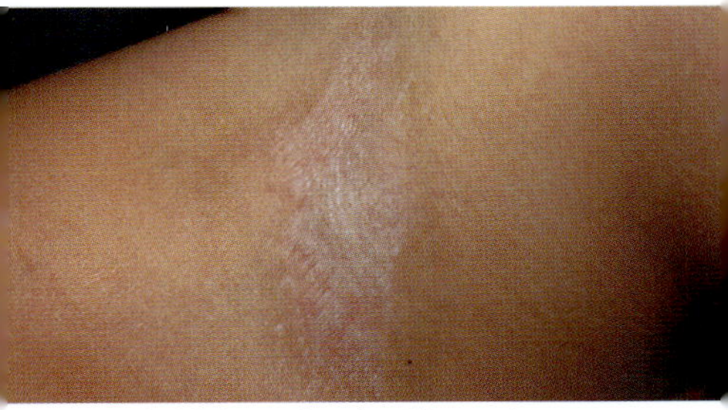

Extragenital lichen sclerosis of the neck. Telangiectasia and fine wrinkling within the white area.

110 WHITE LESIONS

Oculocutaneous albinism (OCA)

DDx ref 105 • 106 • 112

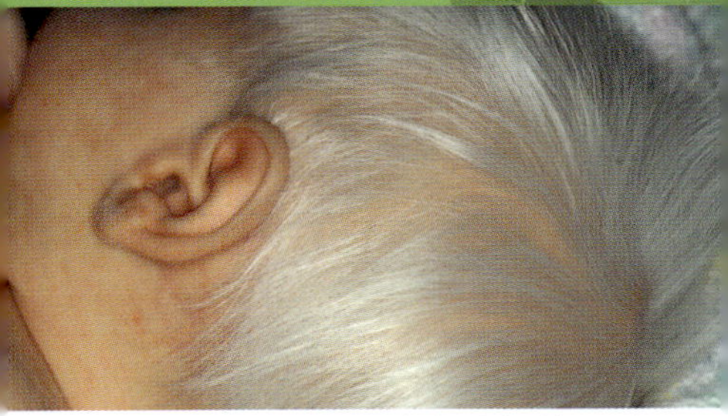

Baby with OCA1A with white hair, pink skin, and severe nystagmus.

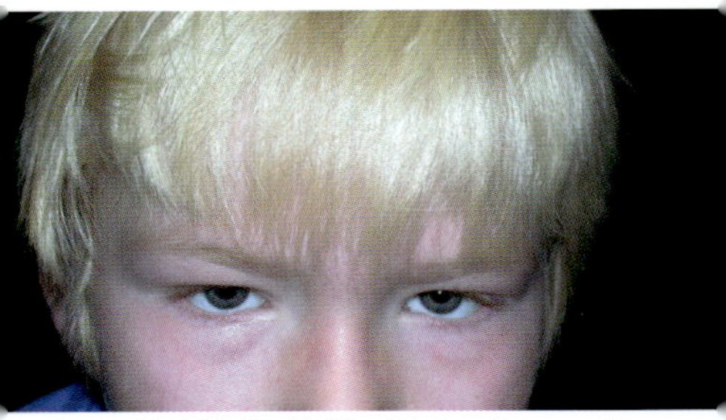

Child with OCA1B with blond hair and some skin pigment.

109 WHITE LESIONS
Lichen sclerosis

DDx ref 105 • 111 • 74

CLINICAL FEATURES

Lichen sclerosis is seen as a hypopigmented plaque in the anogenital areas of grade-school or adolescent girls. It is rarely seen in males. Purpura, vesicles, and telangiectasia may be seen within the plaque. With time, the skin surface may become thinned and wrinkled. Ulcerations and excoriations may be superimposed on the primary plaque lesions. Bruising and bleeding may occur. The anogenital lesions in girls tend to surround both orifices in a figure-of-eight pattern. Itching and burning of skin are frequent complaints. Painful defecation, constipation, bloody stool, and encopresis have been reported. The erosions, bruising, and bleeding in the genital area have been mistaken for child abuse. Some adolescents may improve temporarily, but, if untreated, the condition is one of chronic progression. Squamous cell carcinoma has been reported in long-standing disease in adults. Extragenital lichen sclerosis appears as asymptomatic or slightly pruritic white plaques on the upper back and chest, and occasionally the face and extremities. Coexistence of lichen sclerosis and morphea is observed in children.

TREATMENT

Treatment for anogenital lichen sclerosis is with a superpotent topical steroid ointment twice a day until symptoms resolve. Treatment should be reinstituted immediately if symptoms recur. It is unknown whether or not treatment alters the long-term risk of development of squamous cell carcinoma.

110 WHITE LESIONS
Oculocutaneous albinism (OCA)

DDx ref 105 • 106 • 112

CLINICAL FEATURES

Newborns with white hair, pink skin, photophobia, and ocular nystagmus should bring to mind OCA. There are four classes of OCA. OCA type 1 is autosomal recessive and involves mutations in the gene encoding the tyrosinase enzyme.

Children with OCA1A have no tyrosinase activity and children with OCA1B retain residual tyrosinase activity. There is a temperature-sensitive mutation in OCA1B, where the tyrosinase enzyme fails to function at 35–37°C. Children with OCA1A will never develop pigment, whereas in OCA1B and the other OCAs: OCA2 (p gene defect), OCA3 (TRP-1 gene defect), and OCA4 (MATP defect), some hair and skin pigment will be present at birth and darken with age, including the later appearance of freckles and pigmented nevi. Rarely, albinism may be associated with petechiae and bleeding caused by abnormal platelet aggregation in the Hermansky–Pudlak syndrome, a mutation of B3A subunit of Ap3 gene, the DTNPB1 gene, or the 8HP51, HP53, Hp54, HP56, or BLOC1539 genes. Albino children who suffer frequent infections may have the Chediak–Higashi syndrome with mutations of the CHS1 gene, which results in dysfunctional leukocyte degranulation.

TREATMENT

There is no specific treatment for the pigment loss. Strict sun avoidance and sun protection should be strongly recommended and referral to an ophthalmologist will be needed.

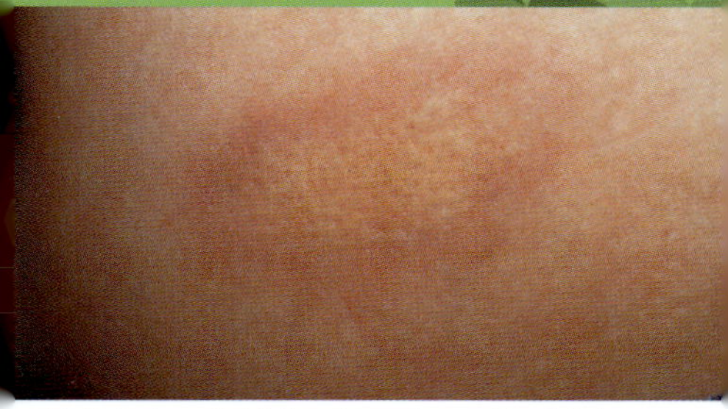

Early lesion of childhood morphea with slightly depressed skin and a lilac border.

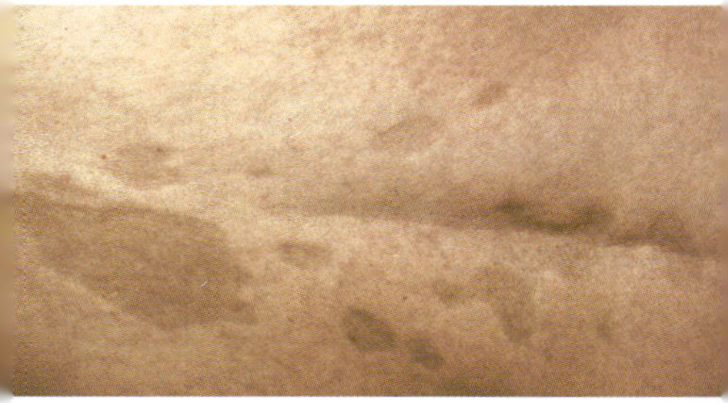

Childhood guttate morphea follows the lines of Blaschko.

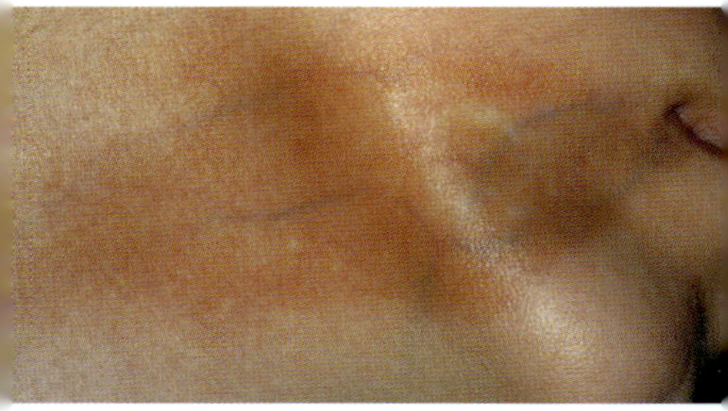

Linear involvement of the jaw and neck in childhood morphea.

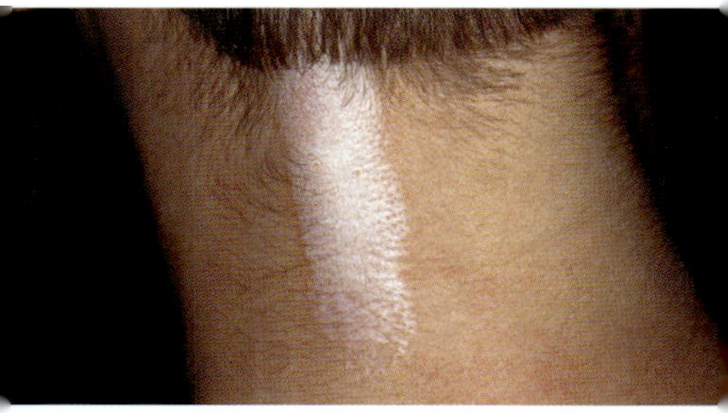

Linear morphea as white immobile plaque on a child's neck.

CLINICAL FEATURES

Childhood morphea is characterized by slightly depressed, immobile areas of skin. Initial lesions are often dusky brown, sometimes with a lilac border, but as lesions evolve they become bound down and white. The skin of early lesions is not immobile.

Two main patterns of childhood morphea are seen, the linear or curvilinear lesions and the oval 'guttate' plaque-type lesions. Some children will exhibit both types. Linear lesions often follow the embryonic lines of Blaschko and are twice as likely on the limbs as the head. Sometimes, linear lesions will be restricted to one half of the body. The linear lesions on the head (*en coup de sabre*) virtually always include loss of scalp and/or eyebrow hair within the affected areas and may progress to bone indentation.

In the Parry–Romberg syndrome, facial hemiatrophy is present but the overlying skin may be lax, not bound down. On a limb, linear lesions that cross a joint will restrict joint movement and may interfere with bone growth. Rarely, the center of the morphea lesion will ulcerate. The guttate morphea lesions usually are multiple and seen on the trunk or proximal extremities. A third of affected children will suffer concomitant arthralgias.

In childhood, peripheral blood eosinophilia and a positive ANA test are sometimes found.

The pathogenesis is unknown. The inflammatory early stage is predominantly lymphocytic, and in the sclerotic stage, dermal collagen replaces the underlying subcutaneous fat, binding the skin down to the subcutaneous fascia. Morphea lesions are active for 2–4 years.

TREATMENT

For childhood morphea, there is no specific treatment or comparative studies of standard treatments.

For early disease, narrowband UVA1 phototherapy with or without calcipotriene ointment may halt progression of morphea. This phototherapy requires a series of treatments that may not be locally available.

For localized disease, topical calcipotriene ointment, and topical imiquimod, have demonstrated improvement.

For bound-down linear lesions or widespread disease, systemic immunosuppressive drugs such as methotrexate or corticosteroids, or both, have been used. Where available, broadband UVA or photochemotherapy (PUVA) have been effective. Childhood morphea is rare and is best managed by experienced pediatric dermatologists or rheumatologists.

112 WHITE LESIONS
Nevus depigmentosus

DDx ref 113 • 104 • 105

Nevus depigmentosus on the lateral trunk of a toddler.

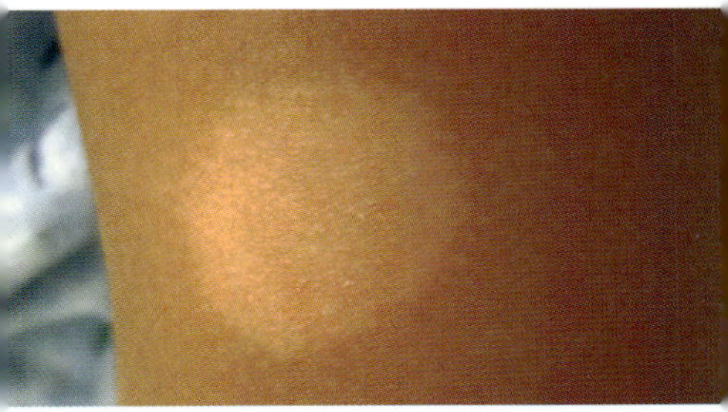

Hypopigmented patch of nevus depigmentosus on the arm of a child. (Reprinted from Paller, AS & Mancini AJ, Hurwitz Clinical Pediatric Dermatology, 4th Edition. Copyright Elsevier 2011.)

113 WHITE LESIONS
Nevus anemicus

DDx ref 112 • 105 • 104

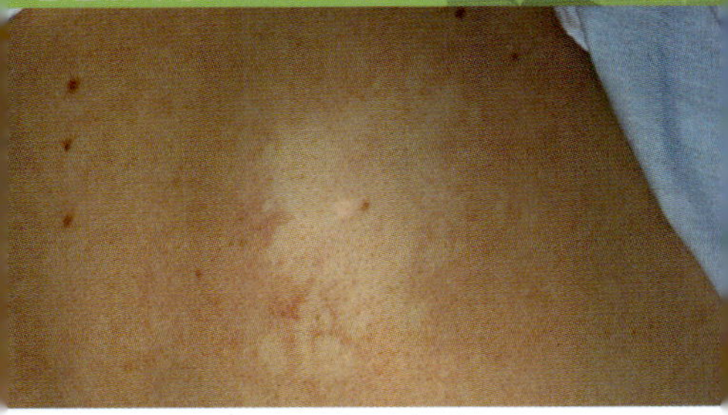

Localized hypopigmented patch of nevus anemicus.

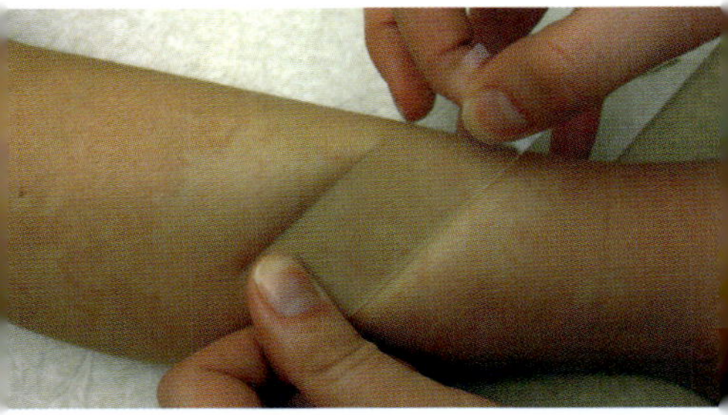

Nevus anemicus. Return of skin to normal color following compression with a glass slide.

112 WHITE LESIONS

Nevus depigmentosus

DDx ref 113 • 104 • 105

CLINICAL FEATURES

Nevus depigmentosus presents as a hypopigmented unilateral patch at birth or within the first few months of infancy. It is quasidermatomal with borders that are sometimes irregular. Whorled patterns following the embryonic lines of Blaschko have been described. Family history of similar lesions is usually negative. Most authorities consider this a birthmark of hypofunctioning melanocytes both in the production and transfer of melanin granules. The skin change persists. Compression of the border will not eliminate color changes as seen in nevus anemicus.

TREATMENT

There is no known effective therapy. Protecting against sunburn in this area with clothing or sunscreen is recommended.

113 WHITE LESIONS

Nevus anemicus

DDx ref 112 • 105 • 104

CLINICAL FEATURES

Nevus anemicus presents as a localized, solitary, hypopigmented macule. Compression of the border will result in equal color of affected and unaffected skin. It is a problem of vascular origin, not melanocytic. It is thought to be a birthmark of blood vessels hyperresponsive to catecholamines via alpha-adrenergic receptors. Injection of alpha-adrenergic blocking agents will temporarily restore the color to that of normal skin.

TREATMENT

There is no effective treatment.

114 DDx ref

WHITE LESIONS
Linear and whorled hypomelanosis (Hypomelanosis of Ito)

112 • 127 • 15

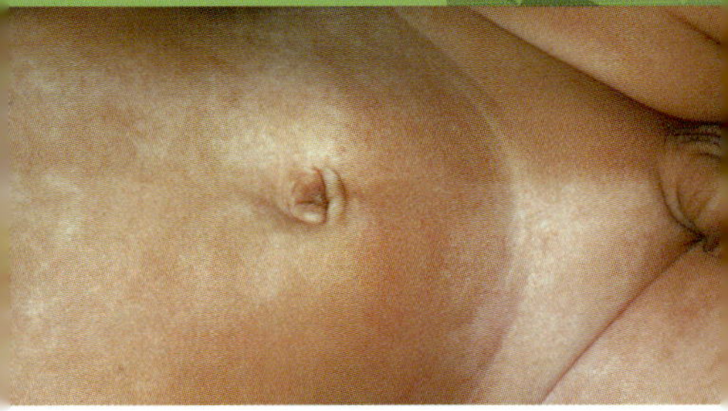

Block-like hypopigmentation terminating at midline in a baby with hypomelanosis of Ito.

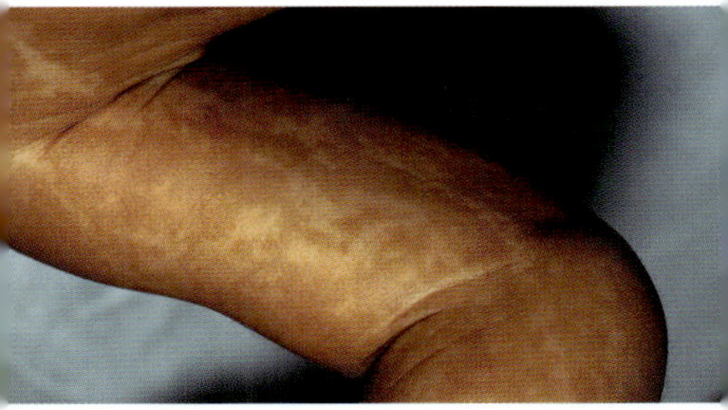

Swirls of hypopigmentation on the arm of an infant with hypomelanosis of Ito.

115 DDx ref

WHITE LESIONS
Halo nevus

105 • 109 • 107

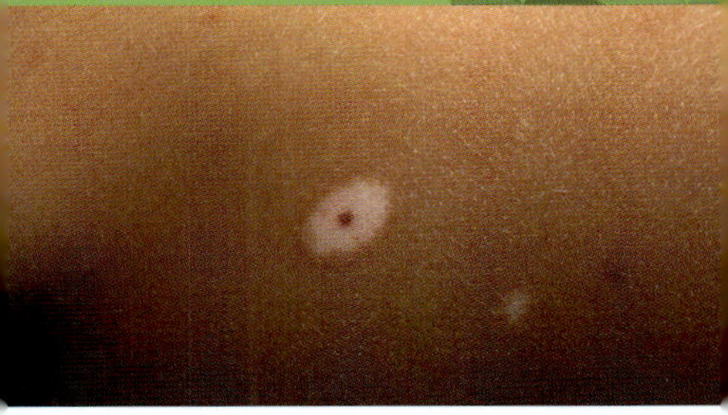

Halo nevus. White depigmented zone surrounds regressing central nevus.

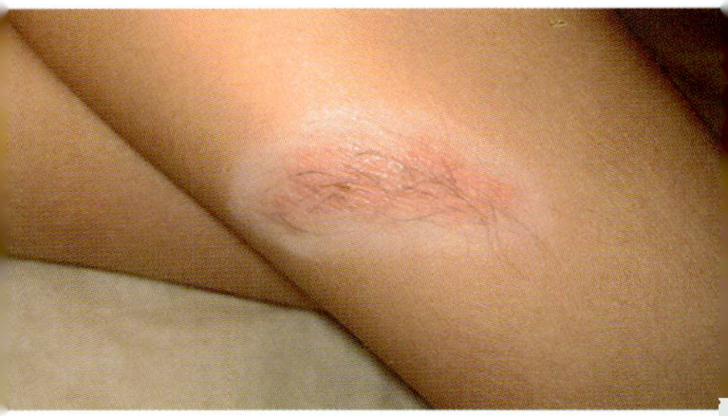

Halo nevus with hypopigmentation surrounding congenital melanocytic nevus.

114 DDx ref

WHITE LESIONS

Linear and whorled hypomelanosis (Hypomelanosis of Ito)

112 • 127 • 15

CLINICAL FEATURES

Hypomelanosis of Ito is a form of genetic mosaicism in which curvilinear swirls of hypopigmented skin are evident from birth.

In very light-skinned newborns, the pigment difference may be so subtle that it is overlooked, but as the baby's melanocytes become more functional in unaffected skin, the color differences become obvious. The hypopigmented swirls may be extensive, covering one half of the body, and sometimes bilateral. They follow the embryonic skin lines of Blaschko. The color difference is best seen on the trunk and extremities, with the swirls terminating abruptly at the midline. Also seen are block-shaped areas of hypopigmentation that also end abruptly at the midline. Changes in color and texture of hair sometimes may be found.

One-third of affected babies may demonstrate associated neurologic, ocular, dental, and skeletal abnormalities. Mental retardation, developmental delays, hypodontia, and skeletal malformations have been described. A detailed history and physical examination including neurologic and ophthalmologic examinations are recommended. Although the result of genetic mosaicism, there is not a single gene defect found, but defects in different genes in different affected children have been implicated.

TREATMENT

There is no effective treatment for the pigmentary changes. Associated abnormalities should guide referral to appropriate specialists.

115 DDx ref

WHITE LESIONS

Halo nevus

105 • 109 • 107

CLINICAL FEATURES

A halo nevus is seen as a white zone surrounding an intradermal nevus or a congenital melanocytic nevus.

A halo around a nevus is a sign of spontaneous regression of a nevus, and over months, traces of the central nevus will disappear and only the round white area remains. With time, the area repigments. Halo nevi may be single or multiple.

A halo nevus in hairy areas may show loss of pigment in the hairs (poliosis).

A child with a halo nevus may also have vitiligo, or develop it later (6 months to 5 years). Halos have been described around malignant melanomas, but this is very rare in childhood.

TREATMENT

There is no need for treatment as the skin areas will eventually repigment. The child with associated vitiligo may require vitiligo therapy.

116 FLAT BROWN LESIONS
Mongolian spots

DDx ref 117 • 118 • 119

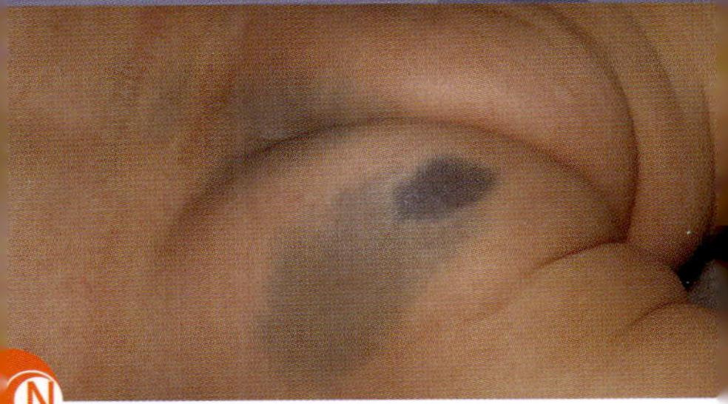

Mongolian spots over the buttocks and lumbosacral skin of a baby.

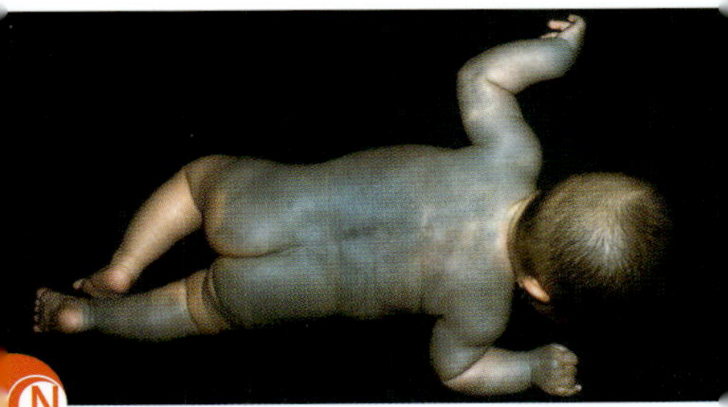

Widespread Mongolian spots of an infant.

117 FLAT BROWN LESIONS
Nevus of Ota

DDx ref 116 • 118 • 119

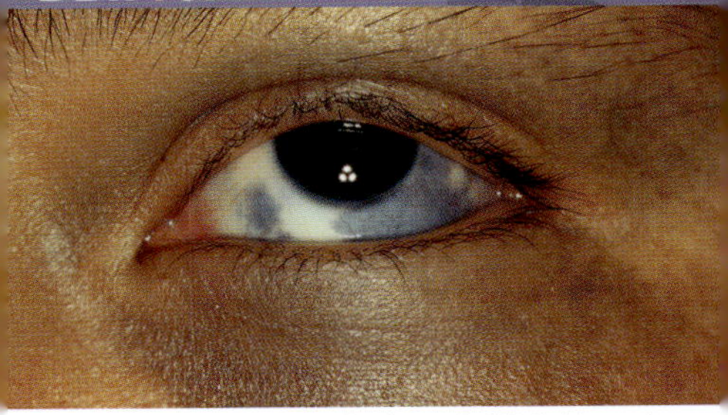

Nevus of Ota. Blue macules in periorbital skin and sclera of a teen.

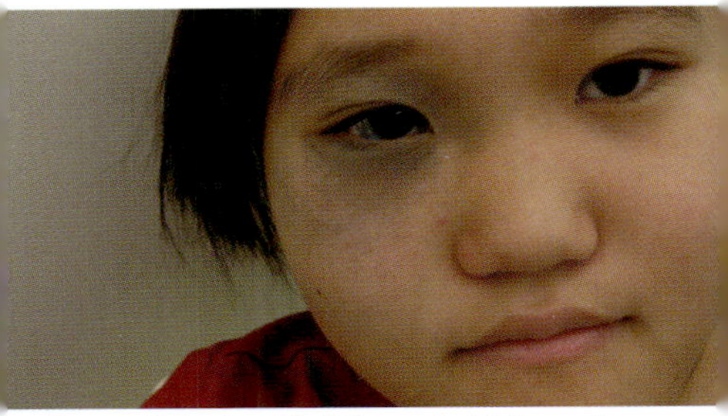

Nevus of Ota. Speckled blue periorbital macule around the right eye of an Asian child.

116 FLAT BROWN LESIONS

Mongolian spots

DDx ref 117 • 118 • 119

CLINICAL FEATURES

The mongolian spot is a blue-black macule found in the lumbosacral region of 90% of Asian, black, and Native American babies.

In some newborns they may be quite extensive, also involving the buttocks, upper back, shoulders, arms, and legs.

The color is due to an increase in spindle-shaped cells filled with melanin located between collagen fibers in the mid to deep dermis. As the epidermal pigment–containing cells mature, the overlying skin darkens and obscures some of the color difference, but mongolian spots are persistent throughout life. Widespread mongolian spots have been associated with Hunter's and Hurler's syndromes as well as GM1 gangliosidosis. They are also seen in children who also have vascular birthmarks and this association is called 'phakomatosis pigmentovascularis type 2'.

TREATMENT

There are no effective treatments. Parents should be advised that some of the color change will be obscured by age 5 years.

117 FLAT BROWN LESIONS

Nevus of Ota

DDx ref 116 • 118 • 119

CLINICAL FEATURES

Nevus of Ota is a macular blue-black, speckled pigmentation involving one side of the face including blue pigment in the sclera of the eye.

In the related nevus of Ito similar blue-black speckled pigmentation is seen around one shoulder and adjacent chest. Most of nevus of Ota and nevus of Ito are present at birth, but some are acquired in childhood.

As in mongolian spots there are spindle-shaped cells containing pigment in the mid to deep dermis.

TREATMENT

Q-switched laser treatments are beneficial in improving the appearance.

118 FLAT BROWN LESIONS

Café-au-lait macules (CALMs)

DDx ref 119 • 121 • 123

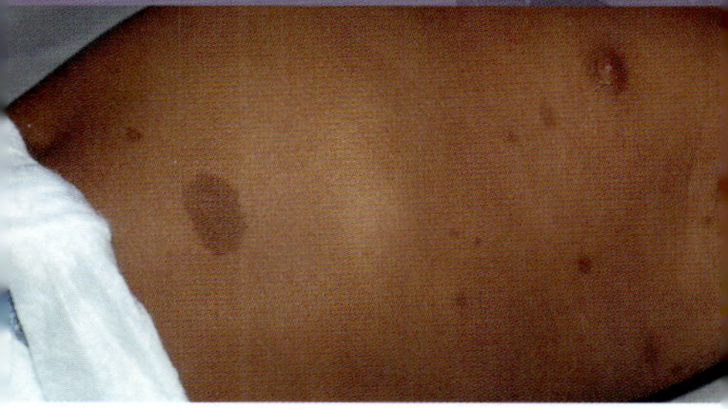

Numerous CALMs in a child with NF1.

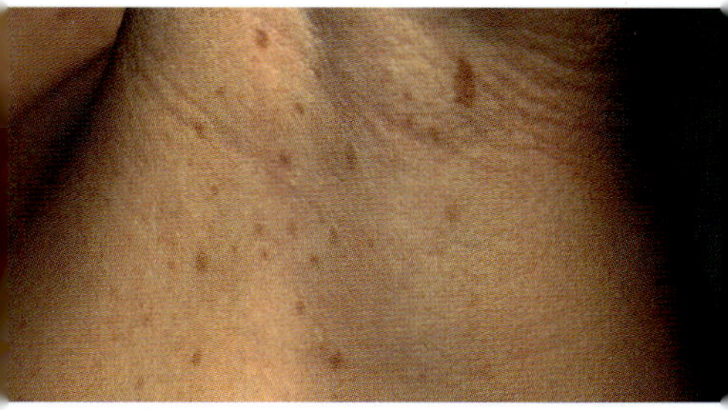

Axillary freckling in a child with NF1.

119 FLAT BROWN LESIONS

Nevus spilus

DDx ref 118 • 121 • 123

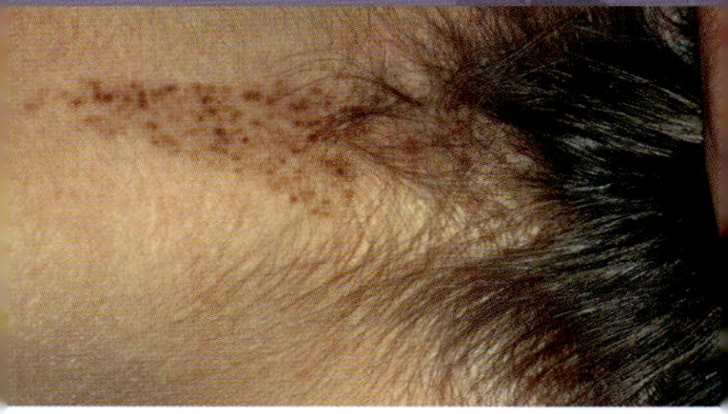

Nevus spilus on posterior neck of a teen.

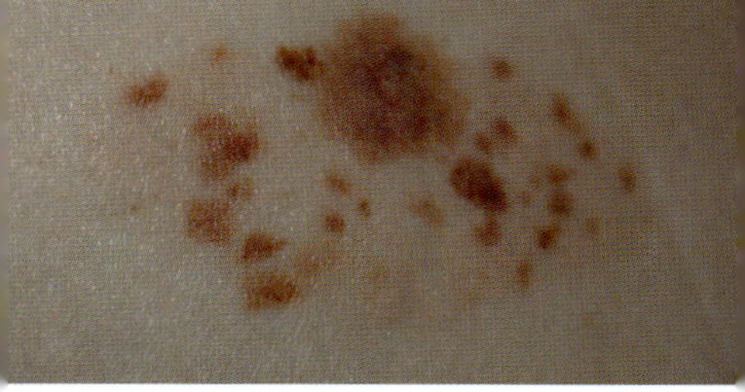

Nevus spilus. The café-au-lait macule is subtle; many brown junctional nevi are present within it.

118 FLAT BROWN LESIONS

Café-au-lait macules (CALMs)

DDx ref 119 • 121 • 123

CLINICAL FEATURES

CALMs are tan, oval macules with distinct borders. Multiple CALMs are an early sign of neurofibromatosis type 1 (NF1). CALMs are rarely present at birth but increase in number with age. One-quarter of healthy teens have at least one CALM, and having two is common.

Six or more CALMs >0.5 cm in diameter is a diagnostic sign of NF1. When combined with one other NF1 criteria [axillary freckling (multiple small CALMs), two or more neurofibromas, one plexiform neurofibroma, iris hamartomas (Lisch nodules), thinning of long bone or sphenoid dysplasia of bone, or a first-degree relative with NF1], the diagnosis of NF1 is presumed.

By age 5 years, most children with NF1 have clinical criteria for diagnosis. NF1 is autosomal dominant due to mutations in the gene encoding neurofibromin, a tumor suppressor gene. Mental deficiency and spinal neurofibromas producing deformities are likely complications. Optic gliomas may occur. Development of neurofibrosarcomas is rare in the child with NF1.

Children with NF2 (mutations in the gene encoding merlin) may have two or three CALMs but rarely more than five. CALMs also are sometimes found in other RASopathies, but usually not more than five. Large, often solitary, block-like CALMs are seen in otherwise normal children or uncommonly in the McCune–Albright syndrome of precocious puberty and fibrous dysplasia of bone. In McCune–Albright syndrome (mutations in GNAS), the CALMs precede the onset of the endocrine and skeletal changes, but the proportion of children presenting with large CALMs who actually will develop McCune–Albright syndrome is unknown and thought to be low, so genetic testing for McCune–Albright syndrome is not recommended for all children with large CALMs. Proteus syndrome, with asymmetrical, distorted areas of tissue overgrowth, and sometimes confused with NF1, rarely has CALMs.

TREATMENT

Facial CALMs may be treated with pigment-selective lasers. With multiple systems involved, children with NF1 should have a referral to a multidiscipline neurofibromatosis clinic or a genetics clinic.

119 FLAT BROWN LESIONS

Nevus spilus

DDx ref 118 • 121 • 123

CLINICAL FEATURES

Nevus spilus, the spotted nevus, is a tan macule with multiple 1–3-mm darker brown papules within it. Nevus spilus is a café-au-lait macule (CALM) with junctional nevi within it.

Usually present from birth, a nevus spilus initially may not have noticeable brown spots within the macule.

More brown spots appear with age. The background color of the CALM can vary from light brown to dark brown and the number of nevi from a few to dozens.

TREATMENT

No treatment is necessary. Rarely, in adults, malignant melanoma has been reported to arise from a nevus spilus.

120 DDx ref

FLAT BROWN LESIONS
Junctional nevi

119 • 122 • 128

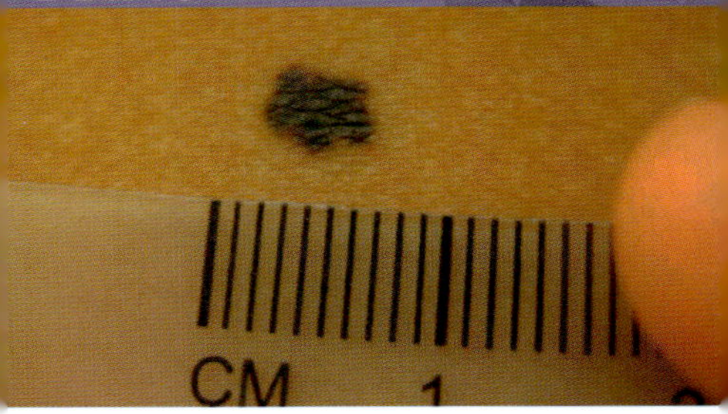

Acquired 4-mm junctional nevus on an infant's back.

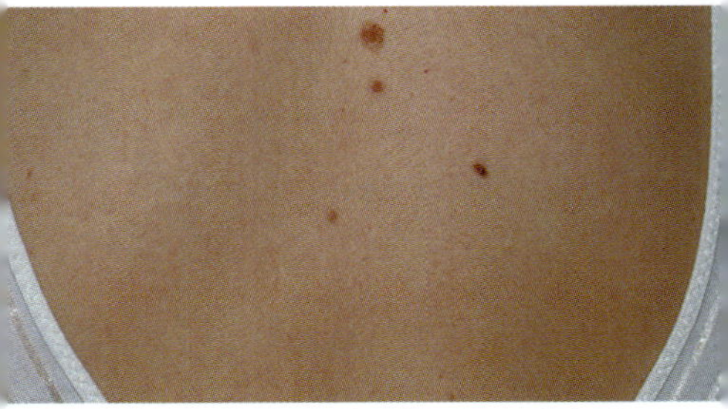

Junctional and compound nevi on a teen's back.

121 DDx ref

FLAT BROWN LESIONS
Freckles

118 • 119 • 122

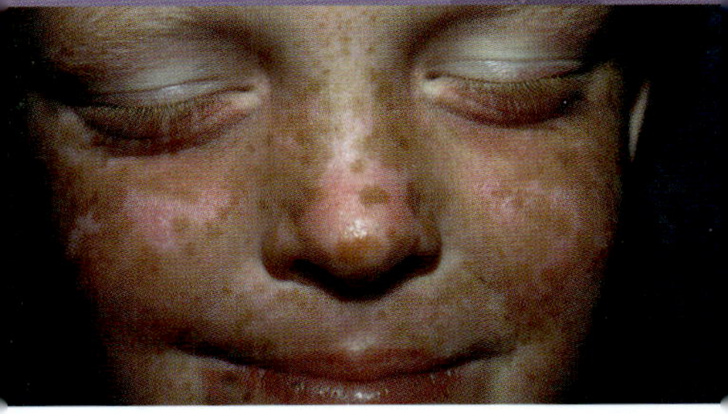

Facial freckles in a child who has sunburned skin between the freckles.

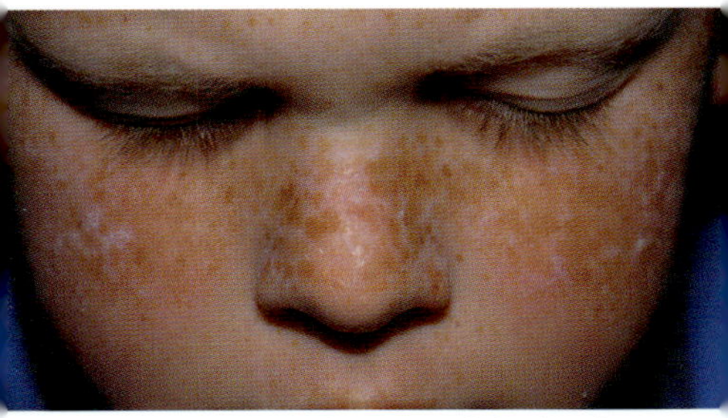

Groups of freckles on the nose and cheeks of a fair-skinned child.

120 FLAT BROWN LESIONS

Junctional nevi

DDx ref 119 • 122 • 128

CLINICAL FEATURES

Junctional nevi are acquired, flat, brown macules. They may appear in the first few months of life and increase in number linearly through the teen years. Of 1-year-old infants, 35% have one junctional nevus; teens have several dozen. The number of nevi is correlated with skin phototype and sun exposure. Junctional nevi are seen predominantly on the lateral upper arms, trunk, and face. An increased number of nevi in childhood has been correlated to an increased risk of developing melanoma in adulthood.

On the extremities, they tend to remain flat, on the face and back; some become raised over time to form compound nevi. A junctional nevus has groups of extra melanocytes at the junction of the epidermis and dermis. With age, more melanocytes appear deeper in the dermis and some nevi will eventually lose their junctional groups of melanocytes with only dermal melanocytes remaining.

On the palms and soles, junctional nevi often appear to have irregular borders because of the swirly pattern of dermal ridges and may be clinically misdiagnosed as melanomas.

On the scalp, they appear with a rim of brown pigment and a lighter center. Sudden change in size or shape of a junctional nevus is usually the result of irritation.

TREATMENT

No treatment is necessary. Surgical removal for cosmetic reasons will result in a scar. Destruction techniques should be avoided because there is no pathology available for study.

121 FLAT BROWN LESIONS

Freckles

DDx ref 118 • 119 • 122

CLINICAL FEATURES

Freckles (ephelides) are acquired 1–5-mm light brown macules seen on sun exposed skin. They first appear at 3–5 years, predominantly on the face and extensor surface of the extremities. Freckles are seen in fair-skinned children with light or red hair as an autosomal dominant trait and are related to polymorphisms in the melanocortin 1 receptor. Freckles contain increased pigment in epidermal basal keratinocytes, but normal numbers of melanocytes. Freckles darken with more sun exposure and lighten with sun protection.

TREATMENT

Freckles are a sign of the need for sun protection, as they are seen in children with an increased likelihood of sunburn, melanoma, and non-melanoma skin cancer. Sun protective clothing and hats, avoidance of midday sun, staying in the shade, and use of high SPF sunscreens should be recommended for children with freckles.

122 DDx ref

FLAT BROWN LESIONS

Lentigines

120 • 121 • 119

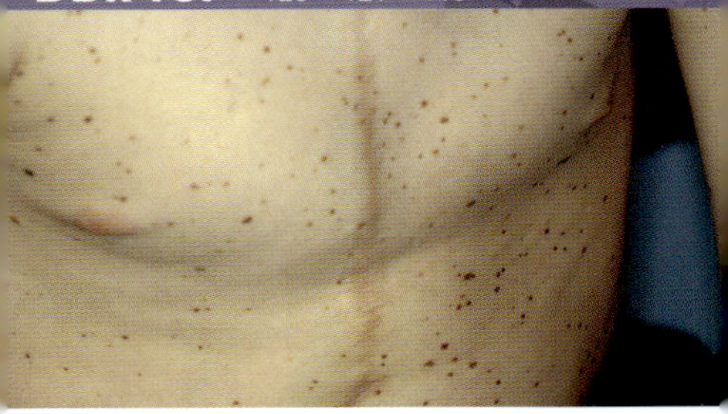

Child with multiple Noonan syndrome with lentigines. Note scar from correction of pulmonary stenosis.

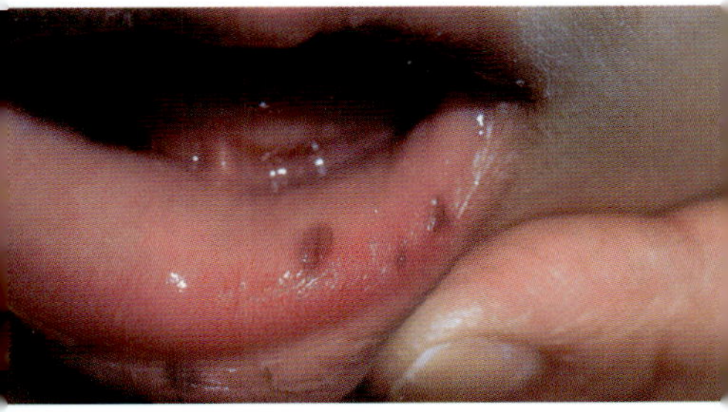

Lip lentigines in teen with Peutz–Jeghers syndrome.

123 DDx ref

FLAT BROWN LESIONS

Becker's nevus

131 • 118 • 119

Becker's nevus over the upper back in a teenage boy.

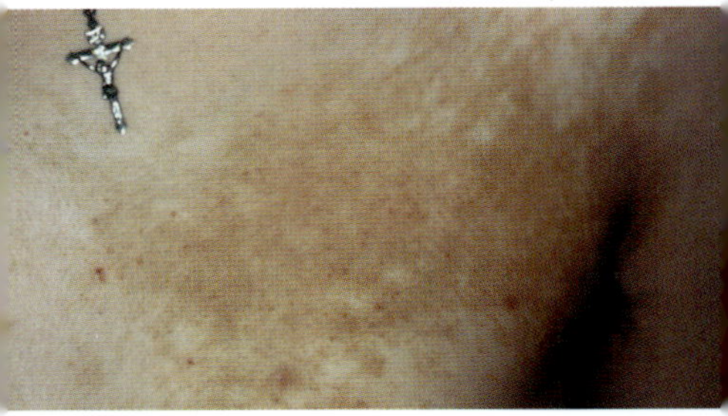

Blotchy brown pigment on the chest of a teenage boy with Becker's nevus.

122 FLAT BROWN LESIONS
Lentigines

DDx ref 120 • 121 • 119

CLINICAL FEATURES

Lentigines are flat, dark brown to black 1–5-mm macules seen anywhere on the skin or occasionally on mucosal surfaces. They first appear between the ages of 5–10 and are not influenced by the sun. Multiple lentigines are found in several syndromes: on the face, trunk, and extremities in Noonan syndrome with lentigines (formerly Moynahan's LEOPARD syndrome – Lentigines, Electrocardiograph abnormalities, Ocular hypertelorism, Pulmonary stenosis, Abnormalities of genitalia, Retardation of growth, and Deafness); in the Carney complex of nevi, myxoid neurofibromas and central facial lentigo; and on the lips in the autosomal dominant Peutz–Jeghers syndrome. In Peutz–Jeghers syndrome, lentigines are associated with multiple bowel polyps and a risk of gastrointestinal and genitourinary carcinomas. Noonan syndrome with lentigines is the result of mutations in the PTPN 11, RAF1, BRAF, or MAP2K1 genes, the Peutz–Jeghers syndrome in PJS, STK11 and LKB1 genes, and the Carney complex with distal arthrogryposis caused by mutations in the PRKARIA and MYH8 genes, respectively. Multiple lentigines, including mucosal lentigines, also can be found in children without associated syndromes.

TREATMENT

The child with multiple lentigines should have a detailed history and physical examination looking for associated problems. Referral to appropriate specialists is guided by the findings. No treatment of the lentigines is necessary, although good results have been seen with pigment selective lasers.

123 FLAT BROWN LESIONS
Becker's nevus

DDx ref 131 • 118 • 119

CLINICAL FEATURES

Becker's nevus is a tan macule with hypertrichosis within the area. The macule often has irregular borders. Often found on the chest and back, Becker's nevus may first be apparent in teenage boys and enlarges after it first appears. There is clinical and histologic overlap with the pilar and smooth muscle hamartoma. Although the smooth muscle hamartoma appears at birth or in early childhood, like Becker's nevus, there is hypertrichosis within increased pigmentation. The conditions share histologic findings of increased numbers of melanocytes at the basal epidermis and increased terminal hairs. The presence of extra arrector pilae smooth muscle cells is only found in pilar and smooth muscle hamartoma. Areas of localized hypertrichosis in infants that are not pigmented may be related. Lesions of Becker's nevus display increased androgen binding, which may explain the male predominance. There is no malignant potential.

TREATMENT

The use of depilatories or hair removal lasers will help remove the unwanted hair. Cosmetic improvement of the pigment has been reported with the Q-switched ruby laser.

124 FLAT BROWN LESIONS

Post-inflammatory hyperpigmentation

DDx ref 125 • 127 • 53

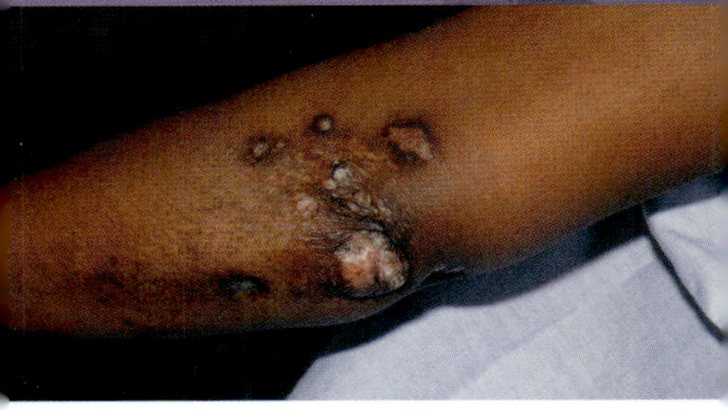

Scarred skin areas with a dark brown rim of hyperpigmentation in a black child with calcinosis cutis secondary to dermatomyositis.

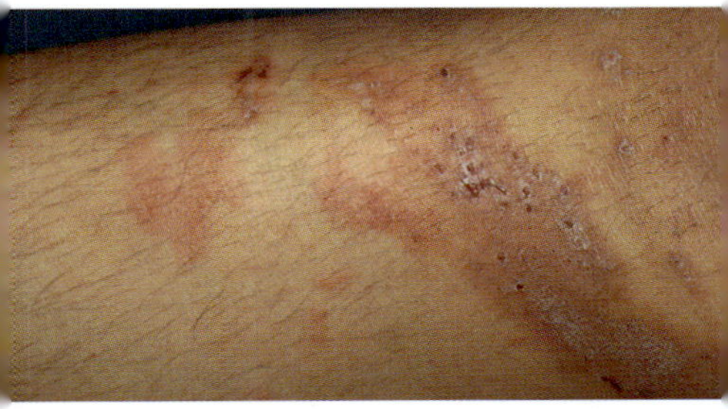

Streaks of post-inflammatory hyperpigmentation on the arm of a teen after a poison oak encounter.

125 FLAT BROWN LESIONS

Phytophotodermatitis

DDx ref 124 • 127 • 123

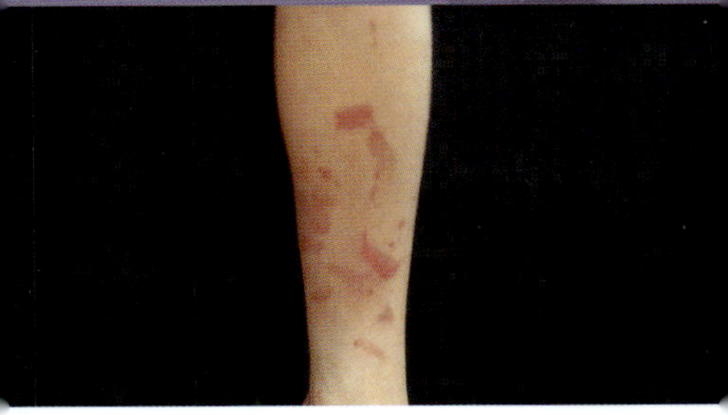

Bizarre patterns of brown pigmentation on the leg of a boy with phytophotodermatitis.

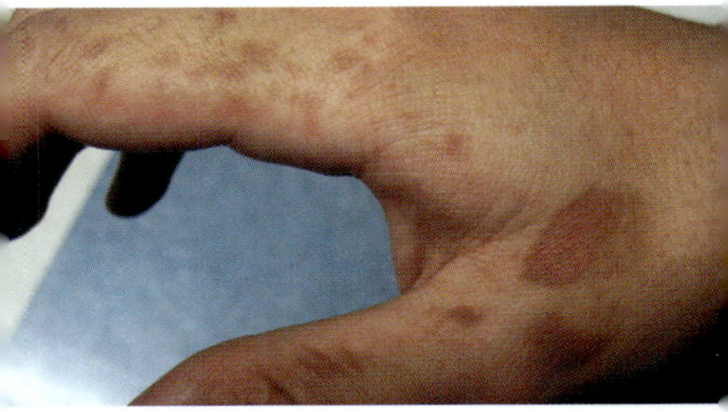

Hyperpigmented streaks on a boy's hand after exposure to wild celery and sunlight.

124 FLAT BROWN LESIONS

Post-inflammatory hyperpigmentation

DDx ref 125 • 127 • 53

CLINICAL FEATURES

Inflammatory skin conditions in dark-skinned children will often heal with residual brown pigmentation. Any pattern may be seen, and in any area of skin. The injury disrupts the epidermal basal layer. Pigment expelled from the epidermis by injury results in collections of pigment within the dermis that are engulfed by macrophages. It requires months to years to eventually clear the extra pigment.

TREATMENT

Bleaching creams containing the combination of 4% hydroquinone, tretinoin, and azelaic acid may lighten the skin if the extra pigment is superficial, but deep dermal involvement will not respond.

125 FLAT BROWN LESIONS

Phytophotodermatitis

DDx ref 124 • 127 • 123

CLINICAL FEATURES

Bizarre patterns of flat, hyperpigmented streaks that may follow redness and occasional blisters characterize phytophotodermatitis. The pigmented streaks persist for months and consist of linear, oval, and drip-like patterns. Many children present only with the streaks without an inflammatory stage. Considerable detective work is required to determine the cause. From the unusual shapes, an exogenous insult should be suspected. The furocoumarin chemical psoralen is responsible. It is found in plants of the celery family, certain grasses, and the juice of limes. The psoralen gets on the skin from the plants but no response occurs, unless there is sun exposure to the affected areas. Therefore, the condition is seen in the spring and summer months or upon return from tropical climates.

TREATMENT

The pigmentation resolves after many months, but in cosmetically important areas, the use of skin bleaching creams such as 4% hydroquinone, tretinoin, or azelaic acid may help. If an inflammatory stage is present, topic corticosteroid creams or ointments twice daily may be used.

126

FLAT BROWN LESIONS

Acanthosis nigricans (AN)

DDx ref 124 • 80 • 79

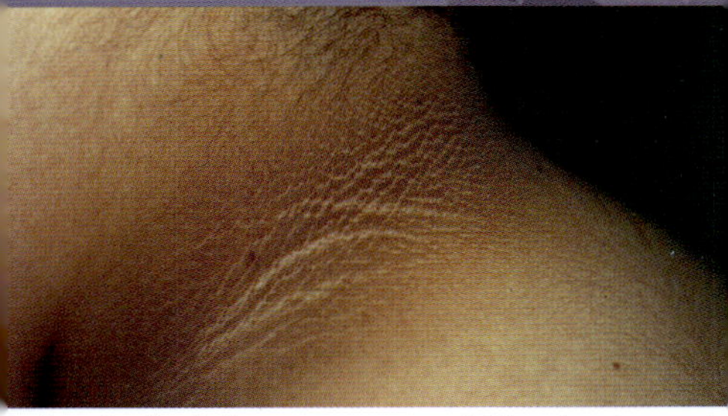

Acanthosis nigricans on an overweight preteen's neck.

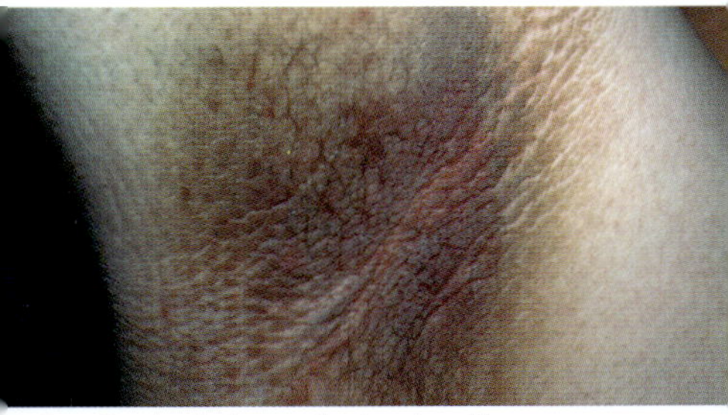

Acanthosis nigricans of a teen's axilla.

127

FLAT BROWN LESIONS

Linear and whorled hyperpigmentation

DDx ref 15 • 125 • 114

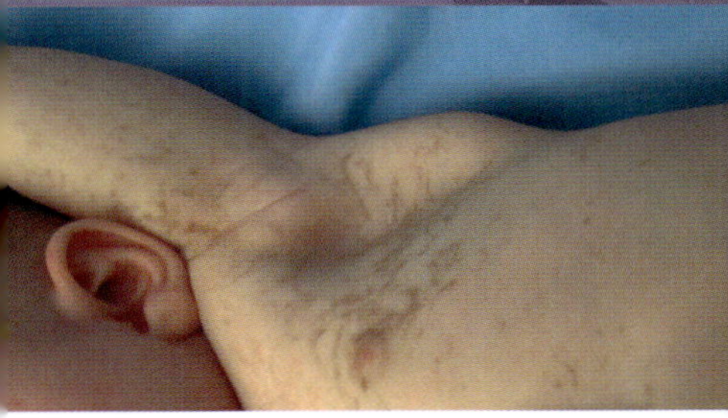

Flat brown whorls over the axilla and arm of an infant with linear and whorled hypermelanosis.

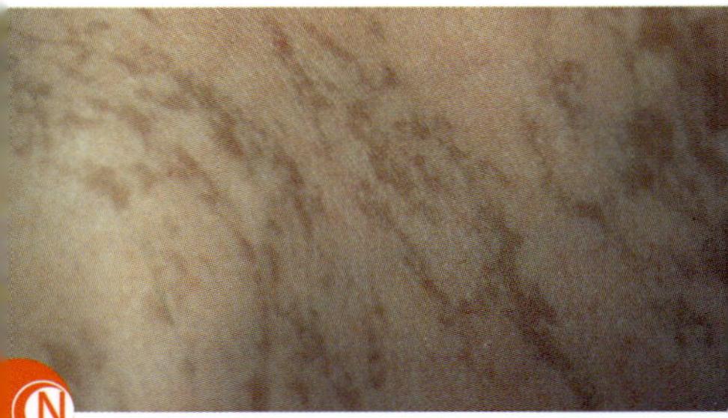

Flat brown whorls over the trunk of a child with linear and whorled hypermelanosis.

126 FLAT BROWN LESIONS

Acanthosis nigricans (AN)

DDx ref 124 • 80 • 79

CLINICAL FEATURES

Hyperpigmentation of folds of skin on the posterior neck, axillae, and groin characterize acanthosis nigricans (AN). AN is predominantly seen in overweight dark-skinned preteens and teens. The surface of the hyperpigmented areas feels soft and velvety and multiple small 1–2-mm skin tags may be found within involved skin. Sometimes, additional skin areas such as elbows, areolae, and knuckles are involved. Parents often complain that the skin is 'dirty' and cannot be washed off. AN is strongly associated with obesity and insulin resistance. Less commonly, it is associated with endocrinopathies such as Cushing's disease or acromegaly, in lipoatrophy, Prader–Willi syndrome, leprechaunism, and craniofacial syndromes that have mutations in the bFGF receptor.

TREATMENT

In overweight teens with AN, improvement has occurred with weight loss, regular exercise, and the use of topical retinoids and low-dose oral metformin. With endocrinopathy-associated AN, correction of the endocrinopathy will help.

127 FLAT BROWN LESIONS

Linear and whorled hyperpigmentation

DDx ref 15 • 125 • 114

CLINICAL FEATURES

Curvilinear and whorled streaks of flat hyperpigmentation that abruptly end at the midline are characteristic. The brown streaks follow the same patterns of the embryonic lines of Blaschko that are seen in incontinentia pigmenti or as white streaks in hypomelanosis of Ito. Linear and whorled hypermelanosis is seen at birth and darkens with age. There is no preceding inflammatory stage as is seen in incontinentia pigmenti. As in all conditions following lines of Blaschko, genetic mosaicism is present and a detailed history and physical examination should be performed to uncover associated abnormalities such as mental retardation and/or seizures, cardiac abnormalities, limb defects, and eye abnormalities.

TREATMENT

Referral to a genetics clinic or multidisciplinary clinic is useful in the child with associated conditions. There is no treatment for the pigmented streaks.

RAISED BROWN LESIONS

Congenital melanocytic nevi

DDx ref 131 • 119 • 134

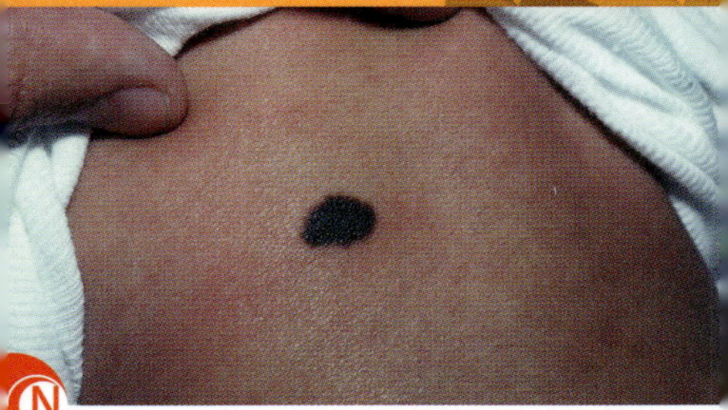

Small congenital melanocytic nevus.

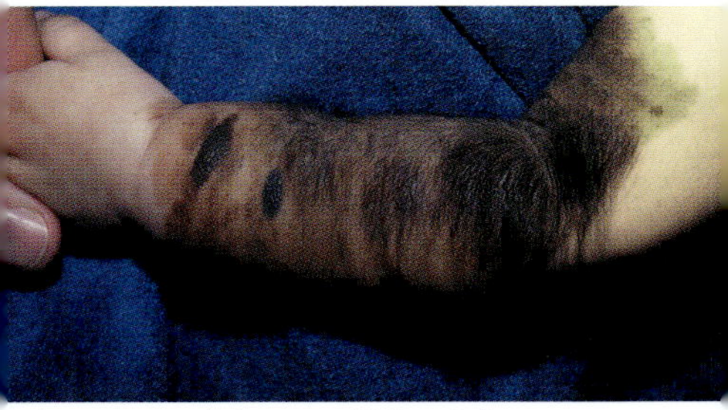

Large congenital nevus with long hairs.

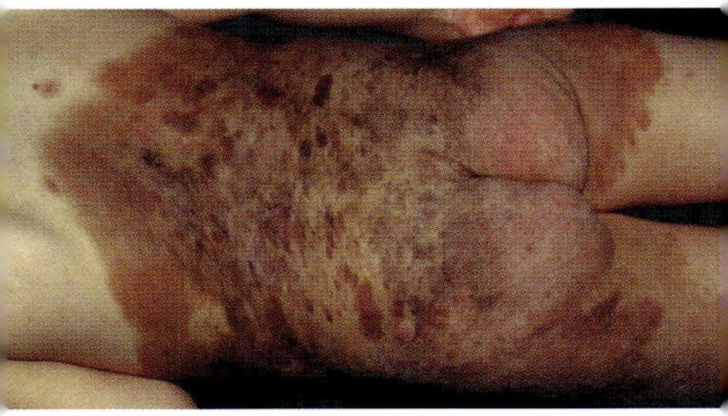

Large congenital melanocytic nevus in the so-called 'bathing suit' distribution.

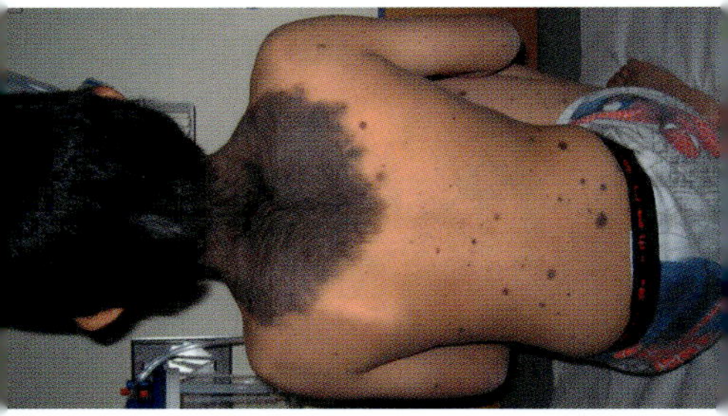

Large congenital melanocytic nevus on a child's back, neck, and scalp.

Congenital melanocytic nevi

DDx ref 131 • 119 • 134

CLINICAL FEATURES

Congenital melanocytic nevi (CMN) are present at birth as flesh-colored to brown or black papules or plaques ranging in size from 1 cm to covering over one-half of the body. Multiple classifications of CMN have been used. All the classifications are based on the size of the lesion. **The most common classification** defines lesions <1.5 cm as small (SCMN), those 1.5–20 cm as medium, and those >20 cm as large (LCMN). There is no clinical or theoretical reason to have a group defined as medium, because the biologic behavior of this group is identical to that of small lesions.

Newer classifications use only small or large categories and define large as >5% of the body surface area or 40 cm or 60 cm diameter of the predicted adult size.

SCMN occur in 1% of newborns. They have minimal if any risk of malignant degeneration.

LCMN occur in 1 in 20 000 live births. LCMN are often not uniform and may contain flat, tan areas, blue-black plaques, and black, long, thick hair. Erosions, ulcerations, and pink proliferative nodules may be seen in neonates but these are not changes that signal malignancy. The risk of malignancy in LCMN is 1–2%.

Numerous smaller nevi developing at skin sites distant from the primary LCMN may also be seen, and more satellite nevi may develop during childhood.

Neurocutaneous melanosis (NCM) is the association of a LCMN overlying the scalp or spine, or more frequently those with multiple rapidly growing satellite lesions with central nervous system (CNS) involvement. Magnetic resonance imaging may be abnormal in up to 25% of these individuals, but symptomatic NCM occurs in only 1–2%. CNS melanoma may occur, but CNS disease without melanoma is more common. Symptomatic NCM is almost always fatal.

TREATMENT

If cosmetically concerning, SCMN can be excised surgically at an age when local anesthesia is all that is necessary. They should not be excised early in life for fear of malignant degeneration. The management of LCMN is controversial. The risk of melanoma is only 1–2% and surgery is often disfiguring and has not been proven to decrease the melanoma risk. It is advisable to take into consideration the potential for cosmetic improvement and surgical risk before recommending attempted removal.

RAISED BROWN LESIONS

Intradermal melanocytic nevi

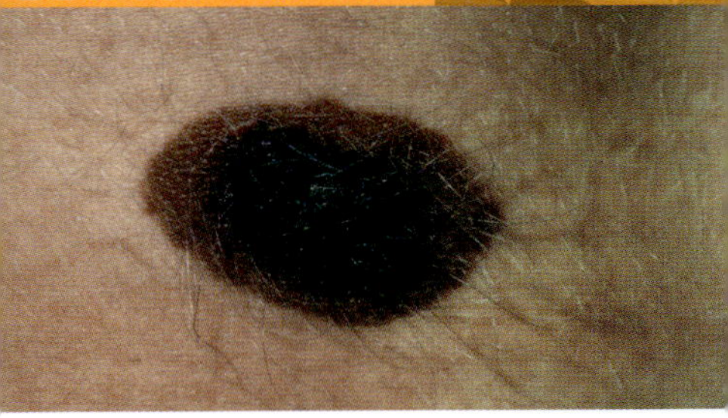

'Fried egg' compound nevus with dark raised center.

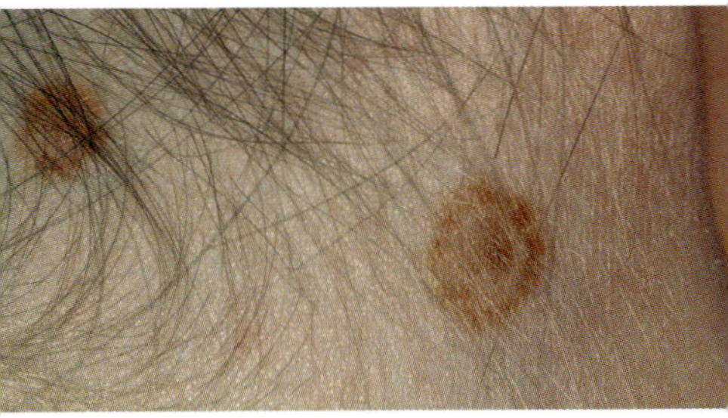

Cockade or target compound nevus with different-colored zones.

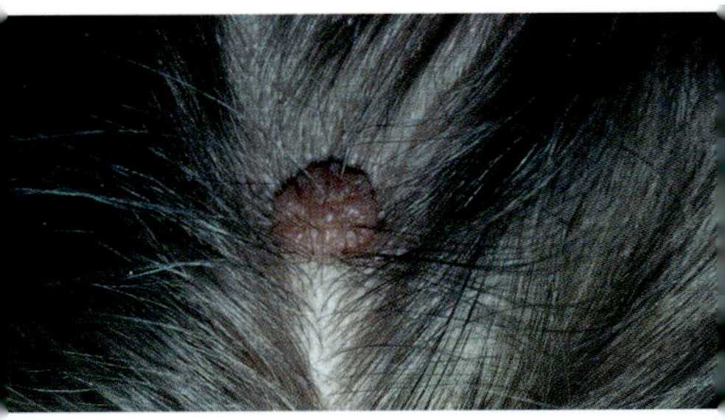

Non-pigmented intradermal nevus of the scalp.

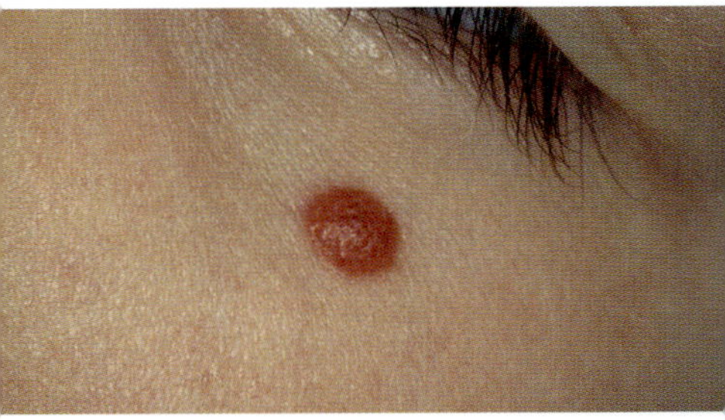

Spitz nevus. Red papule on the face of a child.

CLINICAL FEATURES

The development of acquired melanocytic nevi is related to genetic susceptibility and sun exposure. Melanocytic nevus development in childhood correlates with skin type, hair and eye color, freckles, and sun exposure. Children with light skin, light brown hair, light eye color, multiple freckles, and a history of numerous sunburns develop the highest number of nevi. Children with similar genetic backgrounds who are exposed to more ultraviolet radiation will develop more nevi. Conversely, children with red hair, although light skinned, develop few nevi even with ultraviolet radiation exposure.

The most common type of melanocytic nevus in childhood is the **junctional melanocytic nevus** (see DDx ref 120 Junctional Nevi). Approximately 20% of junctional melanocytic nevi will progress to **compound melanocytic nevi**. These melanocytic nevi have a junctional component of melanocytes as well as a dermal component. Most compound melanocytic nevi appear as dome-shaped, solitary-colored brown to brown-black papules. Several clinical variants of compound melanocytic nevi occur. **The 'fried egg' nevus** presents as a flat, brown papule with a raised, darker center. A variant of the 'fried egg' nevus is the cockade or target nevus. It differs from the 'fried egg' nevus only by the fact that there is a lighter zone between the center and the rim of the nevus. Compound melanocytic nevi may also appear as skin-colored to pink papules with little melanin production. They are seen most commonly in the scalp of light-skinned children. **Dermal melanocytic nevi** are rare prior to adolescence and are melanocytic nevi that have lost their junction component and have only a dermal component remaining.

Atypical melanocytic nevi are usually >5 mm in diameter with a variegated tan-brown color, often on a pink-red background and they have irregular ill-defined borders. They occur in the familial melanoma syndrome and in children with a family history of melanoma who do not have the familial melanoma syndrome. They may also be seen as isolated nevi in the general population.

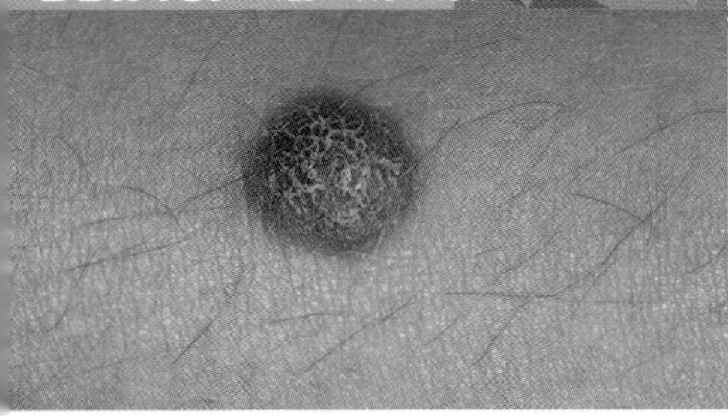

Spitz nevus with fine scale on the surface.

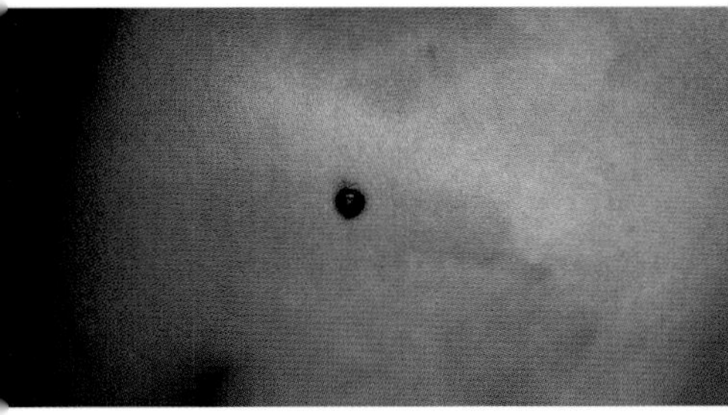

Blue nevus. Blue-black papule on a child's shoulder.

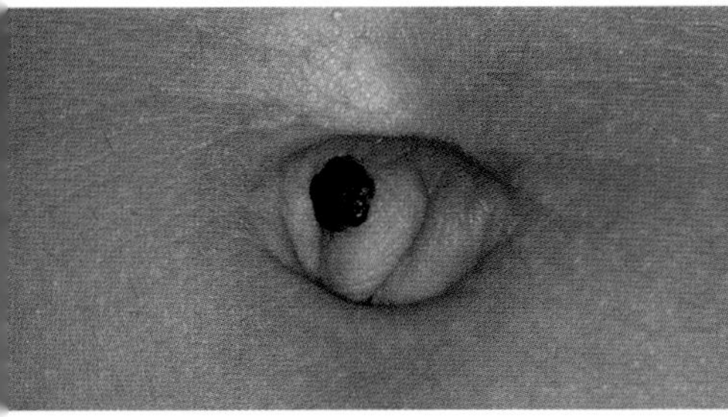

Blue nevus in the umbilicus.

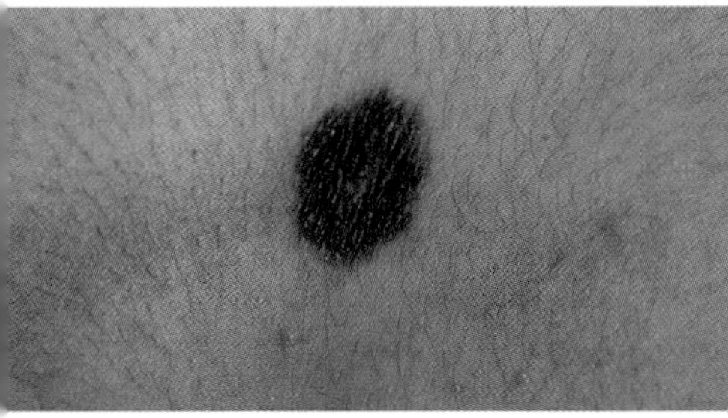

Atypical nevus with irregular borders and pink background.

Blue nevi are blue to blue-black solitary papules. They most commonly occur on the dorsal aspects of the hands and feet. They appear blue because the melanocytic nevus cells are deeper in the dermis than in common dermal nevi. **Spitz nevi (spindle and epithelioid nevi)** are solitary, dome-shaped, red to red-brown papules usually seen on the face or extremities in young children. Spitz nevi may be difficult to distinguish histopathologically from melanoma. The classic red, dome-shaped Spitz nevus in childhood is never a melanoma. The problem arises because many other types of clinical melanocytic nevi will have a histology that is spindle and epithelioid cells with atypia, and these are all called Spitz nevi by the pathologists. The term 'Spitz nevus' should be used only when referring to the classic clinical lesions of childhood. In other circumstances, the lesions should be described as having spindle and epithelioid histology and not called a Spitz nevus.

TREATMENT

Treatment is not required for the majority of melanocytic nevi. Surgical excision should be performed for any lesion with atypical clinical features that could possibly be a melanoma.

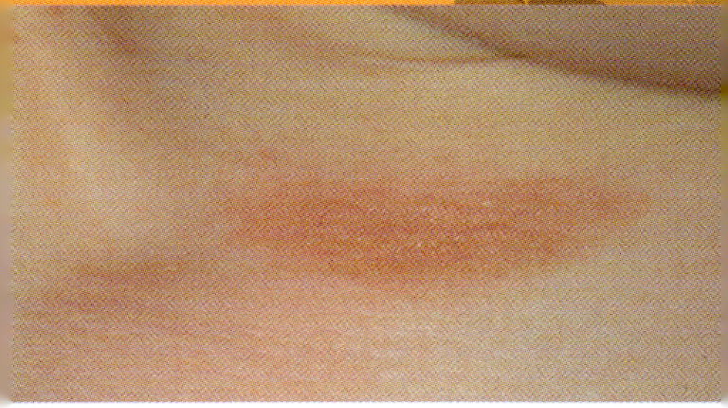

Tan plaque of an infant with solitary mastocytoma.

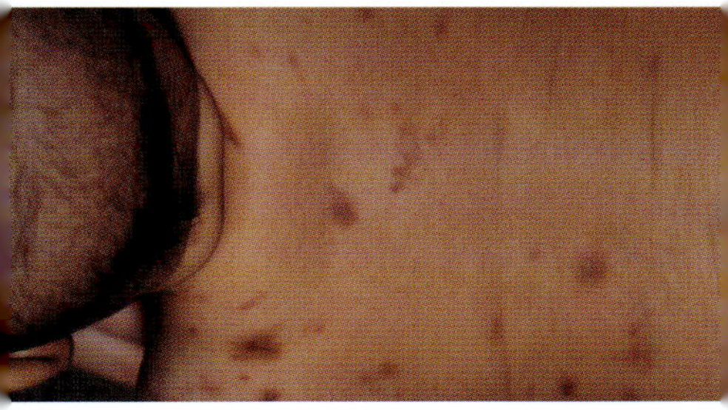

Urticaria pigmentosa. Scattered brown blotchy macules and papules on the trunk of an infant.

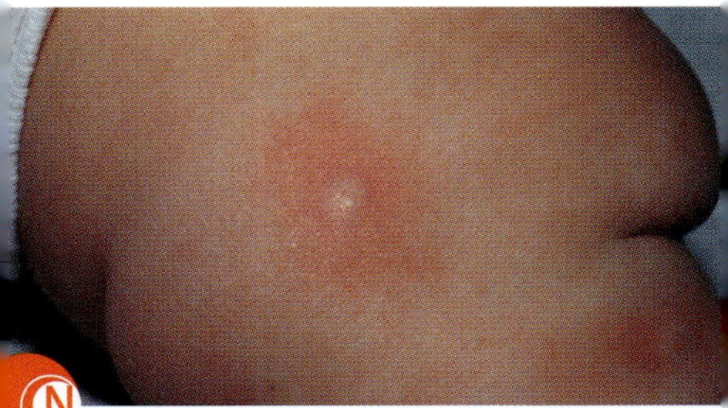

Tense edema and redness within macule of urticaria pigmentosa after stroking (Darier's sign).

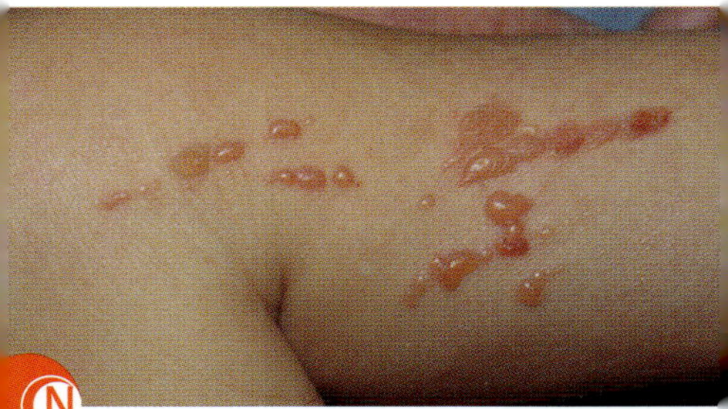

Diffuse cutaneous mastocytosis in an infant. Linear blisters appear along sites of skin stroking.

CLINICAL FEATURES

Solitary mastocytomas are benign accumulations of mast cells. They usually present at birth as solitary yellow-brown papules or plaques. Rubbing or stroking the lesions causes erythema and swelling and sometimes blistering, oozing, and crusting secondary to mast cell mediator release. When blistering, oozing, and crusting occur, they are often confused with impetigo or herpes simplex.

Urticaria pigmentosa (UP) is the name used when children develop multiple mast cell lesions over time. The lesions are blotchy macular, papular, or nodular and may appear before 6 months of age. A few lesions are noted initially, but they continue to increase in number with time. The majority of lesions are located on the trunk, but facial and extremity lesions may be seen. Lesions are initially red and with time, overlying hyperpigmentation develops. As with solitary mastocytomas, urticaria, blistering, oozing, and crusting of individual lesions may occur. Generalized flushing is frequently seen. This is not a sign of systemic mastocytosis. Diarrhea, wheezing, and syncope have been reported, but are rare. There are two subsets of urticaria pigmentosa. The most common type arises within the first year of life; new lesions are rare after age 6 years, with spontaneous resolution during the grade school years. Somatic mutations in c-kit gene are found in 50%. The second subset is caused by germline mutations in the D816V portion of the c-kit gene. These children usually develop their initial lesions later in life and continue to develop new lesions throughout life. They are the children at risk for the development of systemic mastocytosis. Systemic mastocytosis is rare in childhood. However, there is considerable overlap between subsets and it is unknown what proportion of children has genetic disease.

Diffuse cutaneous mastocytosis (DCM) is a rare generalized type of mastocytosis. Urticaria with blister formation is seen early in the neonate. The blisters may be large and peel, leaving eroded bases. Marked dermographism is present. A leathery thickening with yellow-tan skin color develops on truncal skin after the first few months of life. Prolonged hypotension, severe syncopal episodes, and death have been reported. Vomiting, diarrhea, and abdominal pain are common as the child gets older. Gastrointestinal stromal tumors and bone marrow involvement may appear in adults.

TREATMENT

Solitary mastocytomas usually do not require treatment. Recurrent blistering may be treated with intermittent 2-week courses of a super-potent topical steroid. **Most children with UP** are asymptomatic. For children with UP and DCM with frequent urtication and flushing, cetirizine 2.5–10 mg every morning and hydroxyzine 1 mg/kg before bed is usually all that is necessary. More symptomatic children may be treated with twice-weekly narrowband UVB phototherapy.

131 DDx ref

RAISED BROWN LESIONS

Pilar and smooth muscle hamartomas

128 • 130 • 123

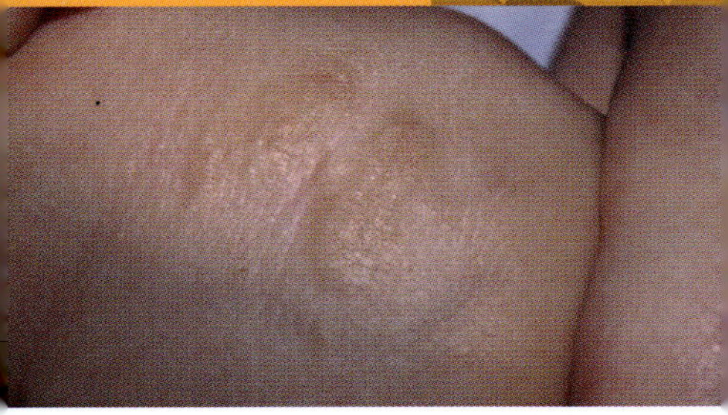

Pilar and smooth muscle hamartoma in a baby as a tan plaque.

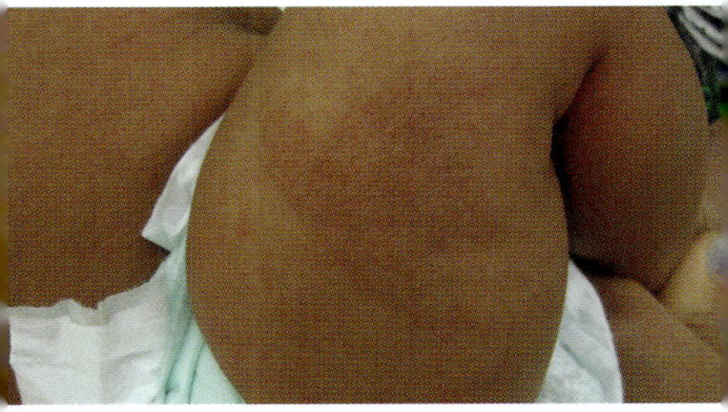

Pilar and smooth muscle hamartoma on the leg of an infant.

132 DDx ref

RAISED BROWN LESIONS

Flat warts (verucca plana)

133 • 74 • 121

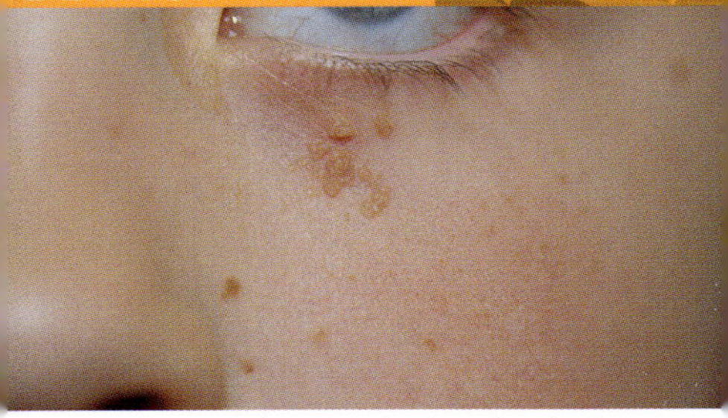

Multiple flat warts (verruca plana) on the cheek.

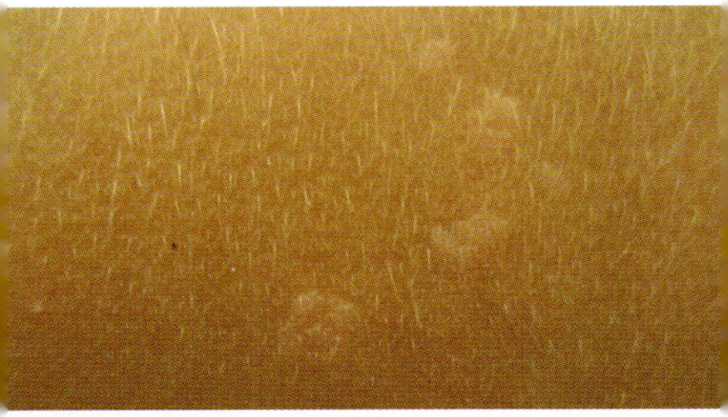

Multiple flat warts on a child's forehead.

131 RAISED BROWN LESIONS

Pilar and smooth muscle hamartomas

DDx ref 128 • 130 • 123

CLINICAL FEATURES

Pilar and smooth muscle hamartomas are developmental anomalies resulting from smooth muscle (arrector pili) associated with hair follicles. They are seen at birth as skin-colored to light brown plaques with overlying hypertrichosis. Rippling of the skin, caused by contraction of the smooth muscle, may occasionally be elicited by gentle stroking. Pilar and smooth muscle hamartomas may occasionally be mistaken for congenital melanocytic nevi. The distinction is important because pilar and smooth muscle hamartomas have no risk for malignant degeneration. Congenital localized hypertrichosis may be a variant. There is clinical and histologic overlap with a Becker's nevus, but they appear later in life and have a male predominance.

TREATMENT

No treatment is necessary.

132 RAISED BROWN LESIONS

Flat warts (verucca plana)

DDx ref 133 • 74 • 121

CLINICAL FEATURES

Flat warts are not flat, but slightly raised flat-topped smooth papules. They are usually a light tan to brown color. They are often grouped and seen on the face and distal extremities in children. The Koebner phenomenon may be seen with lesions occurring in areas of skin trauma. They may be especially widespread on the lower legs of adolescent females who shave their legs.

TREATMENT

Since lesions are frequently so numerous, destructive therapies are usually unsuccessful. Immunologic therapies including topical retinoic acid gels, imiquimod, and *Candida* antigen injection are most often used. Oral isotretinoin and topical glycolic acid 15%/salicylic acid 2% may be beneficial.

133 RAISED BROWN LESIONS

Benign cephalic histiocytosis

DDx ref 132 • 74 • 121

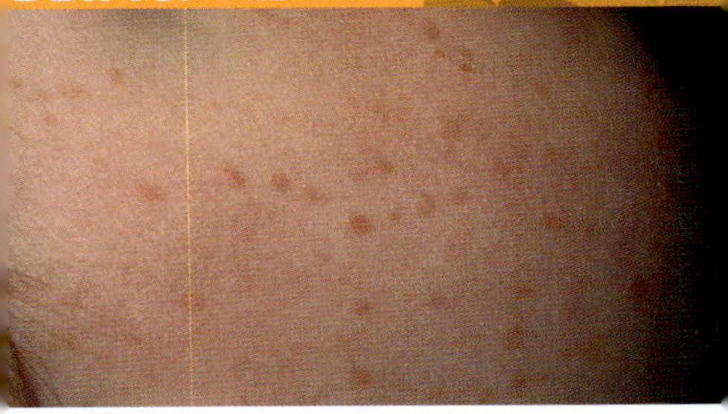

Benign cephalic histiocytosis. Multiple tan flat-topped papules on the face.

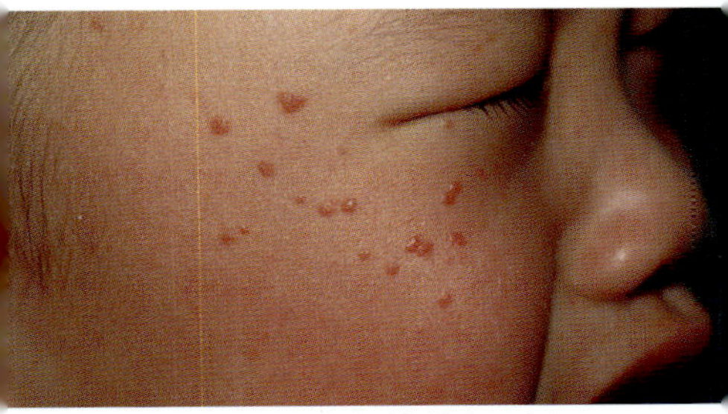

Benign cephalic histiocytosis. Multiple red-tan papules on the face.

134 RAISED BROWN LESIONS

Melanoma

DDx ref 128 • 129 • 120

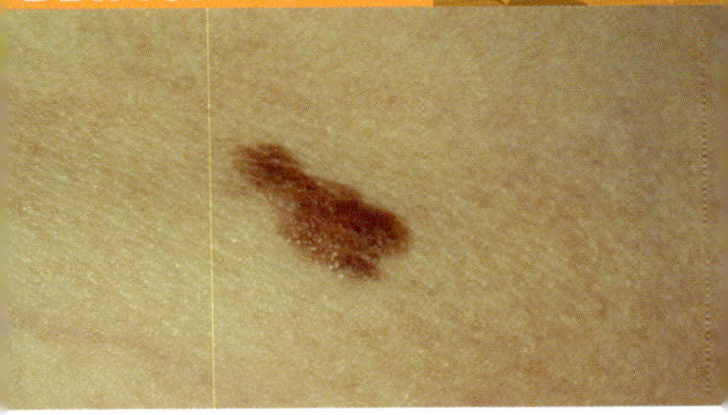

Severely atypical melanocytic nevus with marked abnormalities in symmetry and borders.

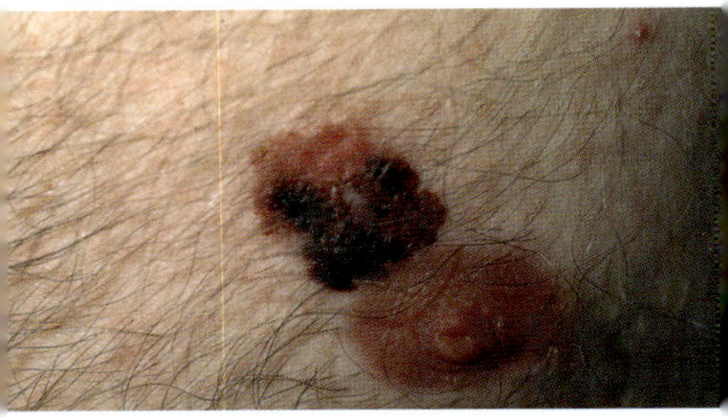

Melanoma on the chest of an adolescent male.

133

DDx ref 132 • 74 • 121

RAISED BROWN LESIONS

Benign cephalic histiocytosis

CLINICAL FEATURES

Benign cephalic histiocytosis presents as light brown to red 2–8-mm papules on the face, most commonly on the cheeks. From a few up to a hundred lesions may be present. It is a non-Langerhans cell histiocytosis. Lesions may also be seen on the neck and trunk. When lesions are present in locations other than the face and neck, one must consider other types of non-Langerhans cell and Langerhans cell histiocytosis in the differential diagnosis. Flat warts should also be considered. The average age of onset is 15 months, but it may be seen in children under 6 months of age. It is rarely if ever seen in children over 6 years old. Lesions spontaneously regress in an average of 2 years.

TREATMENT

Treatment is unnecessary. If concern exists for other types of Langerhans cell or non-Langerhans cell histiocytosis, then a biopsy to obtain a histologic diagnosis should be performed.

134

DDx ref 128 • 129 • 120

RAISED BROWN LESIONS

Melanoma

CLINICAL FEATURES

Melanomas are rare before puberty although are increasing in frequency in adolescents. The ABCDEs of melanoma diagnosis are: **A**symmetry, the lesion is not round, but has an irregular shape; **B**orders, the border is not even, but notched and irregular; **C**olor, areas of red, white, and/or blue within a brown area; **D**iameter, >10 mm; **E**volution, a rapid change in any of these parameters over a few weeks. Many melanocytic nevi in children will have slightly irregular borders. Also, a change from light brown to dark brown is common. It is the appearance of red, white, or blue within a brown lesion that is a worrisome change. The most important clinical feature is rapid, progressive growth, disproportionate to that of the child's other melanocytic nevi. Ulceration and bleeding are far-advanced changes. Risk of melanoma in childhood is correlated to skin type, hair, and eye color, number of melanocytic nevi present, history of excessive sun exposure, and family history of melanoma.

TREATMENT

Any lesion suspected of being a melanoma should be totally surgically excised. If histologically proven to be a melanoma, then referral to a melanoma center is optimal. With a melanoma histologic diagnosis in a prepubertal child, a second pathologic opinion can be most helpful.

135 DDx ref

YELLOW LESIONS
Nevus sebaceous

92 • 136 • 139

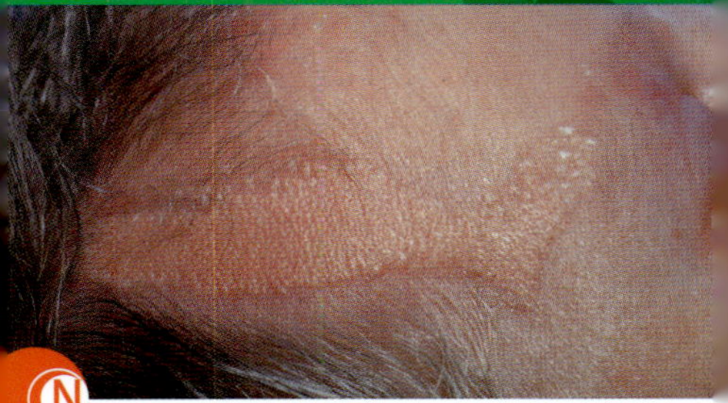

Nevus sebaceous. Linear yellow lesion on the scalp of an infant.

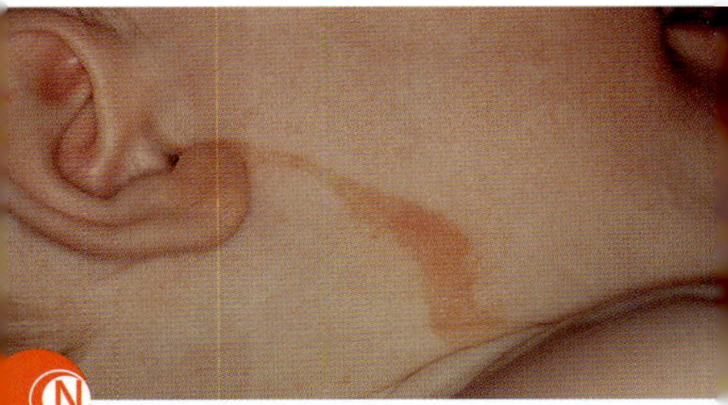

Nevus sebaceous in curvilinear arrangement on the neck and ear of an infant.

136 DDx ref

YELLOW LESIONS
Juvenile xanthogranuloma (JXG)

131 • 129 • 130

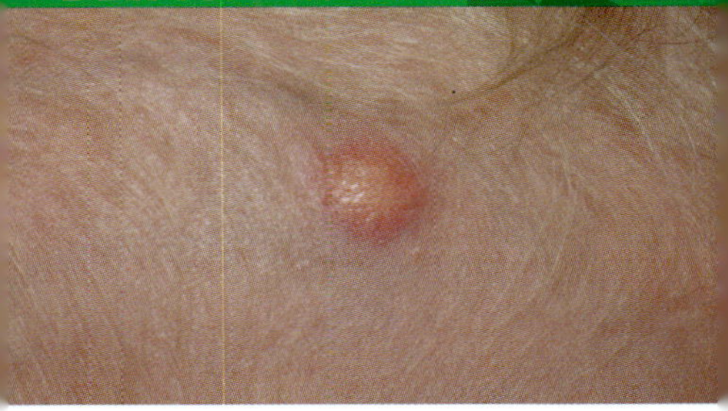

JXG. Orange nodules on an infant's scalp.

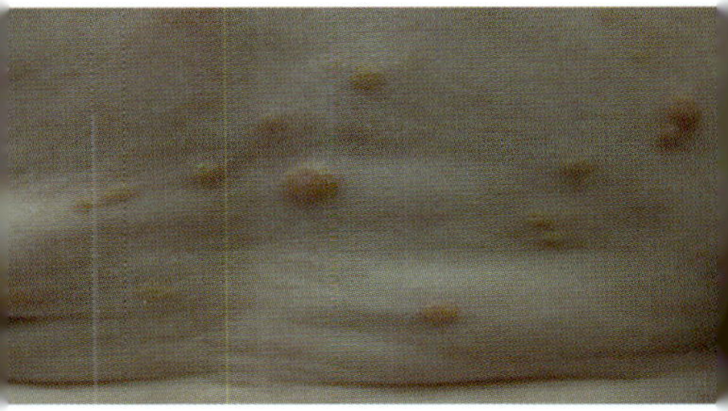

JXG. Multiple yellow-orange nodules on the back of an infant.

135 YELLOW LESIONS

Nevus sebaceous

DDx ref 92 • 136 • 139

CLINICAL FEATURES

Nevus sebaceous presents at birth as slightly raised oval to linear yellow-orange plaques. Greater than 90% will have mutations in the H-Ras gene. The same mutations are also seen in phakomatosis pigmentokeratotica, which includes patients with both nevus sebaceous and nevus spilus. They are seen on the scalp, face, upper chest, and arms. When present on the scalp, they are devoid of hair and are in the differential of congenital circumscribed alopecia. They remain flat until puberty, when the sebaceous glands within the lesion respond to androgenic stimulation causing the lesions to enlarge and thicken with a warty appearance. Tumors may develop after this time in up to 20%, including trichoblastoma (57% of tumors), syringocystadenoma papilliferum (33% of tumors), and basal cell carcinoma (1% of tumors). A second mutation consisting of deletions in the PTCH gene are found in nevus sebaceous at risk for the development of basal cell carcinoma.

TREATMENT

Surgical excision is recommended, but need not be done early in life unless it is performed for cosmetic purposes.

136 YELLOW LESIONS

Juvenile xanthogranuloma (JXG)

DDx ref 131 • 129 • 130

CLINICAL FEATURES

Orange to yellow-brown soft nodules characterize JXG, a benign cutaneous disease. JXGs begin in infancy and may be multiple, often numbering 5–10. Rarely, they are found in newborns. Most lesions involute spontaneously over 2–5 years. JXGs may develop in the iris, mimic retinoblastoma, or cause vision loss. Rarely, JXGs are found in internal organs, including the testes, lung, liver, spleen, and pericardium. The association of multiple JXGs and multiple café-au-lait macules in a child with NF-1 has been associated with an increased risk of juvenile myelomonocytic leukemia (JMML). Within the nodules are increased fibroblasts and lipid-filled macrophages called 'Touton giant cells'.

TREATMENT

Since most lesions spontaneously involute, intervention is unnecessary. In children under age 2 years who have multiple JXGs, referral to an ophthalmologist is recommended.

137
DDx ref

YELLOW LESIONS

Necrobiosis lipoidica diabeticorum (NLD)

111 • 109 • 139

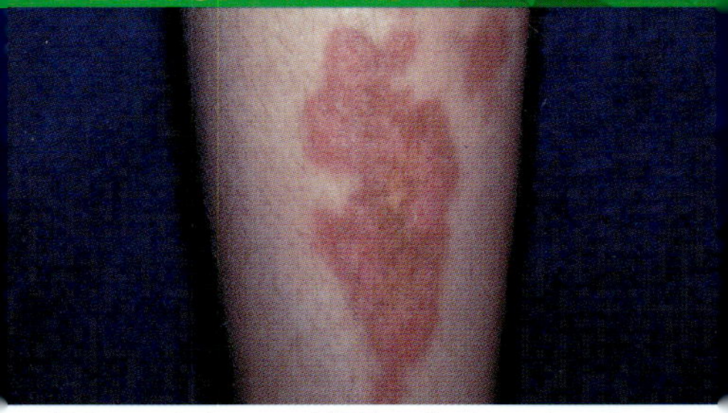

Yellow-red plaques of NLD on the lower leg of a teenage girl with diabetes mellitus.

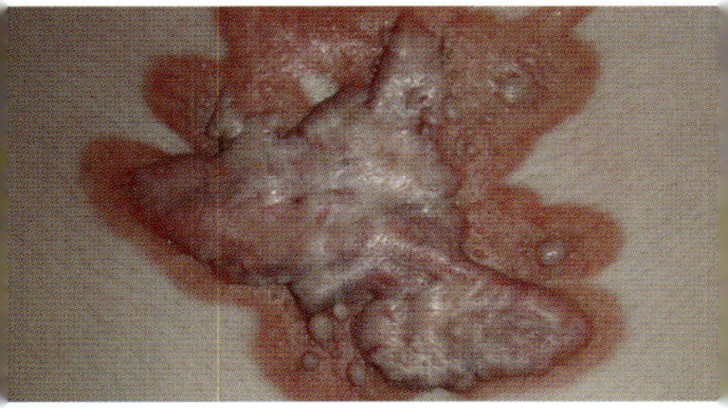

NLD plaque with central scarring from prior ulcerations.

138
DDx ref

YELLOW LESIONS

Focal dermal hypoplasia

15 • 135 • 139

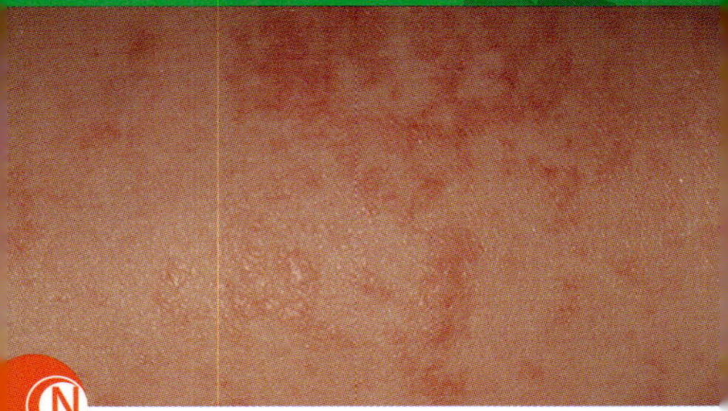

N

Newborn girl with multiple curvilinear red-yellow streaks on the trunk.

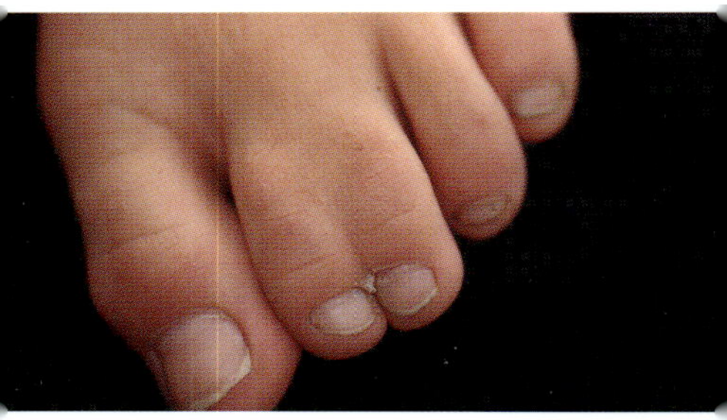

Syndactyly of the toes in an older child with focal dermal hypoplasia.

137 DDx ref

YELLOW LESIONS

Necrobiosis lipoidica diabeticorum (NLD)

111 • 109 • 139

CLINICAL FEATURES

Irregularly shaped yellow plaques with red borders are seen on the lower leg. Sometimes the center of the lesion ulcerates and heals with scarring. The association of NLD and diabetes mellitus is strong, and children with NLD should have an evaluation for diabetes including a serum glucose and an A1c hemoglobin test.

TREATMENT

There are no comparative studies on treatments of NLD. UVA1 phototherapy, hydroxychloroquine, and anti-TNF immunologics have all been reported successful in a limited number of children with NLD. Some improvement has been reported with pentoxifylline.

138 DDx ref

YELLOW LESIONS

Focal dermal hypoplasia

15 • 135 • 139

CLINICAL FEATURES

Curvilinear, red-yellow streaks are seen in newborn girls with focal dermal hypoplasia. The lack of a fibrous dermis within the streaks results in the yellow color of subcutaneous fat being seen. As the baby develops more fat, the color changes from red-yellow to more yellow. Also, some streaks may appear depressed and atrophic, others telangiectatic, and some hypopigmented. Small papillomatous growths may be observed in the periorificial and intertriginous areas. Hair and teeth are sparse, nails are hypoplastic, and lip pits may be seen. Cleft lip, strabismus, colobomas, cataracts, sensorineural hearing loss, and mental retardation have been reported. Syndactyly and polydactyly are found. An X-linked dominant inheritance is described but most cases are sporadic. Mutations of the PORCN gene on the X chromosome (Xp.23) are causative. Deletion of the PORCN gene and contiguous genes has been detected. Most affected children display preferential inactivation of the paternal X chromosome.

TREATMENT

If available, referral to a genetics clinic where a multidisciplinary approach is available, is recommended.

139 DDx ref

CONGENITAL CIRCUMSCRIBED HAIR LOSS

Aplasia cutis congenita

135 • 138 • 139

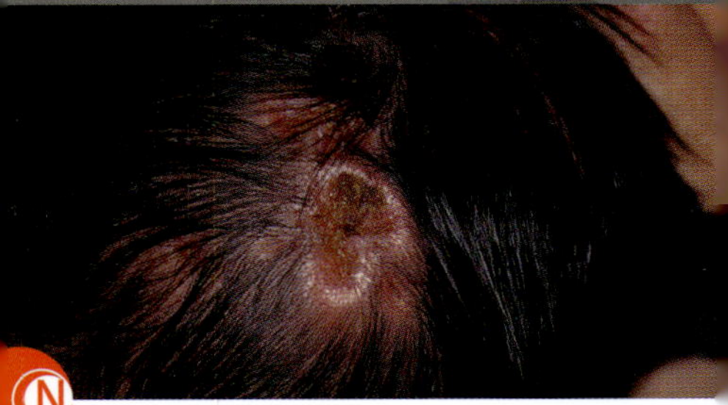

Newborn with ulcerated aplasia cutis congenita of the midline scalp.

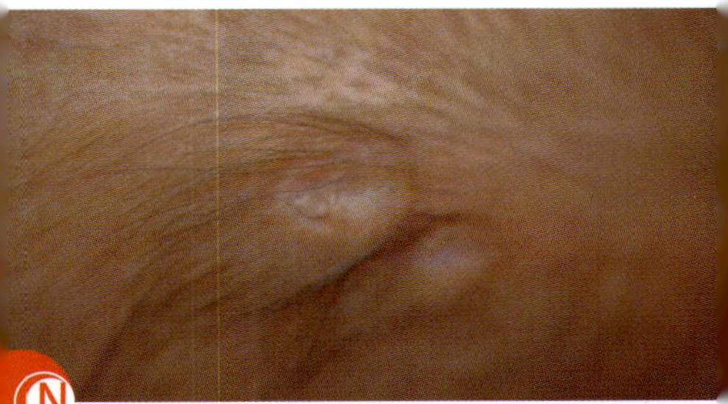

Newborn with a hair collar surrounding aplasia cutis congenita.

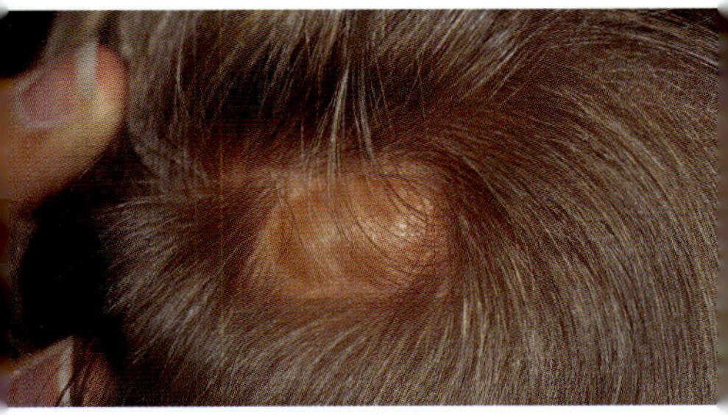

Toddler with a raised scar in the center of a hairless aplasia cutis congenita area.

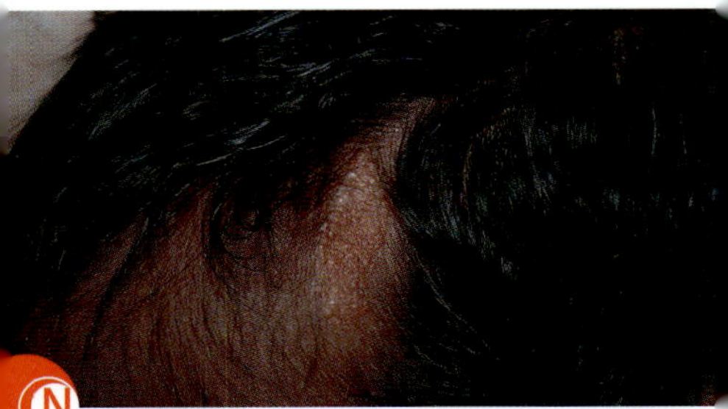

Hairless area of nevus sebaceous in a newborn scalp mimics aplasia cutis congenita.

Aplasia cutis congenita

DDx ref 135 • 138 • 139

CLINICAL FEATURES

Oval, sharply marginated, 1–2-cm hairless ulcerated or scarred areas are usually seen on the midline scalp of newborns due to localized absence of skin. A 'collar' of longer hairs may surround the hairless areas. Sometimes, aplasia cutis congenita is found on the trunk, face, or proximal extremities. It is a developmental defect that occurs 1 per 5000 live births.

An underlying osseous defect is occasionally found. Imaging studies are needed in such babies and in those with associated anomalies. The majority of babies have no other anomalies, but in syndromic aplasia cutis congenita, cleft palate, cleft lip, syndactyly, absence of digits, and heart disease have been associated.

Syndromic aplasia cutis has been linked to mutations in many genes: BMSI in autosomal dominant Aplasia cutis; KCTD1 in Scalp-ear-nipple (SEN) syndrome; ARHGAP31 in Adams–Oliver type 1; Dock 6 in AO-2, RPBS in AO-3; EDGT in AO-4; and Notch 1 in AO-5. Aplasia cutis also is seen in trisomy 13 and deletions of the short arm of chromosome 4 and 19q13.11. Autosomal dominant inheritance has been observed in many families.

Scalp sebaceous nevi are also hairless and can mimic aplasia in newborns.

TREATMENT

If a 'hair' collar is present or the defect large, imaging should be considered. Referral to a neurosurgeon is necessary if skull defects are found. If ulcerated, initially wound dressings and prevention of infection is critical. If there are no underlying skull abnormalities, and after the lesion has scarred, surgical correction can be considered. If the lesion is small, mobilization of the adjacent scalp and simple closure may be feasible.

ACQUIRED CIRCUMSCRIBED HAIR LOSS

Alopecia areata (AA)

DDx ref 141 • 142 • 139

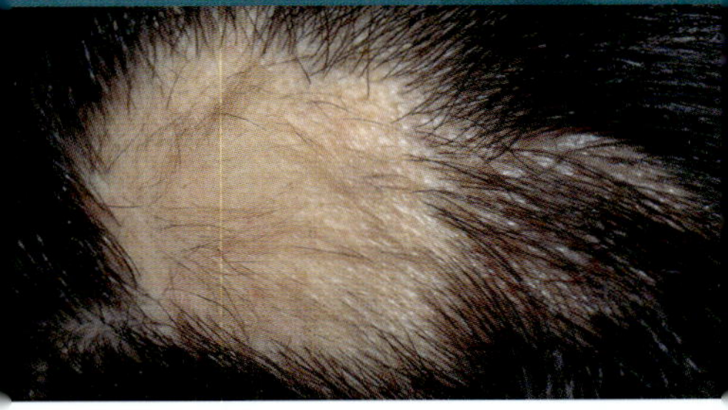

Round patch of complete hair loss without scalp change in a child with AA.

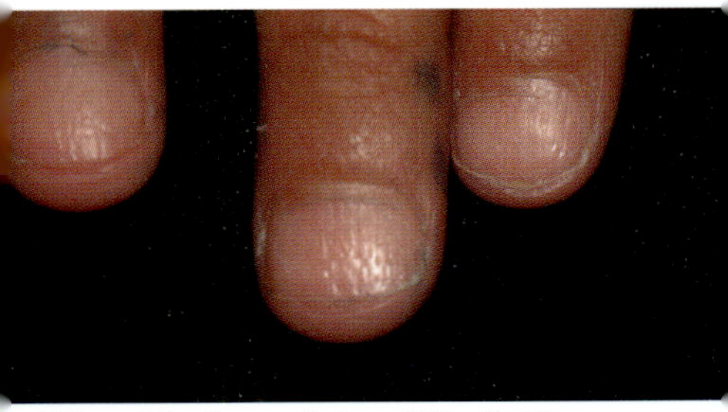

Pitting of the fingernails in a child with AA.

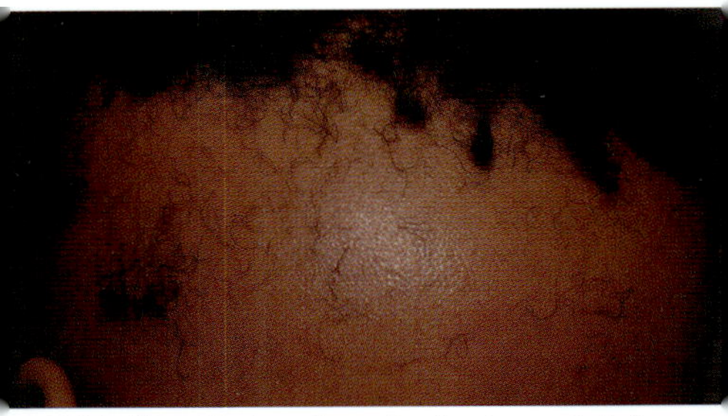

Child with ophiasis pattern of extensive scalp hair loss in the occipital region.

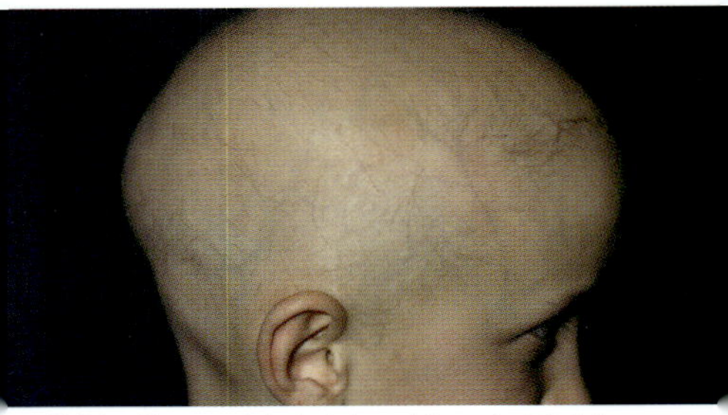

Child with complete hair loss (alopecia totalis).

Alopecia areata (AA)

DDx ref 141 • 142 • 139

CLINICAL FEATURES

Alopecia areata (AA) is an acquired hair loss with the appearance of a circumscribed area completely devoid of hair without scalp change. Most children experience 1–3 areas of hair loss. Scalp hair loss is most common but body hairs, sexual hair, eyebrows, and eyelashes may be lost.

Examination of the nails is mandatory as the presence of nail pitting is useful in making the diagnosis. Nail changes and the absence of broken hairs will help distinguish from tinea capitis or hair pulling. The nail pits are shallow (1–2 mm) and wider than those seen in psoriasis. In a few children, extensive scalp hair loss is seen beginning in the occipital scalp and spreading anteriorly across the hair margins. This is called **ophiasis** and is likely to eventuate in loss of all the scalp hair (alopecia totalis) or all of scalp and body hair (alopecia universalis). There is a rare acute form of rapid hair loss without preceding circumscribed areas.

Alopecia areata may be associated with vitiligo, asthma, allergic rhinitis, atopic dermatitis, and thyroiditis. A positive family history is obtained in 25%. The pathogenesis is unknown but many authorities believe it is an autoimmune process with injury to the growing hair that results in premature conversion from a growing to a resting hair that is shed.

TREATMENT

The child with 1–3 patches of hair loss is likely to spontaneously regrow hair within a year. For the child with extensive hair loss, many forms of topical therapy have induced short-term regrowth, but do not alter the long-term course of AA. Effective topical therapies include super-potent topical steroids, topical pimecrolimus, short contact anthralin, contact sensitizers, and minoxidil. Some authorities use combinations of these therapies. The use of systemic steroids should be discouraged as the hair regrowth is temporary, and will fall out again when the treatment is discontinued. For the child with extensive hair loss, AA support groups are very helpful, and the option of the child to consider wearing a wig may be considered.

ACQUIRED CIRCUMSCRIBED HAIR LOSS

Tinea capitis and kerion

140 • 142 • 87

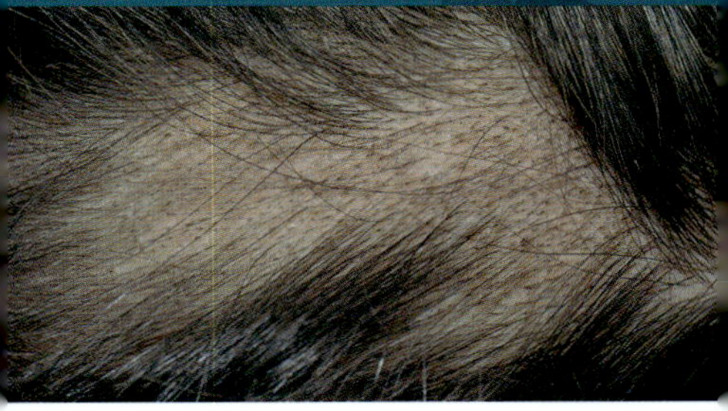

Circumscribed hair loss with hairs broken at the follicular orifice (black dot ringworm).

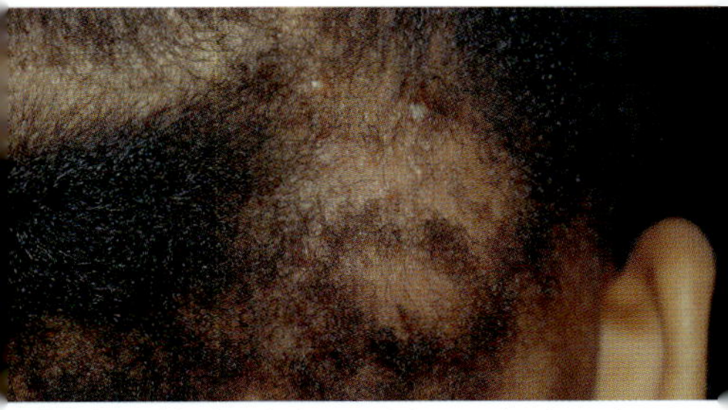

Patches of broken hairs, pustules, and enlarged lymph node in a child with *T. tonsurans* infection.

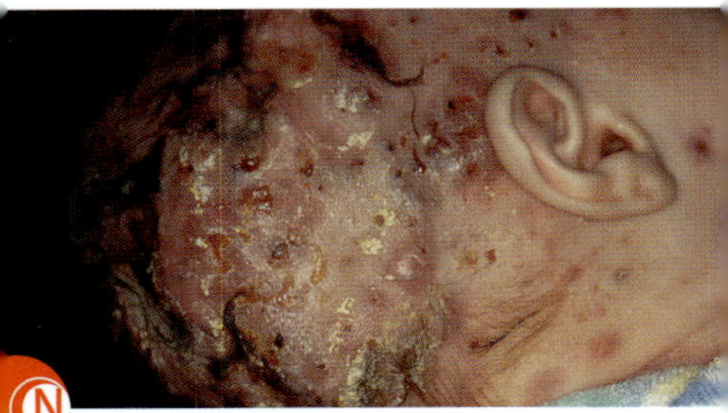

Multiple boggy masses (kerions) and pustules in a newborn with tinea capitis.

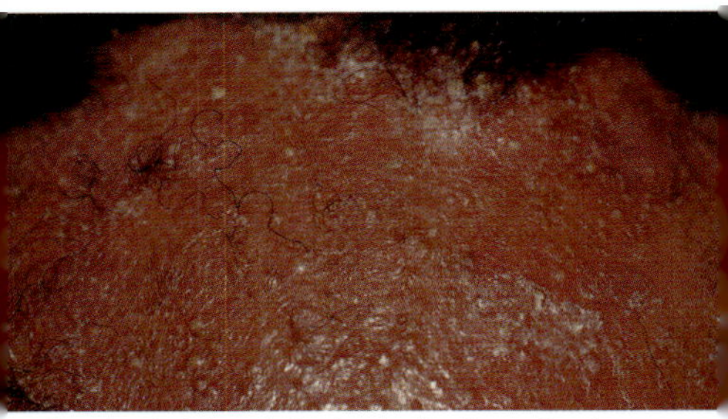

Scarring hair loss following kerion formation in undiagnosed tinea capitis.

Tinea capitis and kerion

DDx ref 140 • 142 • 87

CLINICAL FEATURES

Acquired circumscribed hair loss with broken hairs is characteristic of tinea capitis. The major organisms responsible for tinea capitis are *Trichophyton tonsurans* and *Microsporum canis*.

In *T. tonsurans* infection, hairs are broken at follicular orifices, the so-called 'black dot ringworm'.

In *M. canis* infections, the short hairs appear thickened and white. Initial infection remains noninflammatory for 2–8 weeks with hair loss and broken hairs.

There are four inflammatory stages: (1) diffuse scaling and hair loss in the scalp; (2) multiple scaly patches with pustules in bald areas; (3) a boggy scalp mass called a 'kerion'; and (4) a dermatitis pattern that mimics seborrheic dermatitis with greasy scales. All inflammatory forms have enlargement of regional lymph nodes, especially the occipital lymph nodes.

Kerions may heal with scarring if untreated. In *M. canis* infection, examination with a Wood's lamp reveals yellow-green fluorescence of thickened hairs; *T. tonsurans* does not fluoresce. KOH examination in the noninflammatory stage reveals hyphae and spores within the hair shaft; in an inflammatory stage and diffuse scaling type; the KOH may be negative. Fungal culture remains the mainstay of diagnosis. A dermatophyte test medium makes this a simple procedure. Broken hairs or scale obtained by a sterile curette or cotton swab are inoculated to break the agar surface and the bottle cap left loosened. Dermatophytes turn the agar from yellow to red and a fuzzy growth appears on the surface in 4–6 days. *T. tonsurans* may require 3–4 weeks.

Family members should be screened by fungal culture as 50% of children with tinea capitis due to *T. tonsurans* have an infected family member. *T. tonsurans* is spread by sharing of hats, caps, scarves, combs, or brushes by others in the family; *M. canis* is transmitted by cats and dogs. Tinea capitis can be distinguished from alopecia areata and hair pulling by the presence of scalp inflammation, fluorescent hairs, regional lymphadenopathy, and a positive fungal culture.

TREATMENT

Oral griseofulvin in a micronized form at 20 mg/kg per day for at least 4 weeks after the first negative repeat fungal culture, is the treatment of choice. Griseofulvin should be taken with a fatty meal. Oral terbinafine at 3 mg/kg per day for 4 weeks is slightly better than griseofulvin against *T. tonsurans*, but not very effective against *M. canis*.

Oral fluconazole and itraconazole are alternative therapies. Addition of an antifungal shampoo such as selenium sulfide 2.5% or ketoconazole 2% twice weekly may prevent the spread to others.

Sharing of hats, caps, scarves, combs, or brushes by others in the family should be avoided.

142

ACQUIRED CIRCUMSCRIBED HAIR LOSS

Traction alopecia and hair pulling

DDx ref 140 • 141 • 144

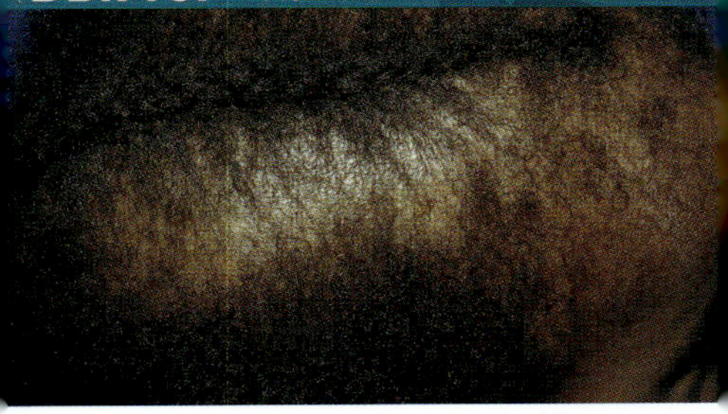

Child with traction alopecia from tight braiding hairstyle.

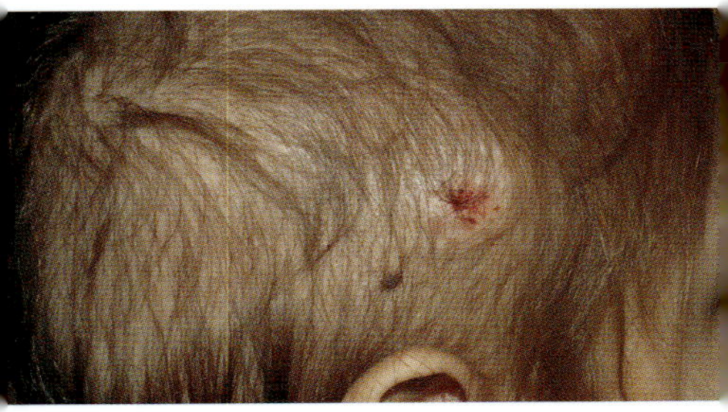

Child with hair pulling and scalp excoriation.

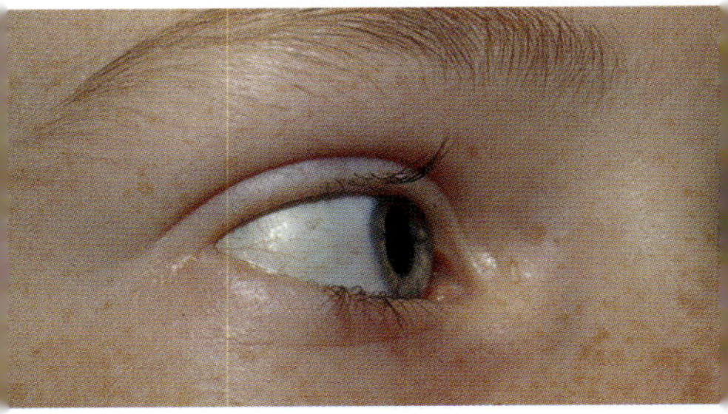

Eyelash pulling in a teenage girl.

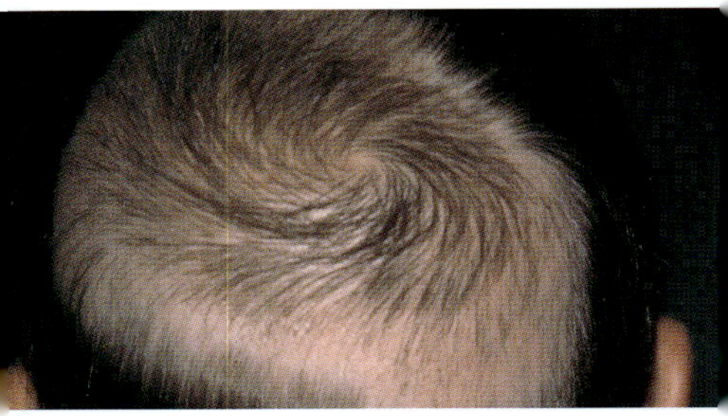

Characteristic 'monk' pattern of hair loss in a teenage boy with impulse control disorder.

DDx ref 140 • 141 • 144

CLINICAL FEATURES

Hairs broken at different lengths and irregular-shaped areas of hair loss are seen in traction alopecia. There are four types: traction alopecia, acute hair pulling, trichotillomania, and hair pulling with psychiatric disease.

Traction alopecia is due to hairstyle with tight braiding or pulling back of hair with tension.

Acute hair pulling is seen more often in toddlers, and the result of hair pulling by a playmate or sibling or self-hair-cutting. Acute hair pulling in the young child often resolves without intervention.

Trichotillomania has a preteen or teenage onset of hair pulling or eyelash pulling and is a sign of an impulse control disorder and may be accompanied by skin-picking as obsessive-compulsive behavior. Eyelash changes reveal broken lashes in an irregular pattern. The scalp may reveal perifollicular petechiae. Microscopic examination of broken hairs or eyelashes will reveal hair-splitting or fragmentation. Trichobezoars from ingestion of the pulled hairs may also be seen. Trichotillomania is often triggered by a traumatic event such as death or severe illness in the family, divorce of parents, or school difficulties. Asking for stresses preceding the hair loss as well as a family history of hair pulling or obsessive-compulsive behavior may be revealing. In some children, a variety of psychologic disorders is associated with hair pulling, including bipolar disease and schizophrenia. Hair pulling can be distinguished from alopecia areata and tinea capitis by hairs broken at different lengths in irregular patterns, the absence of lymphadenopathy or fluorescent hairs, a negative fungal culture, and the presence of excoriations from skin-picking.

TREATMENT

For traction alopecia due to hairstyles, changing to a loose hairstyle will suffice, while educating the family that it will take 6 months to clear. In the teen with impulsive control disorder, using styling mousse on the hair daily will make it too slippery to pull. Identification of stressors in the child's life might result in helpful solutions. A psychiatric referral may be useful in the severely involved.

143 DDx ref

CONGENITAL DIFFUSE HAIR LOSS

Ectodermal dysplasias (ED)

144 • 142 • 138

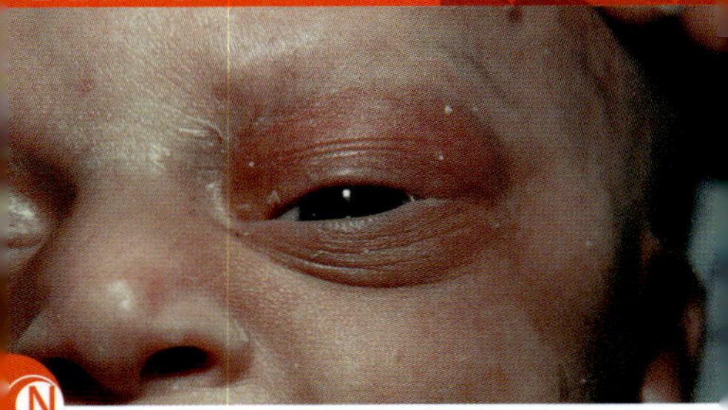

XR hypohidrotic ED. A newborn with absence of eyebrows and lashes and darkened eyelids.

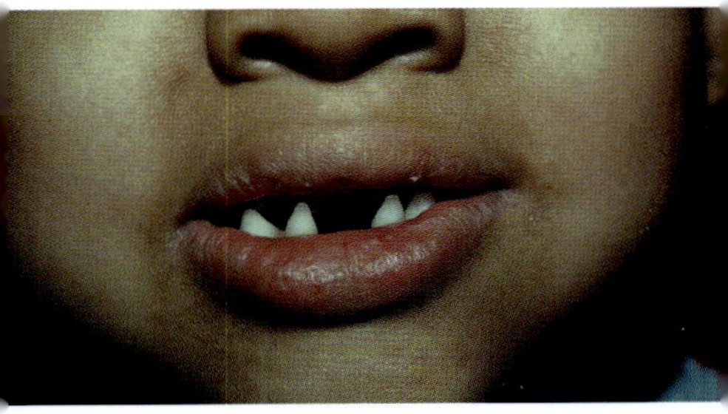

Cone-shaped and missing teeth in a child with XR ED.

144 DDx ref

CONGENITAL DIFFUSE HAIR LOSS

Hair shaft defects

143 • 142 • 141

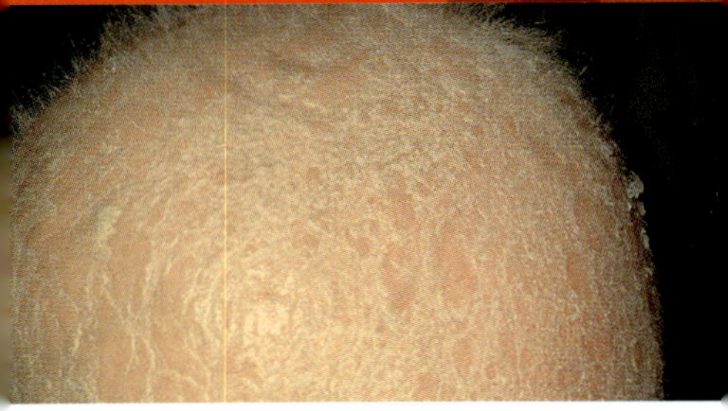

Short, broken scalp hairs in a child with Netherton's syndrome.

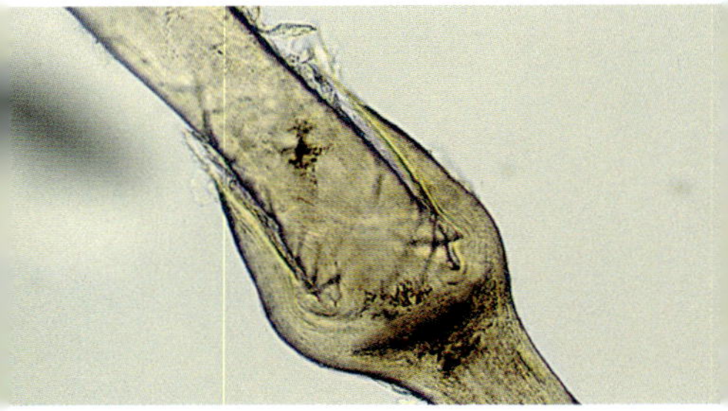

Photomicrograph of a ball and socket hair shaft defect in Netherton's syndrome.

143 CONGENITAL DIFFUSE HAIR LOSS

Ectodermal dysplasias (ED)

DDx ref 144 • 142 • 138

CLINICAL FEATURES

Newborns with sparse or absent hair, eyebrows, and/or eyelashes (congenital diffuse alopecia) should bring to mind the ectodermal dysplasias. There are 170 rare conditions called 'ectodermal dysplasia' and all are developmental defects in hair, teeth, nails, and/or sweat glands. In 89 of these, newborns have sparse scalp hair and never develop normal hair. Many have gene defects of ectodysplasin in the pathway of NF-kappaB signaling. The most common condition is the X-linked recessive hypohidrotic ectodermal dysplasia seen with sparse scalp hair and eyebrows, absence of sweat glands with unexplained fevers, absence of nasal mucous glands, sometimes poorly-formed nails, and when teeth develop, sparse and pegged teeth. A meticulous examination for other developmental defects is needed.

TREATMENT

Referral to a genetics clinic is recommended. There is no treatment for the sparse hair.

144 CONGENITAL DIFFUSE HAIR LOSS

Hair shaft defects

DDx ref 143 • 142 • 141

CLINICAL FEATURES

Short hair in the newborn that does not grow and often leads to the complaint that the child never requires a haircut indicates a hair shaft defect. Plucking hairs and examining under the microscope will help distinguish the structural hair shaft defects. There are six major hair breakage types with Netherton's syndrome of trichorrhexis invaginata (bamboo hairs), ichthyosis, and severe eczema the most common. Netherton's syndrome presents as a red, scaly, hairless newborn. A gene mutation encoding SPINK 5 enzyme creates the defective epidermal barrier. Children with trichorrhexis nodosum have broken hairs that fracture within a hair swelling and the condition is associated with argininosuccinic aciduria, citrullinemia, and Menkes X-linked recessive copper transport deficiency. Developmental retardation is common. Pili torti (twisted hair) may be an isolated finding or associated with syndromes with teeth and nail abnormalities. Monilethrix (beaded hair) is autosomal dominant and due to mutations in hair keratins 81, 83, and 86. Nonphotosensitive trichothiodystrophy (TTD) (banded hair with alternating light and dark areas) is associated with mutations of the C7ORF11 gene, whereas the photosensitive TTD is due to mutations in ERCC2 and ERCC3 helicases or the TGBS gene, and is seen in children that also have physical and developmental retardation.

TREATMENT

There are no effective treatments that will regrow hairs.

ACQUIRED DIFFUSE HAIR LOSS

Telogen and anagen effluvium

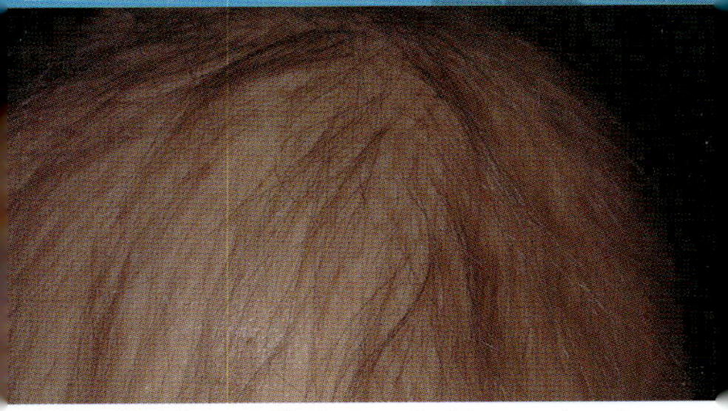

Child with telogen effluvium and widespread scalp hair loss.

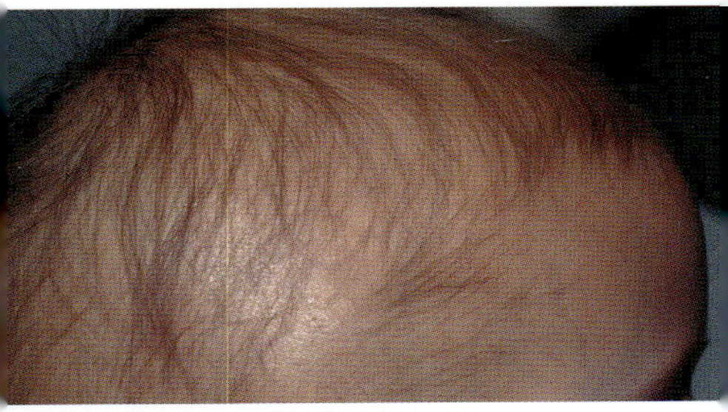

Child with telogen effluvium following hospitalization for febrile illness.

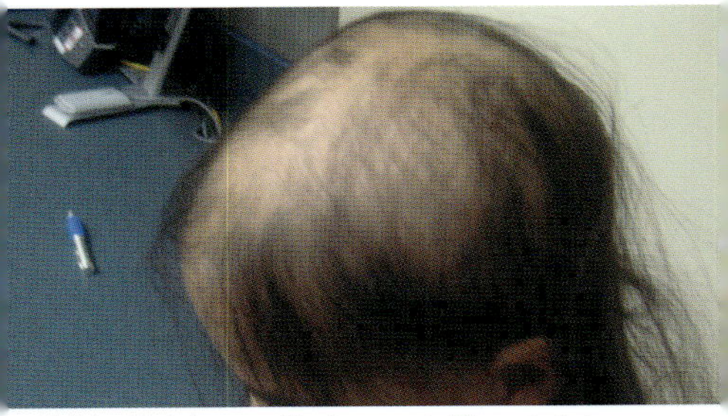

Child with telogen effluvium and diffuse hair loss.

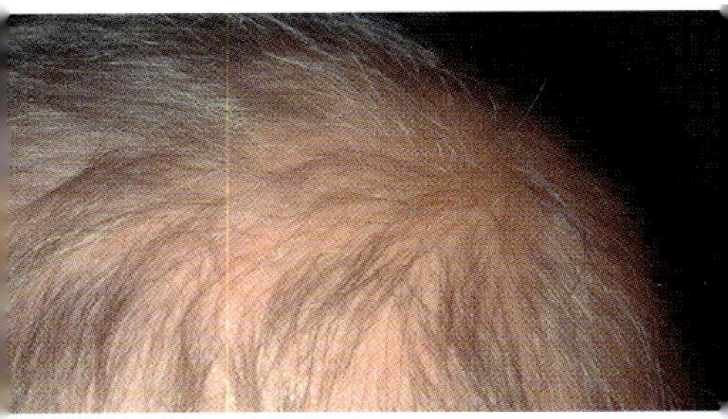

Early telogen effluvium in a child with Down syndrome.

145 ACQUIRED DIFFUSE HAIR LOSS

Telogen and anagen effluvium

DDx ref 140 • 143 • 144

CLINICAL FEATURES

Normally, scalp hair in children cycles asynchronously with 85% in a growing phase (anagen) and 15% resting or about to shed (telogen). Loss of scalp hair in clumps or handfuls is seen in both telogen and anagen effluvium. On examination, light pulling of 50–100 scalp hairs by grasping between the thumb and forefinger at the scalp level easily removes a handful of hairs. The hairs should be examined under the microscope to determine if they are telogen or anagen. Telogen hairs do not have a pigmented bulb and the bulb is about the same thickness as the hair shaft, while anagen hairs have a pigmented bulb that is curled and larger than the hair shaft. The diffuse loss of primarily telogen (resting) hairs occurs 3–4 months following a stressful event. Events include infections with high fevers; surgery; medications such as lithium, beta blockers, retinoids, and oral contraceptives; iron, zinc, biotin, or essential fatty acid deficiencies; psychological stress or postpartum. Telogen effluvium is the result of a sudden conversion of growing hairs to resting hairs from a normal ratio of 85 : 15 to 50 : 50. If the stressful event is removed, regrowth in 6–12 months is expected. Anagen hair loss occurs days to weeks after a severe toxic insult such as chemotherapy, radiotherapy, accidental ingestion of toxic chemicals or plants. Less obvious causes include toxicity from arsenic, thallium, boric acid or mercury, or protein malnutrition. Additionally, there may appear transverse depressions in the nails (Beau's lines) that represent interruption of nail growth. Laboratory screening for heavy metals may be useful in these circumstances. Generally, the hair loss is reversible, provided the precipitating insult has ended. Scalp hair requires 6–12 months for regrowth.

TREATMENT

Infrequent hair combing and wearing of loose hairstyles will help minimize the hair loss until regrowth occurs.

146 THICKENED NAILS

Pachyonychia congenita (PC)

DDx ref 147 • 150 • 68

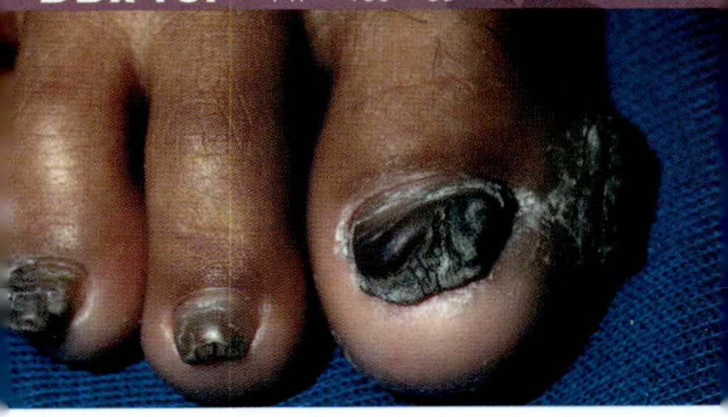

PC with thickening and discoloration of a child's toenails.

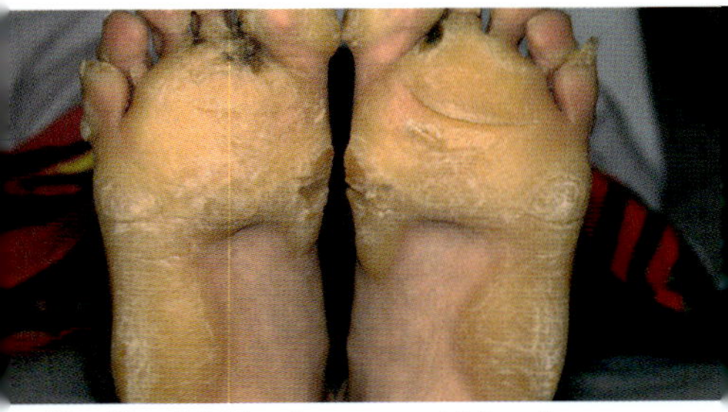

PC with painful keratoses on a child's soles.

147 THICKENED NAILS

Ectodermal dysplasia (nails)

DDx ref 146 • 148 • 149

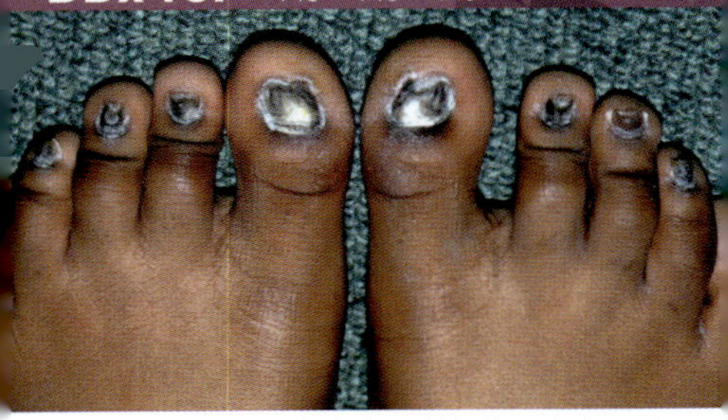

Thick, pigmented nails in hypohidrotic ectodermal dysplasia.

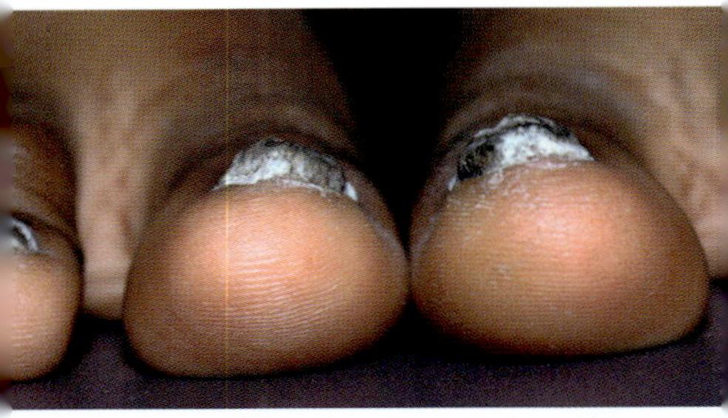

Darkening and thickening of toenails in a child with ectodermal dysplasia.

146 THICKENED NAILS

Pachyonychia congenita (PC)

DDx ref 147 • 150 • 68

CLINICAL FEATURES

Normal newborns have thin short nails. Those born with thick nails should bring to mind pachyonychia congenita. There are five subtypes based on genetic analysis. Mutations in keratin genes 6a and 17 have thickened toenails and fingernails at birth with the nails raised distally and discolored by subungual keratoses. Both types also have palmoplantar keratoses and oral mucosa whitening. K17 defects also have natal teeth and develop skin cysts that are steatocystoma multiplex. Subtypes with mutations of K6b, K6c, or 16 have a later onset within the first 5 years of life and less nail involvement, and K6b and K6c have less keratoderma.

Local keratolytics such as 20% salicylic acid or 40% urea cream applied to the nails will help. Oral retinoids have aided in extreme involvement.

147 THICKENED NAILS

Ectodermal dysplasia (nails)

DDx ref 146 • 148 • 149

CLINICAL FEATURES

Thick nails are found in 25 of the 170 types of ectodermal dysplasia. Distal thickening is most common and discoloration with thickening is also seen. Evidence of nail thickening is usually seen in the newborn period but may develop later. Signs of sparse hair, eyebrows, and eyelashes are seen and sparse and deformed teeth are seen later. Associated skeletal anomalies and cleft lip or palate may be found. Often, the toenails are more affected than fingernails. In some types of ED, nails can be thin and short (see topic 152).

TREATMENT

There are no effective treatments. Improvement may occur with keratolytic preparations such as 20% salicylic acid and 40% urea cream, followed by gentle filing of the nails.

148 DDx ref

THICKENED NAILS

Median nail dystrophy

149 • 147 • 151

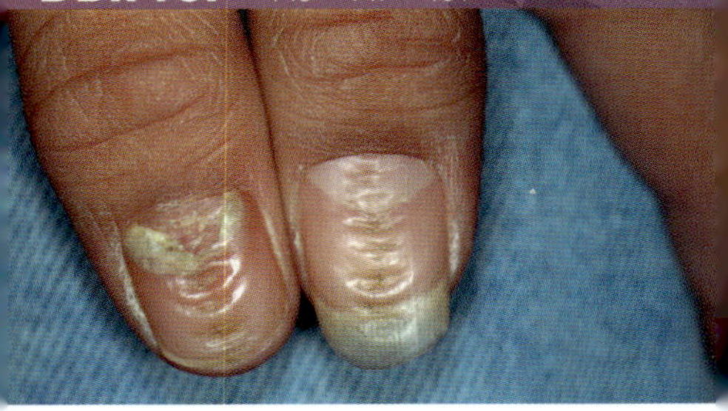

Median nail dystrophy with multiple central grooves on the thumbnails.

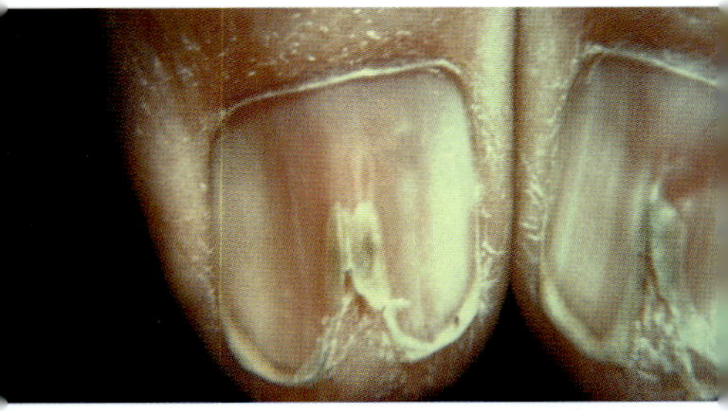

Central thickening and splitting of thumbnails in median nail dystrophy.

149 DDx ref

THICKENED NAILS

Trachyonychia (20 nail dystrophy)

147 • 151 • 150

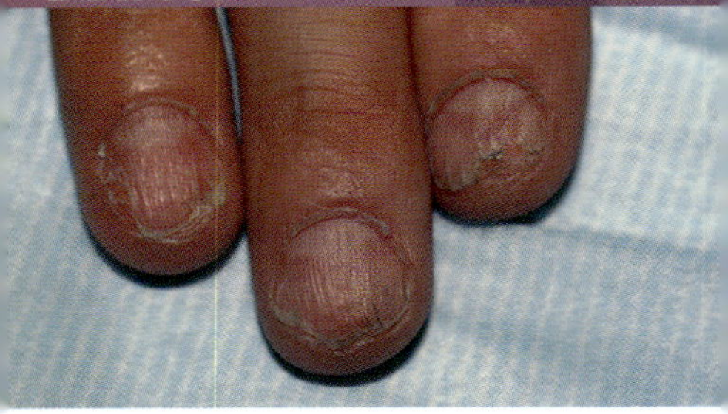

Early trachyonychia with roughness of the fingernails.

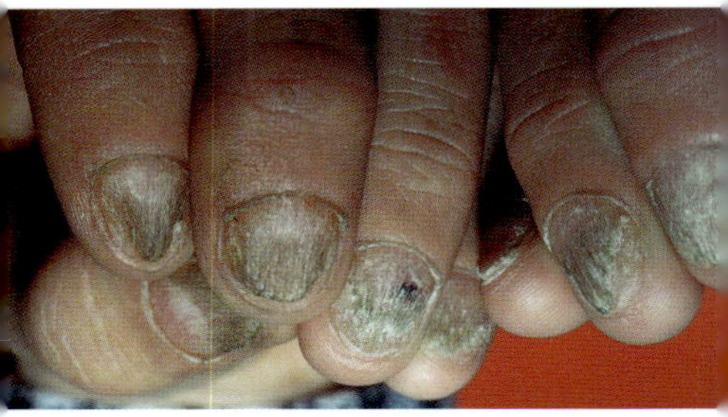

Thickening and roughness of nails in a child with idiopathic trachyonychia.

148 THICKENED NAILS

Median nail dystrophy

DDx ref 149 • 147 • 151

CLINICAL FEATURES

Rubbing of the thumbnail and proximal nail fold of the thumb with the index finger on the same hand results in central transverse grooves of the thumbnail and may eventuate in central thickening and splitting of the thumbnail. Usually both thumbnails are involved; one may be more severely affected than the other. Median nail dystrophy begins as a habit and is usually seen in the preteen or teenage child. The habit often disappears in adult life.

TREATMENT

Breaking the habit may be difficult, although wearing gloves may limit access to the thumbnails. If the habit stops, it requires 6–12 months to revert to normal.

149 THICKENED NAILS

Trachyonychia (20 nail dystrophy)

DDx ref 147 • 151 • 150

CLINICAL FEATURES

Roughening and eventually thickening of the nails' surface is seen in fingernails and sometimes toenails of children. The age of onset is 2–7 years. Although historically called '20 nail dystrophy' it rarely involves all 20 nails. A few affected children will have alopecia areata, although most have idiopathic trachyonychia unassociated with other findings. It is a benign condition that usually resolves within 5 years.

TREATMENT

Topical emollients may improve the roughness. Spontaneous involution is usual.

150 THICKENED NAILS

Psoriasis nails

DDx ref 151 • 146 • 68

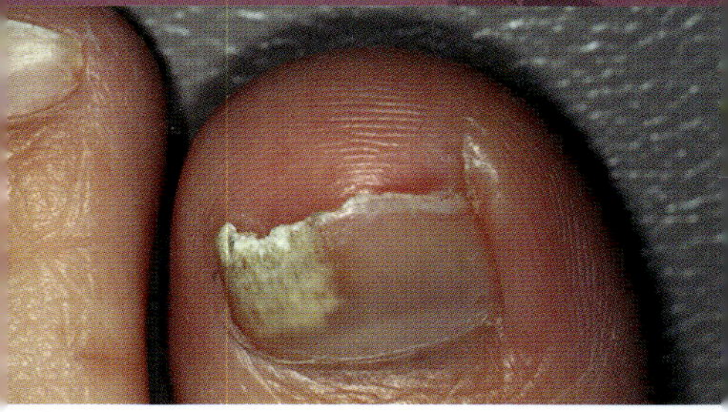

Distal yellowing of a child's nails in psoriasis.

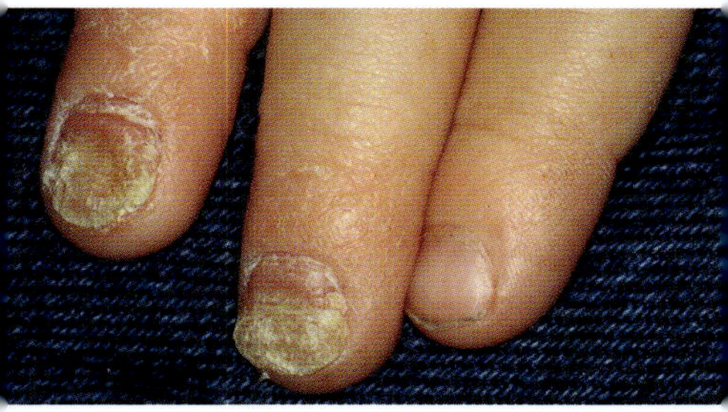

Distal yellow thickening of two nails and one uninvolved nail in psoriasis.

151 THICKENED NAILS

Lichen planus nails

DDx ref 148 • 150 • 68

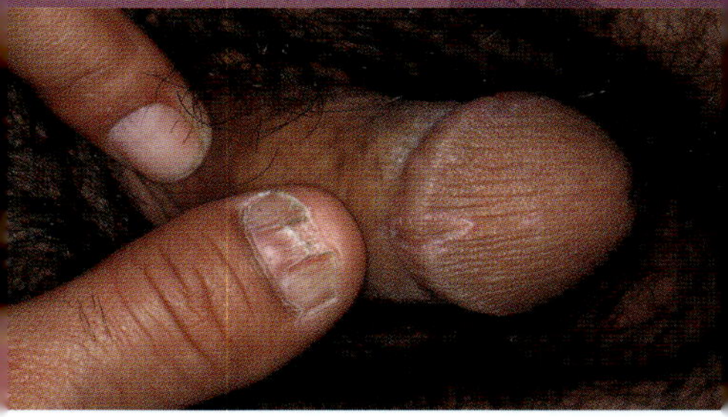

A teenage male with lichen planus of thumbnail and penis.

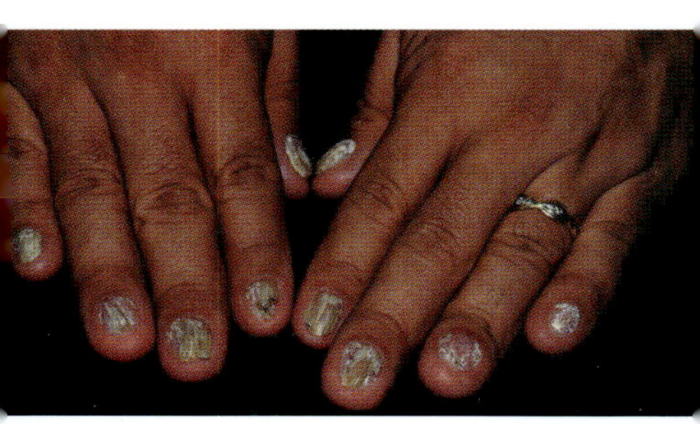

Central thickening of all fingernails in a child with lichen planus.

150

THICKENED NAILS

Psoriasis nails

DDx ref 151 • 146 • 68

CLINICAL FEATURES

In children with psoriasis, nail findings are diagnostically useful, even though they are present in only 15% (see topic 67). Nail pitting is the most frequent, followed by distal yellowing caused by separation of the nail from the nail bed (onycholysis) and, eventually, thick, yellow nails. Fingernails are more involved than toenails and, characteristically, some nails are spared next to others that are involved. Psoriasis, lichen planus, and trachyonychia account for almost all acquired nail thickening. The presence of scaly papules and plaques and the Koebner phenomenon will help distinguish psoriasis. A family history of psoriasis may also help.

TREATMENT

Massaging tazarotene 0.1% gel into the proximal nail fold daily will help clear psoriasis nails. The treatment must be maintained for months. Oral retinoids and oral methotrexate and biologics also are effective, when they are used to treat severe psoriasis and psoriasis with arthritis. It is difficult to justify their use to treat nail disease alone.

151

THICKENED NAILS

Lichen planus nails

DDx ref 148 • 150 • 68

CLINICAL FEATURES

In the child with lichen planus, nail involvement is uncommon. The fingernails may show central thickening and pterygium formation. In severe lichen planus, all 20 nails may be involved and loss of nails seen. To distinguish from psoriasis and trachyonychia, the central nail ridging is useful, as are the purple pruritic plaques and papules and lacy thickening of the buccal mucosa. In some children, nail findings precede cutaneous and mucosal findings. Some 10% of children diagnosed with 20 nail dystrophy may instead have lichen planus.

TREATMENT

There are no comparative studies on treating lichen planus nails. Reports of improvement with potent topical steroids and topical retinoids such as tazarotene are promising.

THIN, SLOW-GROWING, OR LOSS OF NAIL

Ectodermal dysplasia and nail-patella syndrome

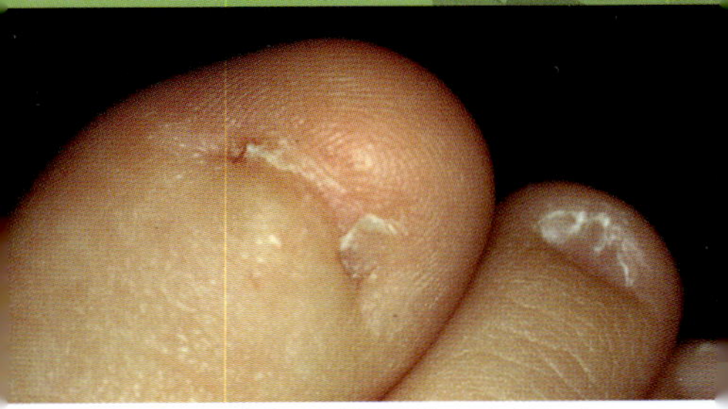

Thin, small toenails in a child with hypohidrotic ectodermal dysplasia.

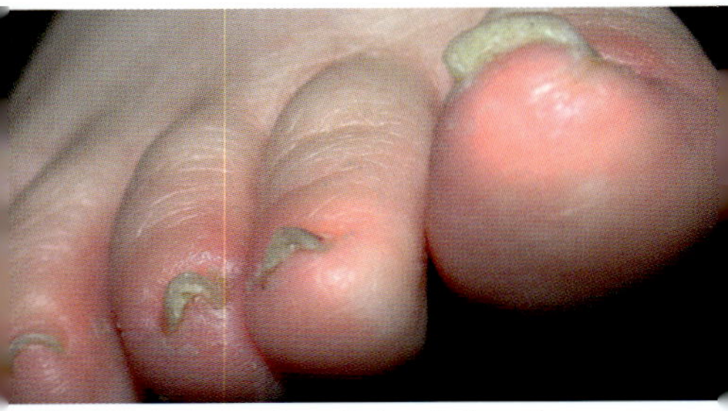

Thin, small, curved toenails in ectodermal dysplasia.

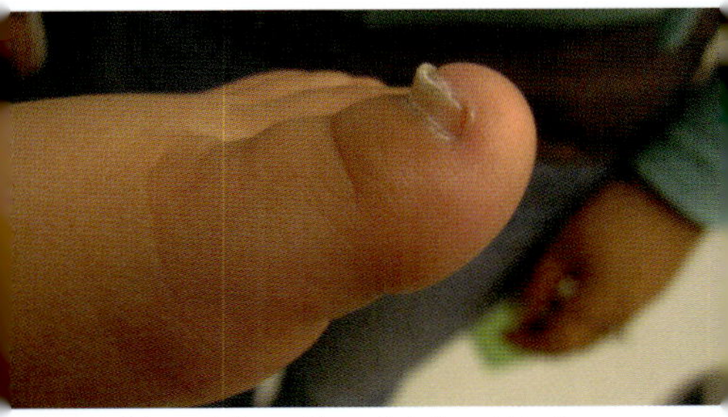

Short, thin malaligned toenail in hypohidrotic ectodermal dysplasia.

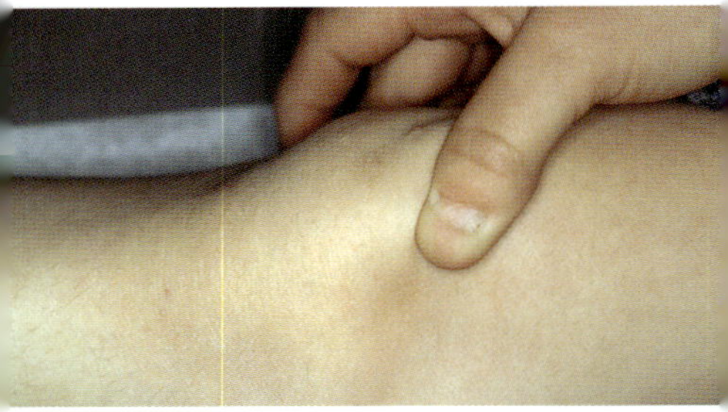

Thin hypoplastic thumbnail and dislocated patella in nail-patella syndrome.

152

Ectodermal dysplasia and nail-patella syndrome

DDx ref 151 • 149 • 150

CLINICAL FEATURES

Thin, small, and/or absent nails are found in 53 of the 170 types of ectodermal dysplasia, including the recessive and dominant types of hypohidrotic ectodermal dysplasia and the ectodermal dysplasias associated with limb abnormalities. Some types of ectodermal dysplasia have thickened rather than thin nails. Also, hypoplastic nails are a feature of the nail-patella syndrome; an autosomal dominant syndrome of small nails, hypoplastic patella, and a nephropathy that may progress to renal failure. Nail-patella is due to mutations in the LMX1B gene. The thumbnails are usually the most severely affected.

TREATMENT

There is no effective treatment.

153 PITTED LESIONS

Ear pits and lip pits

DDx ref 143 • 97 • 139

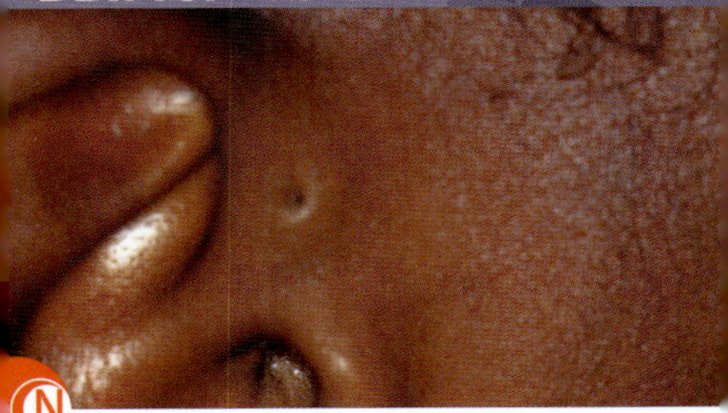

Ear pit in a newborn.

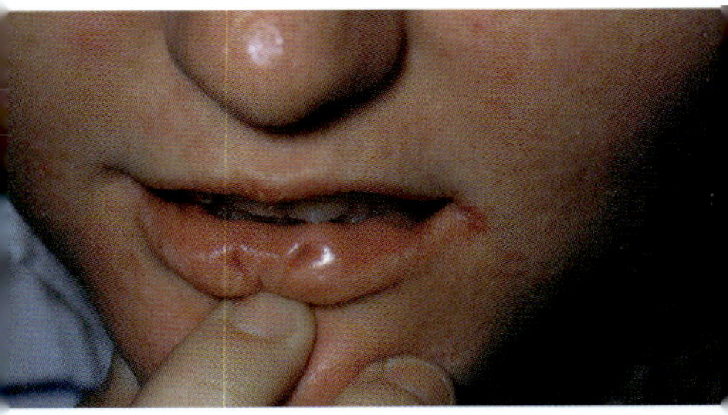

Bilateral lower lip pits present since birth.

154 PITTED LESIONS

Pitted keratolysis

DDx ref 68 • 85 • 91

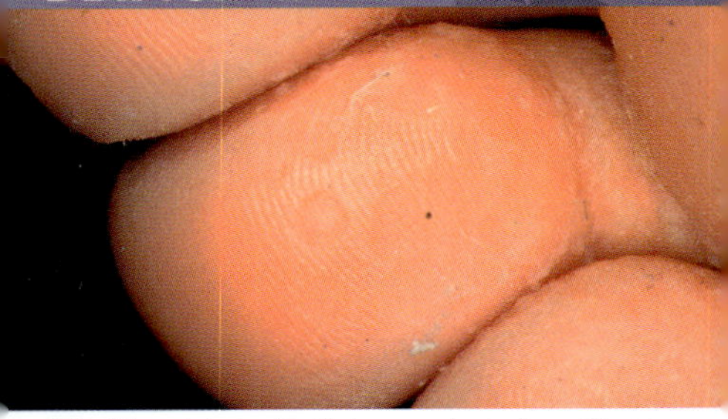

Pitted keratolysis. Multiple, round, shallow pits on the undersurface of a child's toes.

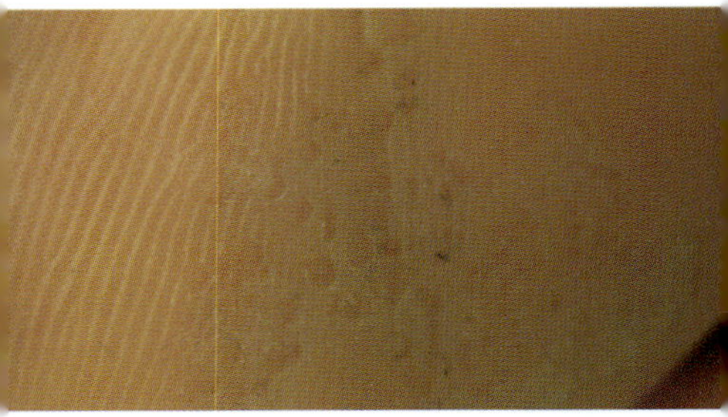

Multiple shallow pits on the forefoot of a child.

153 PITTED LESIONS
Ear pits and lip pits

DDx ref 143 • 97 • 139

CLINICAL FEATURES

Congenital pits are lined with epithelium and usually an isolated finding in the newborn. They are most commonly found in the preauricular or periauricular skin (ear pits) or the mucosal side of commissures of the lips. Ear pits may be associated with congenital cysts or accessory tragi or with craniofacial syndromes. In addition to pits at the angles of the lips, a neonate may have one in the midline of the upper lip or bilateral on either side of the midline of the lower lip. Less common are branchial cleft pits on the lower third of the neck, thyroglossal duct pits at the midline of the upper anterior neck, and bronchogenic pits near the suprasternal notch. All pits have a risk of becoming infected. The appearance of tenderness, redness, and/or drainage should raise suspicion of infection.

TREATMENT

Most pits require no intervention. If infected, then treatment with oral antibiotics is indicated, followed by excision of the pit. Some have long tracts and require a complex surgical approach.

154 PITTED LESIONS
Pitted keratolysis

DDx ref 68 • 85 • 91

CLINICAL FEATURES

Multiple shallow pits on the soles or the undersurface of the toes characterize pitted keratolysis. Excessive sweating of the feet is invariably associated. Sometimes painful in the child, it can also be malodorous. The wearing of occlusive footwear or wet footwear is an aggravating factor. The condition is due to infection with *Corynebacterium* species. They can be seen on Gram-stained scrapings as Gram-positive rods or on silver stains of tissue sections as black rods. Culture is not necessary.

TREATMENT

Topical antibiotics such as erythromycin or clindamycin applied daily to twice daily usually resolve the problem. Washing with antibacterial soaps may help clear the infection. Adjunct therapy such as changing footwear, keeping the feet dry, and use of antiperspirants to reduce sweating may help.

Palmoplantar keratodermas

DDx ref 67 • 69 • 70

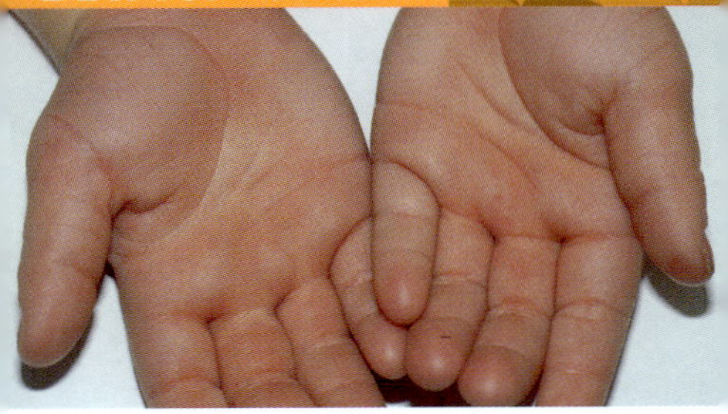

Diffuse palmoplantar keratoderma limited to the palms in a child.

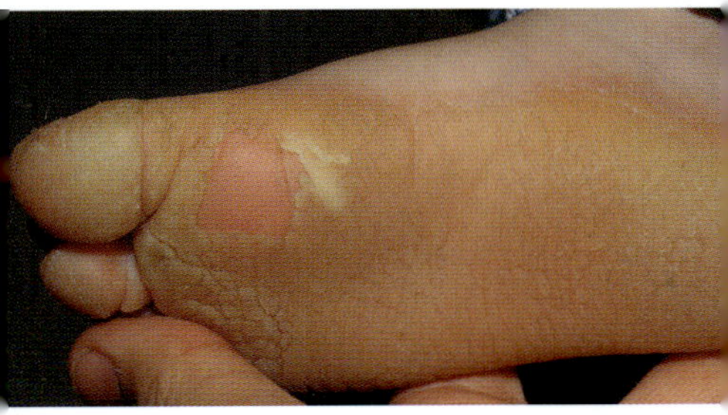

Diffuse palmoplantar keratoderma with spreading and blister formation.

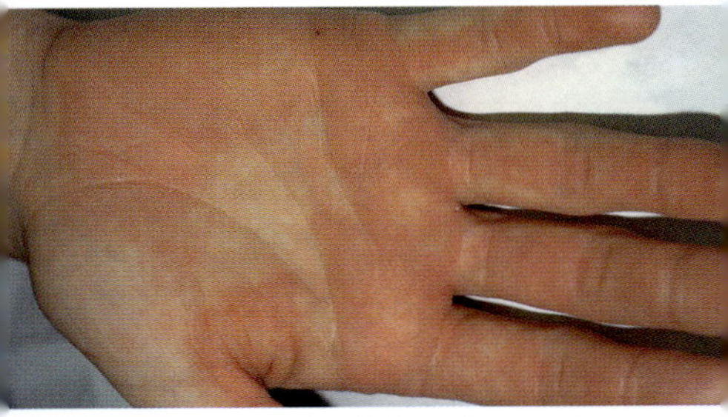

Striate palmoplantar keratoderma in a child.

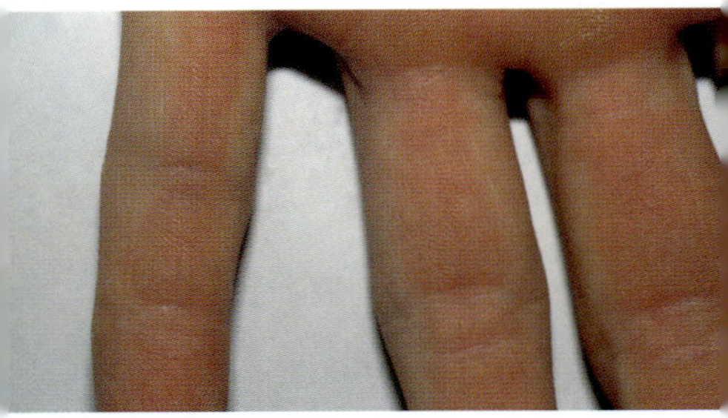

Striate palmoplantar keratoderma of the fingers.

155 Palmoplantar keratodermas

DDx ref 67 • 69 • 70

CLINICAL FEATURES

The hereditary palmoplantar keratodermas (PPK) are a heterogeneous group of conditions with most inherited as an autosomal dominant. The thickening of the palms and soles begins with the first significant friction. The more common PPKs are isolated skin disorders but some may be associated with teeth abnormalities, deafness, cardiac disease, or wooly hair.

Three clinical patterns are seen: a diffuse type; a linear or striate type; and focal or punctuate types. The diffuse type may be epidermolytic (keratin 1 and 9); non-epidermolytic (keratin 9); or mutilating (Vohwinkel-loricrin). The striate types include PPK striate 1 (desmoglein 1); PPK striate 2 (desmoplakin); and PPK striate 3 (keratin 1). Localized types include the focal non-epidermolytic (keratin 16) and the punctate type (AAGAB). There are also other conditions that may have palmoplantar keratoderma, including pachyonychia congenita, tyrosinemia type 2, hidrotic ectodermal dysplasia, pityriasis rubra pilaris, psoriasis, the ichthyoses, Darier's disease, and dominant dystrophic epidermolysis bullosa. **Hyperhidrosis** is seen in most. The palmoplantar thickening may result in pain on walking, may blister, and the affected child may develop secondary infections.

TREATMENT

Topical salicylic acid, urea, lactic acid, or propylene glycol under polyethylene occlusion can be helpful. Topical retinoids are less useful. Oral retinoids should be reserved for the most severe circumstances.

156 DDx ref

PHOTODISTRIBUTION (SUN-INDUCED LESIONS)

Polymorphous light eruption

157 • 79 • 72

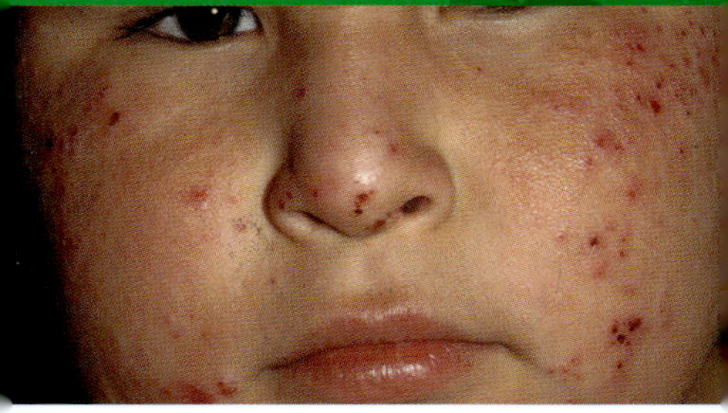

Actinic prurigo with vesicles and crusting of the face in a Native-American boy.

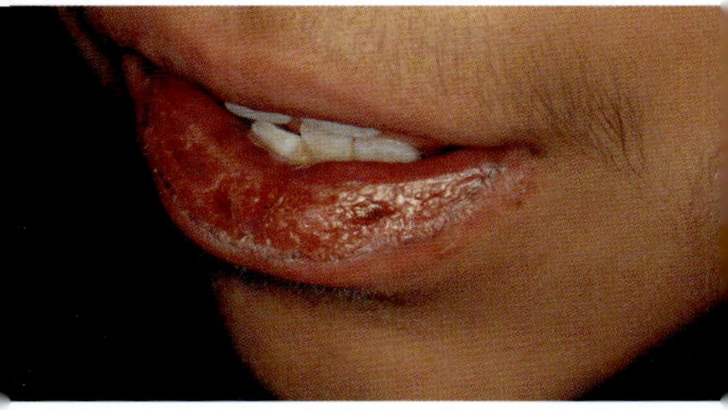

Actinic prurigo with cheilitis in a Native-American boy.

157 DDx ref

PHOTODISTRIBUTION (SUN-INDUCED LESIONS)

Erythropoietic protoporphyria (EPP)

156 • 77 • 72

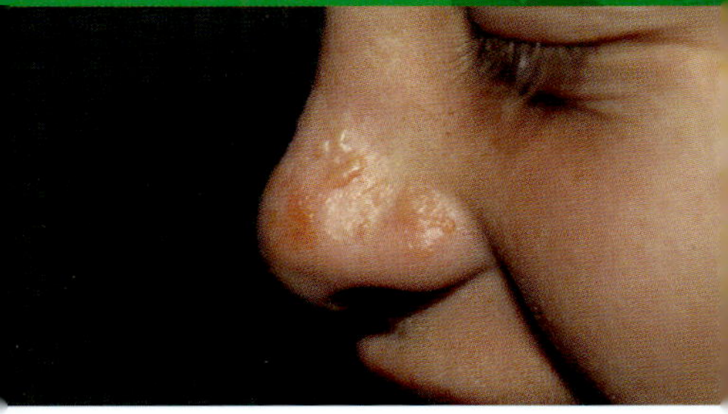

Vesicles on the nose of a child with EPP.

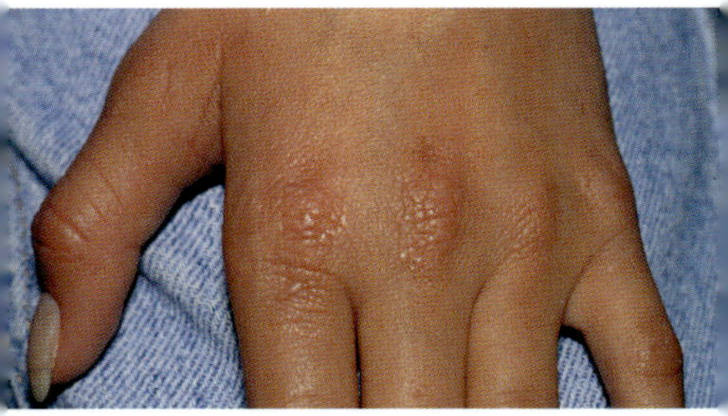

Thickened papules over the dorsal hand of a 12-year-old girl with EPP.

156 DDx ref

PHOTODISTRIBUTION (SUN-INDUCED LESIONS)

Polymorphous light eruption

157 • 79 • 72

CLINICAL FEATURES

The most common form of polymorphous light eruption (PMLE) is the **papular type**. It begins in the spring, with improvement through the summer. Lesions appear within hours to days of sun, last for 7–10 days, and heal without scarring. The eruption consists of discrete erythematous papules and plaques in sun-exposed areas. For unknown reasons, not all sun-exposed areas are involved, but the lesions occur consistently in the same location in a given individual. The majority of patients improve with age.

Actinic prurigo (Hutchinson's summer prurigo) is a dominantly inherited disorder seen predominantly in Native-Americans of North and South America. Most patients are female and the eruption begins before age 5 years. Lesions first develop in the spring and appear as an acute, pruritic dermatitis with edematous papules and vesicles. As the spring progresses, the dermatitis becomes subacute with crusting and lichenification. The eruption usually clears in late summer only to return again the next spring, although some children are so sun-sensitive that they have lesions throughout the year, with worsening in the spring. Chronic cheilitis and conjunctivitis may also be seen.

TREATMENT

Sun avoidance, sun-protective clothing, broad-spectrum sunscreens and mid- to high-potency topical steroids are the mainstay of treatment for both conditions. Thalidomide is effective in actinic prurigo.

157 DDx ref

PHOTODISTRIBUTION (SUN-INDUCED LESIONS)

Erythropoietic protoporphyria (EPP)

156 • 77 • 72

CLINICAL FEATURES

EPP presents in the preschool child as stinging, burning, or itching of the skin, often within minutes of sun exposure. Despite the symptoms, skin changes are frequently not seen. Intense sun exposure may result in facial edema, erythema, urticaria, vesiculation, and crusting. Vesicular injury may cause pitted scarring. Most children will present with chronic changes of slightly thickened skin-colored papules over the dorsa of the hands, nose, and cheeks. Mild anemia may be seen in 25%. Cholelithiasis and abnormal liver function tests occur in 25%. Up to 5% of affected individuals will progress to liver failure, usually after age 30 years. EPP is caused by compound heterozygosity of the gene encoding for ferrochelatase. Lack of ferrochelatase function leads to failure of protoporphyrin incorporation into heme and thus to protoporphyrin accumulation. Visible 409 nm light reacts with the protoporphyrin in the skin, leading to the symptoms. There is also an X-linked EPP with gain of function mutations in ALAS-2.

TREATMENT

Sun-exposure minimization, the wearing of broad-brimmed hats, long-sleeved and long-legged clothing, along with oral beta-carotene is the management of choice. In children, a dosage of 40–120 mg/day resulting in a beta-carotene serum level of 600–800 μg/100 mL is desired. Conventional sunscreens should be used as an adjunct, but are ineffective as the sole treatment. Liver function tests should be monitored and, if abnormal, referral to a liver specialist is required.

ANNULAR ARRANGEMENTS

Annular arrangement

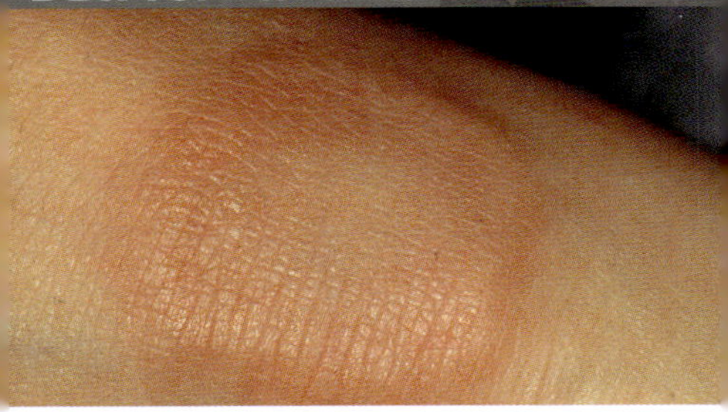

Granuloma annulare. Pink dermal nodules arranged in a circle.

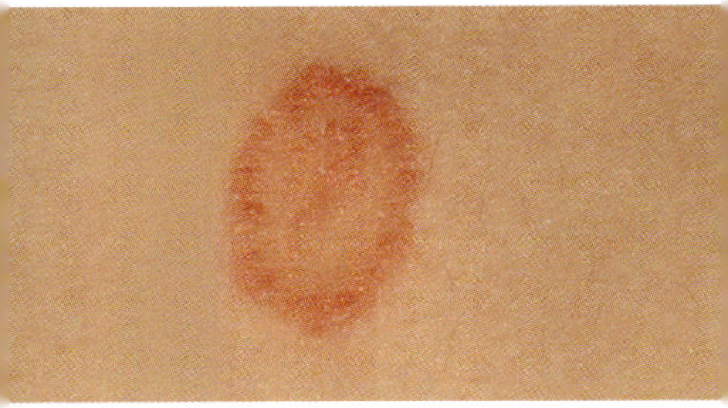

Tinea corporis. Scaly, red border on an annular lesion.

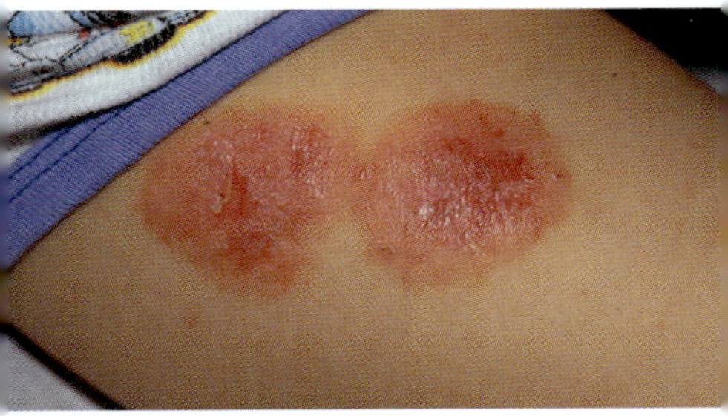

Nummular dermatitis lesions on a child's thigh.

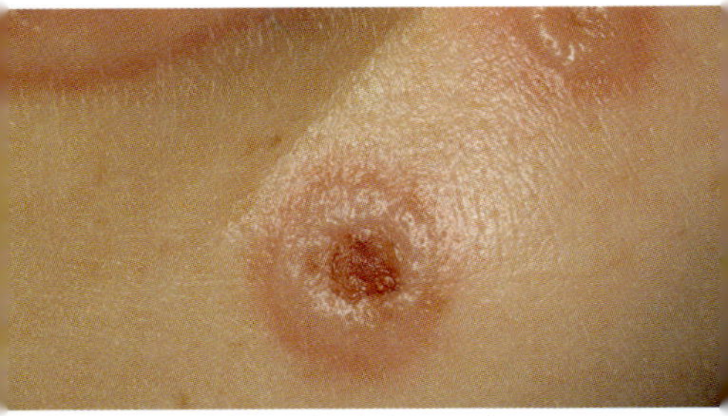

Erythema multiforme. Typical target lesion with central crusted zone.

CLINICAL FEATURES

Many conditions may have **annular (round) skin lesions**, but in children, the most common are nummular eczema, tinea corporis, and granuloma annulare. All are round with clearing in the center, but in nummular dermatitis, there is eczematous change throughout the lesions; in tinea corporis, there is disruption of the skin surface in the form of border scaling; while in granuloma annulare the skin surface is intact pushed up from beneath by the dermal granulomas. Nummular dermatitis-like lesions may also be seen in atopic dermatitis or allergic contact dermatitis. Less common annular conditions include erythema multiforme (EM), characterized by symmetrical round lesions. In EM there are typical target lesions with a dusky or bullous central zone, a red middle zone, and an outer edematous zone. Target lesions also may be seen in lupus erythematosus. Neonatal lupus erythematosus and subacute cutaneous lupus erythematosus also demonstrate annular scaly red plaques, predominantly in sun-exposed skin.

The herald patch of pityriasis rosea is typically annular with slight scale on the border (see topic 66). Similarly, early lesions of psoriasis, of pityriasis lichenoides, of lichen planus, and secondary syphilis can be annular. Rare mechano- and immunobullous diseases can produce an annular border of blisters. This is particularly seen in epidermolysis bullosa simplex of the Dowling–Meara type and in linear IgA dermatosis.

Large urticaria may be round and clear in the center (see topic 48). Urticaria can be distinguished by their transient nature, lasting in one place for a few hours, and the presence of other urticarial lesions that are oval or figurate. Urticaria is frequently misdiagnosed as EM. The target lesions of EM, once present, are fixed in those areas for at least 7 days, whereas urticaria moves to other areas within hours. Also, EM has a central zone of skin injury, but urticaria is clear in the center.

External skin injuries may be round, including self-induced lesions. Areas treated incompletely may also be round, such as warts that clear centrally after cryotherapy or chemical therapy, leaving a round rim of remaining wart.

LINEAR OR CURVILINEAR ARRANGEMENTS

Linear or curvilinear arrangement

92 • 114 • 91

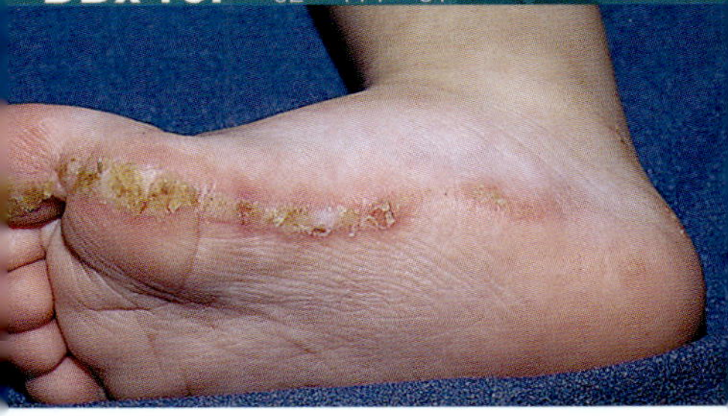

Epidermal nevus as a curvilinear lesion on a child's foot.

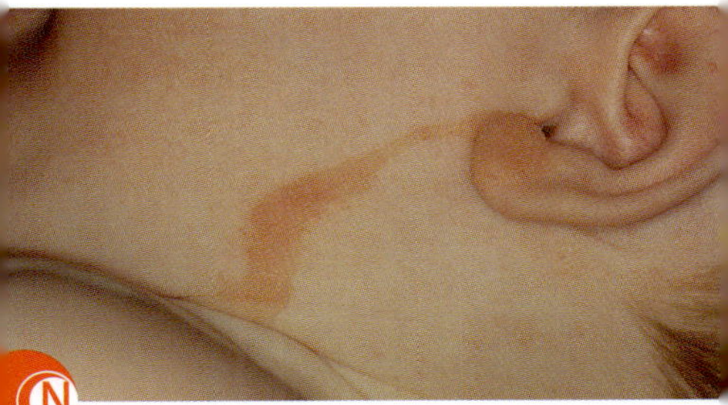

Curvilinear arrangement of nevus sebaceous on a newborn's face.

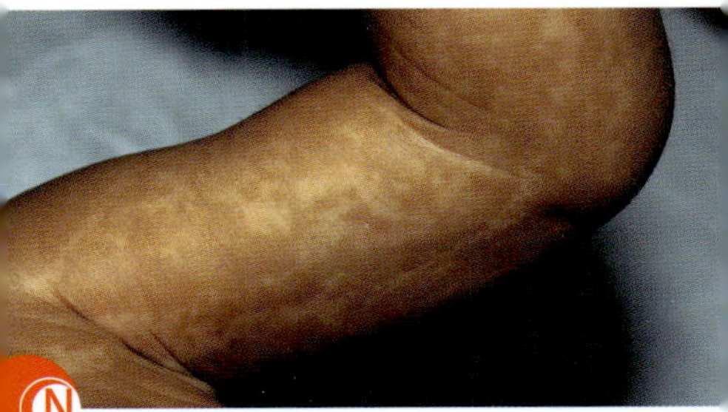

Curvilinear pattern of white lesions in newborn with hypomelanosis of Ito.

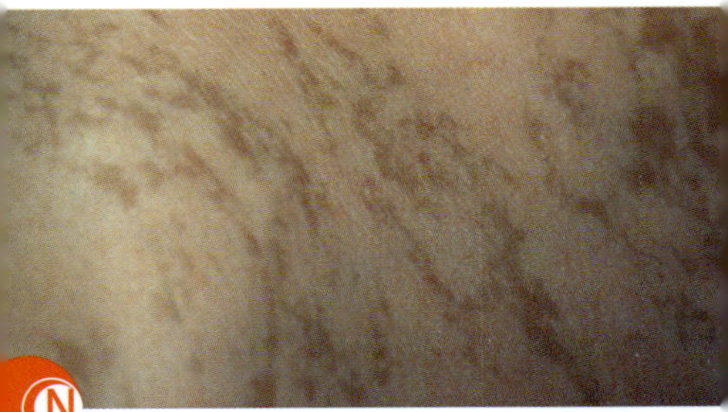

Curvilinear brown streaks in a newborn with linear and whorled hypermelanosis.

CLINICAL FEATURES

An important pattern to recognize is the linear or curvilinear arrangement of lesions, especially in the newborn.

Curvilinear skin lesions on the back assume a V-shape, whereas on the lateral trunk or extremities they assume an S-shape. Lesions end abruptly at the midline. This pattern follows the embryonic lines of Blaschko. Curvilinear patterns reflect genetic mosaicism with two distinct populations of skin cells and are seen in a variety of hereditary skin conditions observed in the newborn. Many conditions that follow the lines of Blaschko pattern have X-linked inheritance such as incontinentia pigmenti, hypohidrotic ectodermal dysplasia, and focal dermal hypoplasia. Others show genomic mosaicism such as hypomelanosis of Ito, linear and whorled hypermelanosis, epidermal nevus, nevus sebaceous, and nevus comedonicus. Frequently, only short segments of the lines of Blaschko are involved, sometimes as a solitary lesion, leaving the appearance of a linear lesion. Sometimes, skin lesions are restricted to lines of Blaschko on one half of the body.

LINEAR OR CURVILINEAR ARRANGEMENTS

Linear or curvilinear arrangement

92 • 114 • 91

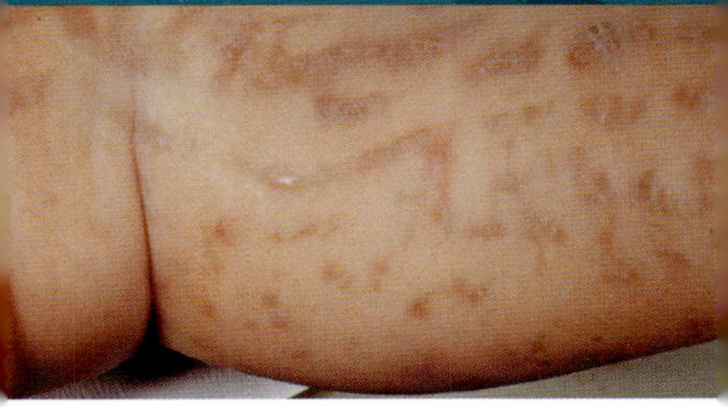

Curvilinear brown streaks in an infant with incontinentia pigmenti.

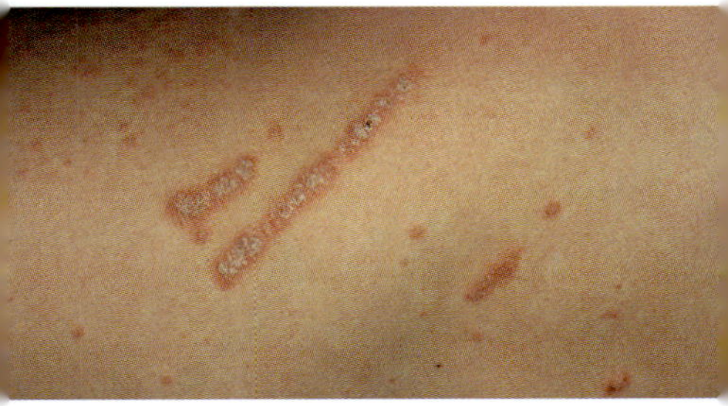

Koebner phenomenon in child with psoriasis.

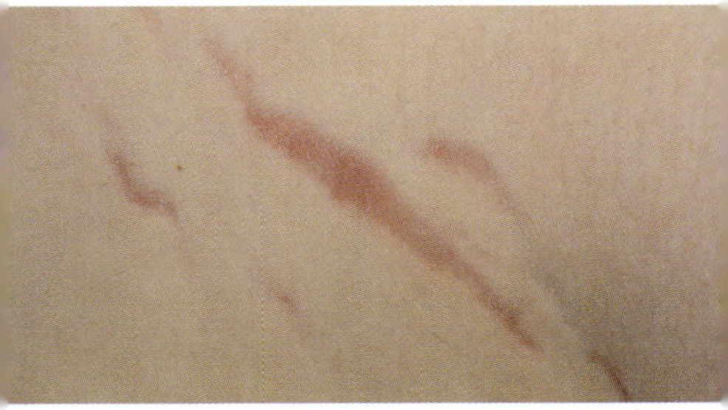

Curvilinear red striae in an adolescent.

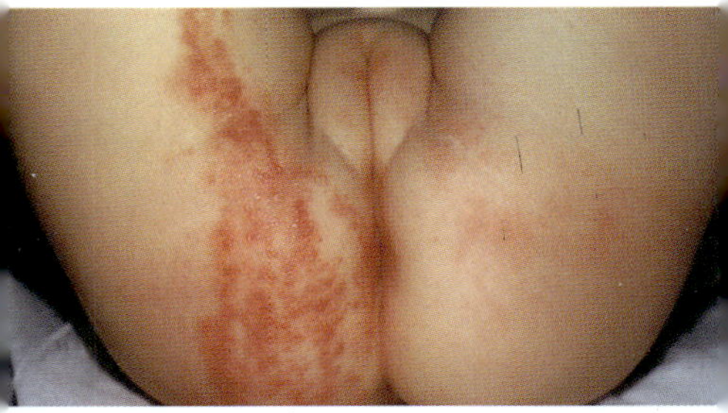

Child with a sudden onset of red streaks in lichen striatus.

Hereditary lesions tend to persist into adult life. One exception is incontinentia pigmenti, where a blistering stage in the newborn is followed by a warty stage and then a brown pigmented stage. The pigment may fade by adolescence, leaving no trace of the condition.

Some acquired conditions that appear after the newborn period can mimic the hereditary conditions. For example, linear lesions can be produced by linear trauma such as a scratch (the Koebner phenomena) in certain skin conditions such as psoriasis, lichen nitidus, and lichen planus. The presence of the Koebner phenomenon can be helpful in the diagnosis of papulosquamous conditions such as psoriasis. A scratch through a region of flat warts will also result in linear flat tan papules. Striae (stretchmarks) can also produce curvilinear lesions. These are particularly common in the adolescent and are related to weight gain or increased muscle mass. Linear morphea and guttate morphea of the trunk may also follow the lines of Blaschko.

The transient acquired condition, **lichen striatus**, mimics unilateral involvement of the lines of Blaschko. The etiology of lichen striatus is unclear.

ELSEVIER

Notices

Knowledge and best practice in this field are constantly changing. As new research and experience broaden our understanding, changes in research methods, professional practices, or medical treatment may become necessary.

Practitioners and researchers must always rely on their own experience and knowledge in evaluating and using any information, methods, compounds, or experiments described herein. In using such information or methods they should be mindful of their own safety and the safety of others, including parties for whom they have a professional responsibility.

With respect to any drug or pharmaceutical products identified, readers are advised to check the most current information provided (i) on procedures featured or (ii) by the manufacturer of each product to be administered, to verify the recommended dose or formula, the method and duration of administration, and contraindications. It is the responsibility of practitioners, relying on their own experience and knowledge of their patients, to make diagnoses, to determine dosages and the best treatment for each individual patient, and to take all appropriate safety precautions.

To the fullest extent of the law, neither the Publisher nor the authors, contributors, or editors, assume any liability for any injury and/or damage to persons or property as a matter of products liability, negligence or otherwise, or from any use or operation of any methods, products, instructions, or ideas contained in the material herein.

ISBN: 9780323396295

Ebook ISBN: 9780323430043

Printed in China

Last digit is the print number: 9 8 7 6 5 4 3 2 1

A Guide to Topical Steroids in Children

Generic name	Brand name
SUPER-POTENT	
Clobetasol propionate	Clobex 0.05% Cormax 0.05% Temovate 0.05% Olux foam
Betamethasone dipropionate	Diprolene 0.05%
POTENT	
Fluocinonide	Lidex 0.05% Vanos 0.1%
Halcinonide	Halog 0.1%
Amcinonide	Cyclocort 0.1%
Diflorasone diacetate	Psorcon 0.05%
Desoximetasone	Topicort 0.05%
MID-STRENGTH	
Fluocinolone acetonide	Synalar 0.025% Derma-Smoothe 0.01%
Triamcinolone acetonide	Kenalog 0.05%
Mometasone furoate	Elocon 0.1%
Hydrocortisone valerate	Westcort 0.2%
Betamethasone valerate	Valisone 0.1%
LOW-STRENGTH	
Prednicarbate	Dermatop 0.1%
Desonide	DesOwen 0.05%
Hydrocortisone butyrate	Locoid 0.1%
WEAK	
Hydrocortisone (all strengths)	

ELSEVIER

www.elsevierhealth.com

ISBN 978-0-323-39629-5

9 780323 396295

Recommended shelving classification:
Dermatology

DDx Deck